References

BOWDEN, C., BRUGGER, A., SWANN, A., et al (1994) Efficacy of divalproex vs lithium and placebo in the treatment of mania. *JAMA*, **271**, 918–924.

—, CALABRESE, J., McELROY, S., et al (2000) A randomised placebo controlled 12-month trial of divalproex and lithium in treatment of outpatients with bipolar I disorder. *Archives of General Psychiatry*, **57**, 481–489.

BRASFIELD, K. (1999) Pilot study of divalproex sodium versus valproic acid drug acquisition costs versus all related costs. *Current Therapeutic Research*, **60**, 138–144.

MIMS (2002) *Monthly Index of Medical Specialities*, January. London: Haymarket.

PERRY, P., BEVER-STILLE, K., ARNDT, S., et al (2000) Correlation of valproate serum concentration and bipolar illness in mania. *Journal of Clinical Psychiatry*, **60**, 232–236.

ZARATE, C., TOHEN, M., NARENDRAN, R., et al (1999) The adverse effect profile and efficacy of divalproex sodium compared with valproic acid: a pharmacoepidemiology study. *Journal of Clinical Psychiatry*, **60**, 232–236.

*Chris Fisher Medical Director, Wendy Broderick Chief Pharmacist, County Durham and Darlington Priority Services NSH Trust, Earls House Hospital, Lanchester Road, Durham DH1 5RD.

Antiepileptic Drugs to Treat Psychiatric Disorders

Abridged Version

Dear Krishna Bala -

Greetings from

Barcelona

Best

Eric

MEDICAL PSYCHIATRY

1. Handbook of Depression and Anxiety: A Biological Approach, *edited by Johan A. den Boer and J. M. Ad Sitsen*
2. Anticonvulsants in Mood Disorders, *edited by Russell T. Joffe and Joseph R. Calabrese*
3. Serotonin in Antipsychotic Treatment: Mechanisms and Clinical Practice, *edited by John M. Kane, H.-J. Möller, and Frans Awouters*
4. Handbook of Functional Gastrointestinal Disorders, *edited by Kevin W. Olden*
5. Clinical Management of Anxiety, *edited by Johan A. den Boer*
6. Obsessive-Compulsive Disorders: Diagnosis • Etiology • Treatment, *edited by Eric Hollander and Dan J. Stein*
7. Bipolar Disorder: Biological Models and Their Clinical Application, *edited by L. Trevor Young and Russell T. Joffe*
8. Dual Diagnosis and Treatment: Substance Abuse and Comorbid Medical and Psychiatric Disorders, *edited by Henry R. Kranzler and Bruce J. Rounsaville*
9. Geriatric Psychopharmacology, *edited by J. Craig Nelson*
10. Panic Disorder and Its Treatment, *edited by Jerrold F. Rosenbaum and Mark H. Pollack*
11. Comorbidity in Affective Disorders, *edited by Mauricio Tohen*
12. Practical Management of the Side Effects of Psychotropic Drugs, *edited by Richard Balon*
13. Psychiatric Treatment of the Medically Ill, *edited by Robert G. Robinson and William R. Yates*
14. Medical Management of the Violent Patient: Clinical Assessment and Therapy, *edited by Kenneth Tardiff*

15. Bipolar Disorders: Basic Mechanisms and Therapeutic Implications, *edited by Jair C. Soares and Samuel Gershon*
16. Schizophrenia: A New Guide for Clinicians, *edited by John G. Csernansky*
17. Polypharmacy in Psychiatry, *edited by S. Nassir Ghaemi*
18. Pharmacotherapy for Child and Adolescent Psychiatric Disorders: Second Edition, Revised and Expanded, *David R. Rosenberg, Pablo A. Davanzo, and Samuel Gershon*
19. Brain Imaging In Affective Disorders, *edited by Jair C. Soares*
20. Handbook of Medical Psychiatry, *edited by Jair C. Soares and Samuel Gershon*
21. Handbook of Depression and Anxiety: A Biological Approach, Second Edition, *edited by Siegfried Kasper, Johan A. den Boer, and J. M. Ad Sitsen*
22. Aggression: Psychiatric Assessment and Treatment, *edited by Emil Coccaro*
23. Depression in Later Life: A Multidisciplinary Psychiatric Approach, *edited by James Ellison and Sumer Verma*
24. Autism Spectrum Disorders, *edited by Eric Hollander*
25. Handbook of Chronic Depression: Diagnosis and Therapeutic Management, *edited by Jonathan E. Alpert and Maurizio Fava*
26. Clinical Handbook of Eating Disorders: An Integrated Approach, *edited by Timothy D. Brewerton*
27. Dual Diagnosis and Psychiatric Treatment: Substance Abuse and Comorbid Disorders: Second Edition, *edited by Henry R. Kranzler and Joyce A. Tinsley*
28. Atypical Antipsychotics: From Bench to Bedside, *edited by John G. Csernansky and John Lauriello*
29. Social Anxiety Disorder, *edited by Borwin Bandelow and Dan J. Stein*
30. Handbook of Sexual Dysfunction, *edited by Richard Balon and R. Taylor Segraves*
31. Borderline Personality Disorder, *edited by Mary C. Zanarini*
32. Handbook of Bipolar Disorder: Diagnosis and Therapeutic Approaches, *edited by Siegfried Kasper and Robert M. A. Hirschfeld*
33. Obesity and Mental Disorders, *edited by Susan L. McElroy, David B. Allison, and George A. Bray*
34. Depression: Treatment Strategies and Management, *edited by Thomas L. Schwartz and Timothy J. Petersen*
35. Bipolar Disorders: Basic Mechanisms and Therapeutic Implications, Second Edition, *edited by Jair C. Soares and Allan H. Young*
36. Neurogenetics of Psychiatric Disorders, *edited by Akira Sawa and Melvin G. McInnis*
37. Attention Deficit Hyperactivity Disorder: Concepts, Controversies, New Directions, *edited by Keith McBurnett, Linda Pfiffner, Russell Schachar, Glen Raymond Elliot, and Joel Nigg*
38. Insulin Resistance Syndrome and Neuropsychiatric Disorders, *edited by Natalie L. Rasgon*
39. Antiepileptic Drugs to Treat Psychiatric Disorders, *edited by Susan L. McElroy, Paul E. Keck, Jr., and Robert M. Post*

ANTIEPILEPTIC DRUGS TO TREAT PSYCHIATRIC DISORDERS

Abridged Version

Edited by

Susan L. McElroy
Lindner Center of HOPE
Mason, Ohio, USA
University of Cincinnati College of Medicine
Cincinnati, Ohio, USA

Paul E. Keck, Jr.
Lindner Center of HOPE
Mason, Ohio, USA
University of Cincinnati College of Medicine
Cincinnati, Ohio, USA

Robert M. Post
Bipolar Collaborative Network
Bethesda, Maryland, USA

informa
healthcare

New York   London

Informa Healthcare USA, Inc.
52 Vanderbilt Avenue
New York, NY 10017

© 2008 by Informa Healthcare USA, Inc.
Informa Healthcare is an Informa business

No claim to original U.S. Government works
Printed in the United States of America on acid-free paper
10 9 8 7 6 5 4 3 2 1

International Standard Book Number-10: 1-4200-9296-0 (Hardcover)
International Standard Book Number-13: 978-1-4200-9296-7 (Hardcover)

**For Corporate Sales and Reprint Permissions call 212-520-2700 or write to: Sales Department,
52 Vanderbilt Avenue, 7th floor, New York, NY 10017.**

Visit the Informa Web site at
www.informa.com

and the Informa Healthcare Web site at
www.informahealthcare.com

Preface

Antiepileptic drugs (AEDs) are increasingly being used in conditions other than epilepsy. Their most common area of "off label" use is in psychiatric and neuropsychiatric disorders. Indeed, several AEDs, namely, divalproex sodium, lamotrigine, and carbamazepine, have United States Food and Drug Administration indications for treating various phases of bipolar disorder. These drugs are now viewed as major treatments for bipolar disorder, with new AEDs often evaluated as potential mood-stabilizing agents.

However, it has become evident that anticonvulsant properties do not automatically predict antimanic or mood-stabilizing effects and that many AEDs have beneficial psychotropic properties, whether or not they have efficacy in bipolar disorder. Thus, while some anticonvulsants may have antimanic or mood-stabilizing effects, others may have anxiolytic, anticraving, or weight-loss properties. Controlled trials that have been conducted suggest that divalproex sodium, lamotrigine, and topiramate may have beneficial effects when used adjunctively with antipsychotics in schizophrenia; that pregabalin may reduce anxiety in generalized anxiety disorder; that topiramate may reduce alcohol and cocaine craving and use in substance use disorders; and that topiramate and zonisamide may have therapeutic effects on eating pathology and weight in eating disorders. These properties need to be properly "profiled" so that they can be used to benefit patients and further advance neuropsychopharmacology research.

Despite the increased clinical use and research with these compounds, the diverse therapeutic effects of AEDs in psychiatric and neuropsychiatric conditions has not been gathered and scrutinized in one source for many years. This book provides an accessible and expert summary of currently available AEDs and their use in these disorders for the mental health professional. The first part of the book (chap. 1) reviews available AEDs, their putative mechanisms of action in epilepsy and other neurological conditions in which they are commonly used (e.g., neuropathic pain and migraine), their use in epilepsy and neuropsychiatric disorders often accompanied by seizures and psychopathology (e.g., traumatic brain injury, autism, and intellectual disability), and their side effects and drug-drug interactions. The second part of the book (chaps. 2–11) is devoted to providing a state-of-the-art update on the use of AEDs in a broad range of psychiatric disorders and disorders with psychiatric features. Specifically, AEDs in the treatment of bipolar and major depressive disorder, schizophrenia, anxiety disorders, substance use disorders, eating and weight disorders, impulse control disorders, personality disorders, sleep disorders, and fibromyalgia are reviewed and summarized. The third part of the book (chap. 12) discusses the mechanisms of action of currently available AEDs potentially underlying their therapeutic properties in psychiatric conditions, with a focus on mood disorders.

Altogether, this book provides a resource for clinicians who treat patients with psychiatric and neuropsychiatric conditions and for researchers studying the expanding role of AEDs in neuropsychopharmacology.

Susan L. McElroy
Paul E. Keck, Jr.
Robert M. Post

Contents

Preface iii
Contributors vii

I. Antiepileptics (AEDs): Overview and Use in Neuropsychiatric Conditions

1. Mechanisms of Action of Antiepileptic Drugs   *1*
Aaron P. Gibson and Nick C. Patel

II. AEDs in Psychiatric Disorders

2. Treatment of Acute Manic and Mixed Episodes   *17*
Paul E. Keck, Jr., Susan L. McElroy, and Jeffrey R. Strawn

3. The Role of Antiepileptic Drugs in Long-Term Treatment of Bipolar Disorder   *27*
Charles L. Bowden and Vivek Singh

4. Antiepileptic Drugs in the Treatment of Rapid-Cycling Bipolar Disorder and Bipolar Depression   *43*
David E. Kemp, Keming Gao, Joseph R. Calabrese, and David J. Muzina

5. Role of Antiepileptic Drugs in the Treatment of Major Depressive Disorder   *65*
Erik Nelson

6. Antiepileptics in the Treatment of Schizophrenia   *75*
Leslie Citrome

7. Antiepileptic Drugs in the Treatment of Anxiety Disorders: Role in Therapy   *95*
Michael Van Ameringen, Catherine Mancini, Beth Patterson, and Christine Truong

8. Antiepileptics in the Treatment of Alcohol Withdrawal and Alcohol Use Relapse Prevention   *139*
Mark A. Frye, Victor M. Karpyak, Daniel Hall-Flavin, Ihsan M. Salloum, Andrew McKeon, and Doo-Sup Choi

9. Antiepileptic Drugs in the Treatment of Drug Use Disorders   *151*
Kyle M. Kampman

10. Antiepileptic Drugs in the Treatment of Impulsivity and Aggression and Impulse Control and Cluster B Personality Disorders   *159*
Heather A. Berlin and Eric Hollander

11. Antiepileptic Drugs and Borderline Personality Disorder   *191*
Mary C. Zanarini

III. Potential Psychotropic Mechanisms of Action of AEDs

12. Psychotrophic Mechanisms of Action of Antiepileptic Drugs in Mood Disorder   *197*
Robert M. Post

Abbreviations 219

Contributors

Heather A. Berlin   Department of Psychiatry, Mount Sinai School of Medicine, New York, New York, U.S.A.

Charles L. Bowden   Department of Psychiatry, University of Texas Health Science Center at San Antonio, San Antonio, Texas, U.S.A.

Joseph R. Calabrese   Bipolar Disorders Center for Intervention and Services Research, Case Western Reserve University, Cleveland, Ohio, U.S.A.

Doo-Sup Choi   Departments of Psychiatry and Psychology and Molecular Pharmacology, Mayo Clinic, Rochester, Minnesota, U.S.A.

Leslie Citrome   New York University School of Medicine, New York, New York, and Clinical Research and Evaluation Facility, Nathan S. Kline Institute for Psychiatric Research, Orangeburg, New York, U.S.A.

Mark A. Frye   Department of Psychiatry and Psychology, Mayo Clinic, Rochester, Minnesota, U.S.A.

Keming Gao   Bipolar Disorders Center for Intervention and Services Research, Case Western Reserve University, Cleveland, Ohio, U.S.A.

Aaron P. Gibson   College of Pharmacy, University of New Mexico, Albuquerque, New Mexico, U.S.A.

Daniel Hall-Flavin   Department of Psychiatry and Psychology, Mayo Clinic, Rochester, Minnesota, U.S.A.

Eric Hollander   Department of Psychiatry, Mount Sinai School of Medicine, New York, New York, U.S.A.

Kyle M. Kampman   University of Pennsylvania School of Medicine, Philadelphia, Pennsylvania, U.S.A.

Victor M. Karpyak   Department of Psychiatry and Psychology, Mayo Clinic, Rochester, Minnesota, U.S.A.

Paul E. Keck, Jr.   Lindner Center of HOPE, Mason, and Department of Psychiatry, University of Cincinnati College of Medicine, Cincinnati, Ohio, U.S.A.

David E. Kemp   Bipolar Disorders Center for Intervention and Services Research, Case Western Reserve University, Cleveland, Ohio, U.S.A.

Catherine Mancini   Department of Psychiatry and Behavioural Neurosciences, McMaster University and Anxiety Disorders Clinic, McMaster University Medical Centre—HHS, Hamilton, Ontario, Canada

Susan L. McElroy   Lindner Center of HOPE, Mason, and Department of Psychiatry, University of Cincinnati College of Medicine, Cincinnati, Ohio, U.S.A.

Andrew McKeon   Department of Neurology, Mayo Clinic, Rochester, Minnesota, U.S.A.

David J. Muzina   Cleveland Clinic Psychiatry and Psychology, Cleveland, Ohio, U.S.A.

Erik Nelson   Department of Psychiatry, University of Cincinnati Medical Center, Cincinnati, Ohio, U.S.A.

Nick C. Patel   College of Pharmacy, University of Georgia, Department of Psychiatry & Health Behavior, Medical College of Georgia, Augusta, Georgia, U.S.A.

Beth Patterson   Anxiety Disorders Clinic, McMaster University Medical Centre—HHS, Hamilton, Ontario, Canada

Robert M. Post   Head, Bipolar Collaborative Network, Bethesda, Maryland, U.S.A.

Ihsan M. Salloum   Department of Psychiatry, University of Miami, Miller School of Medicine, Miami, Florida, U.S.A.

Vivek Singh   Department of Psychiatry, University of Texas Health Science Center at San Antonio, San Antonio, Texas, U.S.A.

Jeffrey R. Strawn   Lindner Center of HOPE, Mason, and Department of Psychiatry, University of Cincinnati College of Medicine, Cincinnati, Ohio, U.S.A.

Christine Truong   Anxiety Disorders Clinic, McMaster University Medical Centre—HHS, Hamilton, Ontario, Canada

Michael Van Ameringen   Department of Psychiatry and Behavioural Neurosciences, McMaster University and Anxiety Disorders Clinic, McMaster University Medical Centre—HHS, Hamilton, Ontario, Canada

Mary C. Zanarini   Laboratory for the Study of Adult Development, McLean Hospital, Belmont and the Department of Psychiatry, Harvard Medical School, Boston, Massachusetts, U.S.A.

1 Mechanisms of Action of Antiepileptic Drugs

Aaron P. Gibson
College of Pharmacy, University of New Mexico, Albuquerque, New Mexico, U.S.A.

Nick C. Patel
College of Pharmacy, University of Georgia, Department of Psychiatry & Health Behavior, Medical College of Georgia, Augusta, Georgia, U.S.A.

INTRODUCTION

Antiepileptic drugs (AEDs) have been utilized in the treatment of various psychiatric disorders for several decades. As early as the 1960s, it was recognized that AEDs had remedial effects on mood and behavior (1–4). Over time and with an accumulating body of evidence, the psychiatric application of AEDs has grown significantly, with a number of these agents being approved for specific disorders and considered mainstays of treatment. The precise mechanisms of action by which AEDs are useful in patients with epilepsy remain largely unknown. Elucidation of AED mechanisms of action in the context of epilepsy has been challenging because agents may have multiple mechanisms of action and there may be differential interaction at the same molecular target between agents. However, a common link among proposed AED mechanisms of action involves the modulation of excitatory and inhibitory neurotransmission via effects on ion channels and certain neurotransmitters. Although an assumption that the putative mechanisms of action of AEDs are similar for both epilepsy and psychiatric disorders may be premature (5), a clearer understanding of the mechanisms of action of AEDs is necessary and may lead to improved predictions about an agent's clinical efficacy and safety profiles across the spectrum of psychiatric disorders. Ultimately, this information may contribute toward targeted treatment interventions with a higher likelihood of response and a subsequent improvement in patient psychosocial functioning.

In this chapter, we summarize the concepts of ion channel and neurotransmitter modulation and review the proposed mechanisms of action of AEDs currently available, as well as those in the development pipeline.

TARGETS FOR ANTIEPILEPTIC DRUGS

Ion Channels

Voltage-dependent sodium (Na^+) and calcium (Ca^{2+}) channels are the primary ion channels associated with the mechanisms of action of a large number of available AEDs. Both ion channels are involved in the regulation of the flow of cations from the extracellular space into the neuron (6) (Fig. 1).

Voltage-dependent Na^+ channels control the intrinsic excitatory activity of the nervous system. At resting membrane potential, Na^+ channels are closed, or inactive. During depolarization, these channels are opened, or activated, and allow for the influx of Na^+ ions. Spontaneous closure of Na^+ channels, termed "inactivation," follows, and it is during this period of time that Na^+ channels cannot be reactivated to evoke another action potential. Repolarization of the membrane potential results in the recovery of Na^+ channels to a resting state (7,8). The duration of

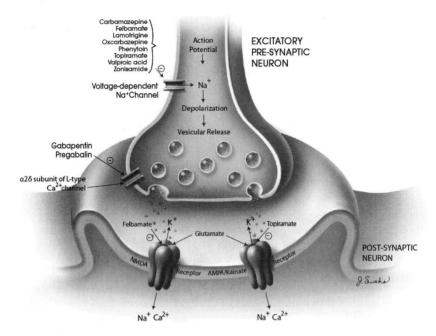

FIGURE 1 Putative mechanisms of action of AEDs at an excitatory synapse in the central nervous system. *Abbreviations*: AEDs, antiepileptic drugs; Na⁺, sodium; Ca²⁺, calcium; K⁺, potassium; NMDA, *N*-methyl-ᴅ-aspartate; AMPA, α-amino-3-hydroxy-5-methyl-isoxazole-4-propionic acid. *Source*: Illustrations courtesy of Jennifer A. Suehs, Biomedical Illustration, Austin, Texas, U.S.A.

Na^+ channel inactivation is brief, permitting sustained high-frequency repetitive firing. Prolongation of the inactive state of these Na^+ channels limits neuronal excitability and confers protection against partial and generalized tonic-clonic seizures (7,8).

Voltage-dependent Ca^{2+} channels are also involved in the excitatory activity of neurons and have been implicated in epileptogenic discharge. Ca^{2+} channels are classified on the basis of the membrane potential at which they are activated: low- and high-threshold (9). Low-threshold T-type Ca^{2+} channels are expressed in thalamic relay neurons, whereas high-threshold Ca^{2+} channels are distributed throughout the nervous system (10). T-type Ca^{2+} channels play a role in the regulation of the T current, which amplifies thalamic oscillations including the characteristic three-per-second spike and wave pattern of absence seizures (11). Some AEDs reduce the flow of Ca^{2+} through T-type channels, thereby reducing the T current (10,11). High-threshold Ca^{2+} channels may also be potential drug targets as these channels have been reported to be associated with neuronal processes important in epileptogenesis. Specifically, the L-type Ca^{2+} channels may modulate the slow after hyperpolarization and the release of neurotransmitters (12,13).

Voltage-dependent potassium (K^+) channels are involved in the repolarization of the membrane potential. Activators of the K^+ channel limit neurons from rapidly firing and may have antiepileptic effects (14).

GABA-Mediated Inhibition

Gamma-aminobutyric acid (GABA) is one of the main inhibitory neurotransmitters and is widely distributed throughout the central nervous system (15). Enhanced GABAergic tone has a broad antiepileptic effect (16) and has served as a principal target for a number of AEDs. Mechanisms by which GABA-mediated inhibition occurs include augmentation of GABA-activated currents and increased GABA supply (Fig. 2).

GABA acts upon three receptor classes: $GABA_A$, $GABA_B$, and $GABA_C$ (17,18). $GABA_A$ receptors are ligand-operated ion channels that increase the influx of chloride anions (Cl^-) following postsynaptic GABA binding. This, in turn, results in hyperpolarization of the neuron. The role of ionotropic $GABA_A$ receptors in the context of AED mechanisms of action is well established, specifically allosteric modulation related to benzodiazepines and barbiturates. $GABA_B$ receptors are G-protein coupled metabotropic receptors that, when activated, lead to increased K^+ conductance, decreased Ca^{2+} entry, and suppression of the release of other neurotransmitters (15,19). It has been suggested that GABA binding to the $GABA_B$ receptor may result in activation of K^+ channels through a second messenger pathway involving arachidonic acid (20). Although the role of $GABA_B$ receptors is currently limited to potential treatments for absence seizures, enhanced GABA binding or allosteric receptor facilitation at these receptors may indeed have antiepileptic effects in other types of seizure activity (18). The significance of $GABA_C$ receptors, which are also ligand-operated ion channels, in the brain is unclear (17).

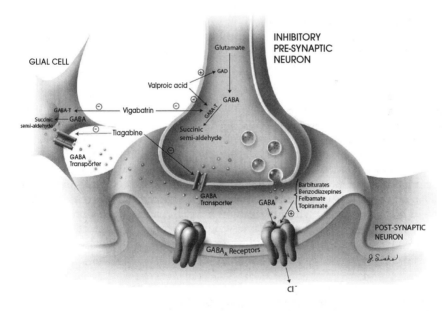

FIGURE 2 Putative mechanisms of action of AEDs at an inhibitory synapse in the central nervous system. *Abbreviations*: AEDs, antiepileptic drugs; Cl^-, chloride; GABA, γ-aminobutyric acid; GAD, glutamic acid decarboxylase, GABA-T, GABA transaminase. *Source*: Illustrations courtesy of Jennifer A. Suehs, Biomedical Illustration, Austin, Texas, U.S.A.

In inhibitory presynaptic terminals, synthesis of GABA from glutamic acid is dependent on glutamic acid decarboxylase (GAD). Following vesicular release and subsequent receptor activation, GABA is removed from the synaptic cleft by GABA reuptake transporters into presynaptic terminals and glial cells. Thereafter, GABA is recycled for release from presynaptic terminals or metabolized into succinic acid semialdehyde by GABA transaminase (GABA-T) (21,22). Increased availability of GABA resulting from increased GABA production by GAD, inhibition of reuptake transporters, or inhibition of GABA-T forms the basis of antiseizure actions of some newer AEDs.

Glutamate-Mediated Excitation

In contrast to GABA, glutamate is the major excitatory neurotransmitter in the brain (21), and decreased glutamatergic tone may have antiepileptic effects. Glutamate has activity at the following ionotropic glutamate receptors: N-methyl-D-aspartate (NMDA), α-amino-3-hydroxy-5-methyl-isoxazole-4-propionic acid (AMPA), and kainate (Fig. 1). These ligand-operated ion channels allow for the flow of Na^+ and Ca^{2+}. The NMDA receptor subtype is associated with slower kinetics compared with the AMPA/kainate receptor subtypes. Antagonism at NMDA and AMPA receptors are targets for AEDs, although few available AEDs act via these particular mechanisms (23).

Glutamate also has activity at metabotropic glutamate (mGlu) receptors, which have effects on neuronal excitability through G-protein-linked modifications of enzymes and ion channels. The mGlu receptors are predominantly presynaptic and have been classified into three groups (I, II, and III). Furthermore, these receptors have been shown to modify glutamatergic and GABAergic neurotransmission. Antagonists of group I mGlu receptors and agonists of groups II and III mGlu receptors may confer anticonvulsant properties (23,24).

Serotonergic Neurotransmission

Recent developments suggest that serotonin may have a role in epileptogenesis. Specifically, serotonin depletion in the brain may lower the seizure threshold, increasing the susceptibility to audiogenically, chemically, and electrically induced seizures. Current evidence indicates that activation of the serotonin-2C (5-HT$_{2C}$) receptor may be a potential mechanism for antiepileptic effects (25). Mutations of the 5-HT$_{2C}$ receptor genes have been shown to be associated with increased risk of seizure (26,27), while administration of known 5-HT$_{2C}$ agonists has reduced seizure activity (28,29). In addition, selective serotonin reuptake inhibitors have been reported to have anticonvulsant properties, perhaps through potentiation of serotonergic activity (30,31).

MECHANISMS OF ACTION OF ANTIEPILEPTIC DRUGS

The mechanisms of action of AEDs are diverse, affecting one or more of the potential targets detailed above. In this section, we review the proposed mechanisms of action of first- and second-generation AEDs, as well as those related to compounds in development. Table 1 summarizes the mechanisms of action of available AEDs.

TABLE 1 Summary of Principal Mechanisms of Action of First- and Second-Generation Antiepileptic Drugs

AED	Na$^+$ channel blockade	Ca^{2+} channel blockade	K$^+$ channel activation	Enhanced GABA-mediated inhibition	Reduced glutamate-mediated excitation	Other
First-Generation						
Carbamazepine	+	+	+			
Valproate	+			+		
Phenytoin	+					
Benzodiazepines				+		
Barbiturates				+		
Ethosuximide		+				
Acetazolamide						+
Second-Generation						
Felbamate	+	+		+	+	
Topiramate	+	+		+	+	
Gabapentin		+		+		
Zonisamide	+	+				
Lamotrigine	+	+				
Levetiracetam						+
Oxcarbazepine	+	+	+			
Pregabalin		+				
Tiagabine				+		
Vigabatrin				+		

Abbreviations: AED, antiepileptic drug; Ca^{2+}, calcium; GABA, γ-aminobutyric acid; K$^+$, potassium; Na$^+$, sodium.

First-Generation Antiepileptic Drugs
First-generation AEDs include carbamazepine, valproate, phenytoin, benzodiazepines, barbiturates, ethosuximide, and acetazolamide.

Carbamazepine
Carbamazepine (CBZ) limits the sustained, high-frequency repetitive firing of neurons through the stabilization of inactivated Na$^+$ channels in a voltage-, frequency-, and time-dependent fashion (32). The effectiveness of CBZ in extending the inactive phase of Na$^+$ channels and inhibiting action potentials may be higher during periods of neuronal excitability as Na$^+$ channels may be more susceptible to blockade. It has also been reported that CBZ may have activity at K$^+$ channels, thereby increasing K$^+$ conductance (33), and may inhibit L-type Ca^{2+} channels (34). The CBZ metabolite 10,11-epoxycarbamazepine also contributes to CBZ's overall antiepileptic effects by limiting repetitive neuronal firing (35). Given these pharmacological properties, CBZ is widely used for the treatment of partial seizures and primary generalized tonic-clonic seizures.

CBZ has also been shown to have effects on GABA$_A$ (36) and GABA$_B$ (37,38) receptors, inhibits the increase in intracellular free Ca^{2+} induced by NMDA and glycine (39), and inhibits glutamate release (40). Furthermore, it has been reported that CBZ may act as an antagonist of adenosine A$_1$ receptors (41) and "peripheral-type" benzodiazepine receptors (42), attenuate cAMP production (43), induce the release of serotonin (40,44,45), and decrease the release of the excitatory amino acid aspartate (42). It is unclear whether these additional pharmacological effects of CBZ contribute to its antiepileptic profile.

Valproate
Much of the attention regarding the broad antiepileptic effects of valproate (VPA) has focused on its mechanisms of action on the GABAergic system. Specifically, VPA has been shown to elevate whole-brain GABA levels and potentiate response by inhibiting GABA-T and activating GAD (16). VPA may enhance GABA release via activity at presynaptic $GABA_B$ receptors, and may block GABA reuptake (46). The GABAergic effects of VPA may indeed be specific to certain regions of the brain (16).

At therapeutically relevant concentrations, VPA has been reported to suppress sustained, high-frequency repetitive neuronal firing through blockade of voltage-dependent Na^+ channels (35). VPA may reduce peak conductance and slow the recovery of Na^+ channels from fast inactivation, although these proposed actions remain controversial (47–49). VPA may also reduce T-type Ca^{2+} channel currents, although this effect is considered modest (50). Other potential mechanisms involved in the antiepileptic effects of VPA are the inhibition of NMDA-evoked depolarizations (51,52) and decreased release of aspartate (53).

Phenytoin
Similar to CBZ, phenytoin (PHT) is effective for partial and generalized seizures as it limits the repetitive firing of action potentials mediated through Na^+ channel blockade (54). This action is both voltage- and frequency-dependent; PHT binds with greater affinity to channels in the inactive state, and reductions in neuronal firing are increased after depolarization and decreased after hyperpolarization (54,55). PHT may also modulate postsynaptic, high voltage-activated Ca^{2+} currents (56), possibly contributing to its antiseizure activity. Other effects of PHT include potentiation of GABA at the $GABA_A$ receptor (36), attenuation of glutamatergic neurotransmission (57,58), and inhibition of Ca^{2+}/calmodulin-regulated protein phosphorylation and neurotransmitter release (59).

Benzodiazepines
Benzodiazepines (BZDs) have broad-spectrum AED activity, with demonstrated efficacy in partial and generalized tonic-clonic seizures, as well as status epilepticus. Clonzepam, diazepam, and lorazepam are among the most commonly used BZDs for seizure treatment. The antiseizure properties of BZDs result primarily from their positive allosteric activation of postsynaptic $GABA_A$ receptors and subsequent increase in the frequency of Cl^- channel opening and augmentation of GABA-activated currents. BDZs do not affect the mean open time or conductance of the Cl^- channel (60). In the absence of GABA, however, BZDs are unable to directly activate $GABA_A$ receptors (61). In addition to their established effects on the GABAergic system, there is evidence suggesting that high concentrations of BZDs inhibit currents carried by Na^+ and Ca^{2+} channels (62,63). This action indicates that BZDs, like CBZ, VPA, and PHT, can reduce sustained, high-frequency repetitive neuronal firing.

Barbiturates
The principal molecular target of barbiturates, including phenobarbital (PB) and pentobarbital (PTB), is the $GABA_A$ receptor. These agents are similar to BZDs in

that the antiepileptic effects result from enhanced effects of GABA-evoked Cl⁻ currents. In contrast to BZDs, PB and PTB increase the mean open time of Cl⁻ channels, but do not affect the frequency of Cl⁻ channel openings or conductance of these channels (60,64). Furthermore, PB and PTB can directly activate $GABA_A$ receptors without the presence of GABA (61). Secondary mechanisms by which PB and PTB may exert antiseizure activity include blockade of voltage-dependent Na^+ channels at high concentrations (62), blockade of high-voltage-activated Ca^{2+} channels (65), and inhibition of the AMPA/kainate glutamate receptor subtype (66).

Ethosuximide
Ethosuximide (ESM) is protective against absence seizures because it reduces T-type Ca^{2+} currents in thalamic relay neurons (11). ESM has also been reported to have effects on Na^+ and K^+ currents (67,68), and $GABA_A$ receptors (69). However, it is unclear whether these secondary mechanisms are associated with ESM's antiepileptic properties.

Acetazolamide
While acetazolamide (AZM) has been used as an adjunct for the treatment of partial and generalized seizures for several decades, its precise mechanism of action related to antiepileptic effects remains unclear. Because AZM is a potent carbonic anhydrase inhibitor (70), it has been postulated that an increase in carbon dioxide concentrations in neurons and an increase in pH and a decrease in bicarbonate concentrations in neuroglia may confer its antiseizure activity (71). As a result of these ionic and acid-base changes, extracellular K^+ concentrations decrease, leading to reduced neuronal excitability (72). Extracellular pH levels also decrease, leading to NMDA receptor blockade (73) and enhanced $GABA_A$ receptor response (74).

Second-Generation Antiepileptic Drugs
Second-generation AEDs include felbamate, topiramate, gabapentin, zonisamide, lamotrigine, levetiracetam, oxcarbazepine, pregabalin, tiagabine, and vigabatrin.

Felbamate
Felbamate (FBM) possesses clinical efficacy across a wide spectrum of seizure types, which is attributed to its multiple mechanisms of action (75). FBM is unique in that it is the first to have direct action on the NMDA glutamate receptor subtype. Clinically relevant concentrations of FBM have been shown to inhibit NMDA/glycine-stimulated increases in intracellular Ca^{2+} (76) and block NMDA receptor–mediated excitatory postsynaptic potentials (77). Although some studies suggest that FBM block of NMDA receptors occurs at the glycine recognition site (78,79), other studies indicate that this may not be the site at which FBM interacts (80,81). FBM may also inhibit AMPA/kainate receptors (82).

In addition to its glutamatergic effects, FBM potentiates GABA responses via barbiturate-type action on $GABA_A$ receptors (80,83). FBM may stabilize the inactive state of voltage-dependent Na^+ channels, reducing sustained, high-frequency repetitive firing of neurons (84). Furthermore, FBM may reduce high-voltage-activated Ca^{2+} channels (85).

The clinical use of FBM has been limited due to postmarketing surveillance reports of fatal aplastic anemia and hepatoxicity (75).

Topiramate

Topiramate (TPM) has multiple mechanisms of action and is protective against partial and generalized tonic-clonic seizures (86). TPM reduces Na^+ and Ca^{2+} currents through prolongation of the inactivation of Na^+ channels (87) and inhibition of L-type Ca^{2+} channels (88), respectively. These effects are believed to be associated with TPM's ability to reduce sustained repetitive firing and spontaneous bursting (89).

TPM interacts with both the GABA and glutamate neurotransmitter systems. TPM potentiates GABA response by acting at a site on the $GABA_A$ receptor to enhance Cl^- influx and increase Cl^- currents (90). The $GABA_A$ receptor site at which TPM acts is different from that at which BZDs act because flumazenil, a BZD antagonist, does not reverse the effects of TPM (91). TPM also blocks the AMPA/ kainate glutamate receptor subtype (92).

Interestingly, TPM is a weak inhibitor of carbonic anhydrase (93). It is unlikely that this property contributes much to TPM's antiepileptic profile as it does for AZM, a potent carbonic anhydrase inhibitor.

Gabapentin

Gabapentin (GBP) is a synthetic GABA analogue that is recommended as adjunct treatment of partial seizures with or without secondary generalization (94). GBP does not act at $GABA_A$ or $GABA_B$ receptors despite its structural similarities with GABA (95), nor does it affect GABA reuptake or synthesis (61). GBP has been shown to promote GABA release (96), although the precise mechanism of this is unknown. It has been reported that GBP enhances nipecotic acid–promoted non-vesicular release of GABA (97).

GBP has not been found to have direct actions on voltage-dependent Na^+ channels. However, GBP may modulate Ca^{2+} currents through high-affinity binding at the $\alpha_2\delta$-subunit of the L-type voltage-dependent Ca^{2+} channels (98). The relevance of this pharmacological property in the context of GBP's antiepileptic effects remains unclear.

Zonisamide

Zonisamide (ZNS) is a broad-spectrum AED that is effective against localization-related and generalized epilepsies, and appears to be potent in progressive myoclonic epilepsy syndromes (99). Effects on ion channels are believed to be the principal mechanisms involved in ZNS's antiseizure activity; specifically, ZNS inhibits voltage-dependent Na^+ channels and T-type Ca^{2+} channels (100,101).

Other potential pharmacological actions of ZNS possibly conferring antiepileptic properties include weak inhibition of carbonic anhydrase (102), inhibition of monoamine release and metabolism (103,104), inhibition of K^+-evoked glutamate release (105), and free radical scavenging (106).

Lamotrigine

Lamotrigine (LTG) was initially developed as a folate antagonist on the basis of the presumed correlation between antifolate and antiepileptic properties (107).

However, LTG shares a pharmacological profile similar to that of CBZ and PHT and possesses a broad spectrum of clinical efficacy for generalized tonic-clonic, partial, and absence seizures. LTG inhibits sustained repetitive neuronal firing by prolonging the inactivated state of Na^+ channels in a voltage-, use-, and frequency-dependent manner (108,109). LTG may exhibit selectivity for neurons that synthesize glutamate and aspartate (110). In addition to its effects on Na^+ channels, LTG reduces Ca^{2+} currents through a voltage-dependent block of Ca^{2+} channels (111,112).

Levetiracetam

Levetiracetam (LEV) is a recent AED effective against partial seizures with or without secondary generalization (113). The mechanism of action of LEV is unknown, as this agent does not interact with either Na^+, Ca^{2+}, or K^+ channels or the GABAergic or glutamatergic systems. It is believed that LEV does interact with a specific synaptic membrane-binding site because LEV is displaced from this site by ESM, pentylenetetrazol, and bemegride (114). Recently, the binding site of LEV was identified as SV2A, a synaptic vesicle protein. Although the molecular action of SVA2 is unclear, there is a strong correlation between the affinities of agents that act at SVA2 and antiseizure potency (115).

Oxcarbazepine

Oxcarbazepine (OXC) is effective against partial and generalized tonic-clonic seizures (61). Structurally related to CBZ, OXC displays similar mechanisms of action, including inhibition of voltage-dependent Na^+ and Ca^{2+} channels (116,117) and increased K^+ conductance (116). The block of high-threshold Ca^{2+} currents by OXC may reduce presynaptic glutamate release (117,118). OXC does have an active monohydroxy metabolite, known as licarbazepine, which may contribute to its antiepileptic properties.

Pregabalin

Similar to GBP, pregabalin (PGL) is a GABA analogue and is effective against partial seizures (119). The putative mechanism of action of PGL is the binding to voltage-dependent Ca^{2+} channels at the $\alpha_2\delta$-subunit and modulation of Ca^{2+} influx. PGL also reduces the synaptic release of several neurotransmitters, including noradrenaline and glutamate, possibly accounting for its ability to reduce neuronal excitability (120).

Tiagabine

Tiagabine (TGB) is an analogue of nipecotic acid, a GABA uptake antagonist. TGB exhibits potent inhibition of neuronal and glial GABA uptake transporters, specifically the GABA transporter-1 (121). This pharmacological action results in higher GABA levels in the synaptic cleft and possibly, a subsequent prolongation of the duration of the peak inhibitory postsynaptic current (122). TGB is effective as an adjunct for partial seizures with or without secondary generalization (123).

Vigabatrin

Vigabatrin (VGB) is a structural analogue of GABA that demonstrates protection against partial seizures with or without secondary generalization (124). VGB is an irreversible inhibitor of GABA-T, particularly in neurons (125). Inhibition of GABA-T leads to elevated brain GABA levels and enhancement of inhibitory neurotransmission. VGB may also block glial cell uptake of GABA (126).

Future Antiepileptic Drugs

Some compounds in the AED pipeline have been based on the structures of existing AEDs and target conventional molecular targets. These include: CBZ analogues racemic licarbazepine and (S)-licarbazepine acetate; VPA-like agents valrocemide, valnoctamide, propylisopropyl acetamide, and isovaleramide; selective partial BZD receptor agonists such as TPA023 and ELB139; FBM analogue flurofelbamate and another carbamate, RWJ-333369; and, LEV analogues brivaracetam and seletracetam (127).

Other compounds in the pipeline capitalize on novel mechanisms of action potentially conferring antiepileptic effects. Lacosamide is a functional amino acid that may allosterically inhibit NMDA receptors. Talampanel is a 2,3-benzodiazepine selective noncompetitive AMPA receptor antagonist, while NS1209 is a water-soluble, competitive AMPA receptor antagonist. Retigabine and ICA-27243 are KCNQ K^+ channel openers with and without $GABA_A$ receptor modulation, respectively. Finally, ganaxolone is a neuroactive steroid that modulates $GABA_A$ receptors, and rufinamide is a triazole that is believed to have Na^+ channel–blocking activity (127).

CONCLUSION

Available and future AEDs exhibit a variety of mechanisms of action that may be attributed to antiseizure activity. Oftentimes, multiple pharmacological actions have been suggested for one agent. In the treatment of epilepsy, an AED's pharmacological profile may reliably predict its spectrum of clinical efficacy, as well as certain side effects. It is unknown whether an AED's mechanisms of action relevant to epilepsy are indeed relevant to its psychotropic effects. As AEDs have and will continue to be valuable in the treatment armamentarium of psychiatric disorders, a better understanding of their pharmacology may help guide the field to determine which psychiatric disorders or symptoms where particular agents could be of benefit.

REFERENCES

1. Dalby MA. Antiepileptic and psychotropic effect of carbamazepine (Tegretol) in the treatment of psychomotor epilepsy. Epilepsia 1971; 12(4):325–334.
2. Lambert PA, Carraz G, Borselli S, et al. Neuropsychotropic action of a new anti-epileptic agent: depamide. Ann Med Psychol (Paris) 1966; 124(5):707–710.
3. Okuma T, Kishimoto A, Inoue K, et al. Anti-manic and prophylactic effects of carbamazepine (Tegretol) on manic depressive psychosis. A preliminary report. Folia Psychiatr Neurol Jpn 1973; 27(4):283–297.
4. Okuma T, Kishimoto A. A history of investigation on the mood stabilizing effect of carbamazepine in Japan. Psychiatry Clin Neurosci 1998; 52(1):3–12.
5. Ovsiew F. Antiepileptic drugs in psychiatry. J Neurol Neurosurg Psychiatry 2004; 75 (12):1655–1658.
6. Barchi RL. Ion channel mutations affecting muscle and brain. Curr Opin Neurol 1998; 11(5):461–468.
7. Errington AC, Stohr T, Lees G. Voltage gated ion channels: targets for anticonvulsant drugs. Curr Top Med Chem 2005; 5(1):15–30.

8. Ragsdale DS, Avoli M. Sodium channels as molecular targets for antiepileptic drugs. Brain Res Brain Res Rev 1998; 26(1):16–28.

9. Hoffman F, Biel M, Flockerzi V. Molecular basis for Ca2+ channel diversity. Annu Rev Neurosci 1994; 17:399–418.

10. Stefani A, Spadoni F, Bernardi G. Voltage-activated calcium channels: targets of antiepileptic drug therapy? Epilepsia 1997; 38(9):959–965.

11. Coulter DA, Huguenard JR, Prince DA. Characterization of ethosuximide reduction of low-threshold calcium current in thalamic neurons. Ann Neurol 1989; 25(6):582–593.

12. Blalock EM, Chen KC, Vanaman TC, et al. Epilepsy-induced decrease of L-type Ca2+ channel activity and coordinate regulation of subunit mRNA in single neurons of rat hippocampal 'zipper' slices. Epilepsy Res 2001; 43(3):211–226.

13. Otoom S, Hasan Z. Nifedipine inhibits picrotoxin-induced seizure activity: further evidence on the involvement of L-type calcium channel blockers in epilepsy. Fundam Clin Pharmacol 2006; 20(2):115–119.

14. Porter RJ, Rogawski MA. New antiepileptic drugs: from serendipity to rational discovery. Epilepsia 1992; 33(suppl 1):S1–S6.

15. Olsen RW, Avoli M. GABA and epileptogenesis. Epilepsia 1997; 38(4):399–407.

16. Loscher W. Valproate: a reappraisal of its pharmacodynamic properties and mechanisms of action. Prog Neurobiol 1999; 58(1):31–59.

17. Chebib M. GABAC receptor ion channels. Clin Exp Pharmacol Physiol 2004; 31(11):800–804.

18. Sperk G, Furtinger S, Schwarzer C, et al. GABA and its receptors in epilepsy. Adv Exp Med Biol 2004; 548:92–103.

19. Gage PW. Activation and modulation of neuronal K+ channels by GABA. Trends Neurosci 1992; 15(2):46–51.

20. Misgeld U, Bijak M, Jarolimek W. A physiological role for GABAB receptors and the effects of baclofen in the mammalian central nervous system. Prog Neurobiol 1995; 46(4):423–462.

21. Meldrum BS. Update on the mechanism of action of antiepileptic drugs. Epilepsia 1996; 37(suppl 6):S4–S11.

22. Tillakaratne NJ, Medina-Kauwe L, Gibson KM. Gamma-Aminobutyric acid (GABA) metabolism in mammalian neural and nonneural tissues. Comp Biochem Physiol A Physiol 1995; 112(2):247–263.

23. Meldrum BS. Glutamate as a neurotransmitter in the brain: review of physiology and pathology. J Nutr 2000; 130(suppl 4S):S1007–S1015.

24. Moldrich RX, Chapman AG, De Sarro G, et al. Glutamate metabotropic receptors as targets for drug therapy in epilepsy. Eur J Pharmacol 2003; 476(1–2):3–16.

25. Isaac M. Serotonergic 5-HT2C receptors as a potential therapeutic target for the design antiepileptic drugs. Curr Top Med Chem 2005; 5(1):59–67.

26. Applegate CD, Tecott LH. Global increases in seizure susceptibility in mice lacking 5-HT2C receptors: a behavioral analysis. Exp Neurol 1998; 154(2):522–530.

27. Heisler LK, Chu HM, Tecott LH. Epilepsy and obesity in serotonin 5-HT2C receptor mutant mice. Ann N Y Acad Sci 1998; 861:74–78.

28. Gobert A, Rivet JM, Lejeune F, et al. Serotonin (2C) receptors tonically suppress the activity of mesocortical dopaminergic and adrenergic, but not serotonergic, pathways: a combined dialysis and electrophysiological analysis in the rat. Synapse 2000; 36(3):205–221.

29. Hutson PH, Barton CL, Jay M, et al. Activation of mesolimbic dopamine function by phencyclidine is enhanced by 5-HT (2C/2B) receptor antagonists: neurochemical and behavioral studies. Neuropharmacology 2000; 39(12):2318–2328.

30. Pasini A, Tortorella A, Gale K. The anticonvulsant action of fluoxetine in substantia nigra is dependent upon endogenous serotonin. Brain Res 1996; 724(1):84–88.

31. Favale E, Audenino D, Cocito L, et al. The antcionvulsant effect of citalopram as an indirect evidence of serotonergic impairment in human epileptogenesis. Seizure 2003; 12(5):316–318.

32. Macdonald RL. Antiepileptic drug actions. Epilepsia 1989; 30(suppl 1):S19–S28 (discussion S64–S18).

33. Zona C, Tancredi V, Palma E, et al. Potassium currents in rat cortical neurons in culture are enhanced by the antiepileptic drug carbamazepine. Can J Physiol Pharmacol 1990; 68(4):545–547.

34. Ambrosio AF, Silva AP, Malva JO, et al. Carbamazepine inhibits L-type Ca2+ channels in cultured rat hippocampal neurons stimulated with glutamate receptor agonists. Neuropharmacology 1999; 38(9):1349–1359.
35. McLean MJ, Macdonald RL. Carbamazepine and 10,11-epoxycarbamazepine produce use- and voltage-dependent limitation of rapidly firing action potentials of mouse central neurons in cell culture. J Pharmacol Exp Ther 1986; 238(2):727–738.
36. Granger P, Biton B, Faure C, et al. Modulation of the gamma-aminobutyric acid type A receptor by the antiepileptic drugs carbamazepine and phenytoin. Mol Pharmacol 1995; 47(6):1189–1196.
37. Motohashi N, Ikawa K, Kariya T. GABAB receptors are up-regulated by chronic treatment with lithium or carbamazepine. GABA hypothesis of affective disorders? Eur J Pharmacol 1989; 166(1):95–99.
38. Zhang JD, Saito K. Carbamazepine facilitates effects of GABA on rat hippocampus slices. Zhongguo Yao Li Xue Bao 1997; 18(3):230–233.
39. Hough CJ, Irwin RP, Gao XM, et al. Carbamazepine inhibition of N-methyl-D-aspartate-evoked calcium influx in rat cerebellar granule cells. J Pharmacol Exp Ther 1996; 276(1): 143–149.
40. Waldmeier PC, Baumann PA, Wicki P, et al. Similar potency of carbamazepine, oxcarbazepine, and lamotrigine in inhibiting the release of glutamate and other neurotransmitters. Neurology 1995; 45(10):1907–1913.
41. Biber K, Walden J, Gebicke-Harter P, et al. Carbamazepine inhibits the potentiation by adenosine analogues of agonist induced inositolphosphate formation in hippocampal astrocyte cultures. Biol Psychiatry 1996; 40(7):563–567.
42. Post RM, Weiss SR, Chuang DM. Mechanisms of action of anticonvulsants in affective disorders: comparisons with lithium. J Clin Psychopharmacol 1992; 12(1 suppl):S23–S35.
43. Chen G, Pan B, Hawver DB, et al. Attenuation of cyclic AMP production by carbamazepine. J Neurochem 1996; 67(5):2079–2086.
44. Dailey JW, Reith ME, Yan QS, et al. Carbamazepine increases extracellular serotonin concentration: lack of antagonism by tetrodotoxin or zero Ca2+. Eur J Pharmacol 1997; 328(2-3):153–162.
45. Dailey JW, Reith ME, Yan QS, et al. Anticonvulsant doses of carbamazepine increase hippocampal extracellular serotonin in genetically epilepsy-prone rats: dose response relationships. Neurosci Lett 1997; 227(1):13–16.
46. Fraser CM, Sills GJ, Butler E, et al. Effects of valproate, vigabatrin and tiagabine on GABA uptake into human astrocytes cultured from fetal and adult brain tissue. Epileptic Disord 1999; 1(3):153–157.
47. Albus H, Williamson R. Electrophysiologic analysis of the actions of valproate on pyramidal neurons in the rat hippocampal slice. Epilepsia 1998; 39(2):124–139.
48. Remy S, Urban BW, Elger CE, et al. Anticonvulsant pharmacology of voltage-gated Na+ channels in hippocampal neurons of control and chronically epileptic rats. Eur J Pharmacol 2003; 17(12):2648–2658.
49. Vreugdenhil M, van Veelan CW, van Rijen PC, et al. Effect of valproic acid on sodium currents in cortical neurons from patients with pharmaco-resistant temporal lobe epilepsy. Epilepsy Res 1998; 32(1–2):309–320.
50. Kelly KM, Gross RA, Macdonald RL. Valproic acid selectively reduces the low-threshold (T) calcium current in rat nodose neurons. Neurosci Lett 1990; 116(1-2):233–238.
51. Gean PW, Huang CC, Hung CR, et al. Valproic acid suppresses the synaptic response mediated by the NMDA receptors in rat amygdalar slices. Brain Res Bull 1994; 33(3): 333–336.
52. Zeise ML, Kasparow S, Zieglgansberger W. Valproate suppresses N-methyl-D-aspartate-evoked, transient depolarizations in the rat neocortex in vitro. Brain Res 1991; 544(2): 345–348.
53. Chapman AG, Croucher MJ, Meldrum BS. Anticonvulsant activity of intracerebroventricularly administered valproate and valproate analogues. A dose-dependent correlation with changes in brain aspartate and GABA levels in DBA/2 mice. Biochem Pharmacol 1984; 33(9):1459–1463.
54. McLean MJ, Macdonald RL. Multiple actions of phenytoin on mouse spinal cord neurons in cell culture. J Pharmacol Exp Ther 1983; 227(3):779–789.

55. Schwarz JR, Grigat G. Phenytoin and carbamazepine: potential- and frequency-dependent block of Na currents in mammalian myelinated nerve fibers. Epilepsia 1989; 30(3):286–294.
56. Schumacher TB, Beck H, Steinhauser C, et al. Effects of phenytoin, carbamazepine, and gabapentin on calcium channels in hippocampal granule cells from patients with temporal lobe epilepsy. Epilepsia 1998; 39(4):355–363.
57. Tunnicliff G. Basis of antiseizure action of phenytoin. Gen Pharmacol 1996; 27(7):1091–1097.
58. Wamil AW, McLean MJ. Phenytoin blocks N-methyl-D-aspartate responses of mouse central neurons. J Pharmacol Exp Ther 1993; 267(1):218–227.
59. DeLorenzo RJ. Calmodulin systems in neuronal excitability: a molecular approach to epilepsy. Ann Neurol 1984; 16(suppl): S104–S114.
60. Twyman RE, Rogers CJ, Macdonald RL. Differential regulation of gamma-aminobutyric acid receptor channels by diazepam and phenobarbital. Ann Neurol 1989; 25(3):213–220.
61. White HS. Comparative anticonvulsant and mechanistic profile of the established and newer epileptic drugs. Epilepsia 1999; 40(suppl 5):S2–S10.
62. McLean MJ, Macdonald RL. Benzodiazepines, but not beta carbolines, limit high frequency repetitive firing of action potentials of spinal cord neurons in cell culture. J Pharmacol Exp Ther 1988; 244(2): 789–795.
63. Skerritt JH, Werz MA, McLean MJ, et al. Diazepam and its anomalous p-chloro-derivative Ro 5-4864: comparative effects on mouse neurons in cell culture. Brain Res 1984; 310(1): 99–105.
64. Macdonald RL, Rogers CJ, Twyman RE. Barbiturate regulation of kinetic properties of the GABAA receptor channel of mouse spinal neurones in culture. J Physiol 1989; 417: 483–500.
65. Rogawski MA, Porter RJ. Antiepileptic drugs: pharmacological mechanisms and clinical efficacy with consideration of promising developmental stage compounds. Pharmacol Rev 1990; 42(3):223–286.
66. Marszalec W, Narahashi T. Use-dependent pentobarbital block of kainate and quisqualate currents. Brain Res 1993; 608(1):7–15.
67. Crunelli V, Leresche N. Block of thalamic T-type Ca(2+) channels by ehtosuximide is not the whole story. Epilepsy Curr 2002; 2(2):53–56.
68. Leresche N, Parri HR, Erdemli G, et al. On the action of the anti-absence drug ethosuximide in the rat and cat thalamus. J Neurosci 1998; 18(13):4842–4853.
69. Kaminski RM, Tochman AM, Dekundy A, et al. Ethosuximide and valproate display high efficacy against lindane-induced seizures in mice. Toxicol Lett 2004; 154(1–2):55–60.
70. Reiss WG, Oles KS. Acetazolamide in the treatment of seizures. Ann Pharmacother 1996; 30(5):514–519.
71. Woodbury DM, Engstrom FL, White HS, et al. Ionic and acid-base regulation of neurons and glia during seizures. Ann Neurol 1984; 16(suppl): S135–S144.
72. Schwartzkroin PA. Cellular electrophysiology of human epilepsy. Epilepsy Res 1994; 17 (3):185–192.
73. Traynelis SF, Cull-Candy SG. Proton inhibition of N-methyl-D-aspartate receptors in cerebellar neurons. J Physiol 1990; 345(6273):347–350.
74. Krishek BJ, Amato A, Connolly CN, et al. Proton sensitivity of the GABA (A) receptor is associated with the receptor subunit composition. J Physiol 1996; 492(pt 2):431–443.
75. Pellock JM. Felbamate. Epilepsia 1999; 40(suppl 5):S57–S62.
76. Taylor LA, McQuade RD, Tice MA. Felbamate, a novel antiepileptic drug, reverses N-methyl-D-aspartate/glycine-stimulated increases in intracellular Ca2+ concentration. Eur J Pharmacol 1995; 289(2):229–233.
77. Corradetti R, Pugliese AM. Electrophysiological effects of felbamate. Life Sci 1998; 63 (13):1075–1088.
78. McCabe RT, Wasterlain CG, Kucharczyk N, et al. Evidence for anticonvulsant and neuroprotectant action of felbamate mediated by strychnine-insensitive glycine receptors. J Pharmacol Exp Ther 1993; 264(3):1248–1252.
79. White HS, Harmsworth WL, Sofia RD, et al. Felbamate modulates the strychnine-insensitive glycine receptor. Epilepsy Res 1995; 20(1):41–48.
80. Rho JM, Donevan SD, Rogawski MA. Mechanism of action of the anticonvulsant felbamate: opposing effects on N-methyl-D-aspartate and gamma-aminobutyric acid A receptors. Ann Neurol 1994; 35(2):229–234.

81. Subramaniam S, Rho JM, Penix L, et al. Felbamate block of the N-methyl-D-aspartate receptor. J Pharmacol Exp Ther 1995; 273(2):878–886.
82. De Sarro G, Ongini E, Bertorelli R, et al. Excitatory amino acid neurotransmission through both NMDA and non-NMDA receptors is involved in the anticonvulsant activity of felbamate in DBA/2 mice. Eur J Pharmacol 1994; 262(1–2):11–19.
83. Rho JM, Donevan SD, Rogawski MA. Barbiturate-like actions of the propanediol dicarbamates felbamate and meprobamate. J Pharmacol Exp Ther 1997; 280(3):1383–1391.
84. Taglialatela M, Ongini E, Brown AM, et al. Felbamate inhibits cloned voltage-dependent Na+ channels from human and rat brain. Eur J Pharmacol 1996; 316(2–3):373–377.
85. Stefani A, Calabresi P, Pisani A, et al. Felbamate inhibits dihydropyridine-sensitive calcium channels in central neurons. J Pharmacol Exp Ther 1996; 277(1):121–127.
86. Privitera MD. Topiramate: a new antiepileptic drug. Ann Pharmacother 1997; 31(10): 1164–1173.
87. Zona C, Ciotti MT, Avoli M. Topiramate attenuates voltage-gated sodium currents in rat cerebellar granule cells. Neurosci Lett 1997; 231(3):123–126.
88. Zhang X, Velumian AA, Jones OT, et al. Modulation of high-voltage-activated calcium channels in dentate granule cells by topiramate. Epilepsia 2000; 41(suppl 1):S52–S60.
89. DeLorenzo RJ, Sombati S, Coulter DA. Effects of topiramate on sustained repetitive firing and spontaneous recurrent seizure discharges in cultured hippocampal neurons. Epilepsia 2000; 41(suppl 1): S40–S44.
90. White HS, Brown SD, Woodhead JH, et al. Topiramate enhances GABA-mediated chloride flux and GABA-evoked chloride currents in murine brain neurons and increases seizure threshold. Epilepsy Res 1997; 28(3):167–179.
91. White HS, Brown SD, Woodhead JH, et al. Topiramate modulates GABA-evoked currents in murine cortical neurons by a nonbenzodiazepine mechanism. Epilepsia 2000; 41(suppl 1): S17–S20.
92. Gibbs JW, Sombati S, DeLorenzo RJ, et al. Cellular actions of topiramate: blockade of kainate-evoked inward currents in cultured hippocampal neurons. Epilepsia 2000; 41 (suppl 1):S10–S16.
93. Shank RP, Gardocki JF, Vaught JL, et al. Topiramate: preclinical evaluation of structurally novel anticonvulsant. Epilepsia 1994; 35(2):450–460.
94. Morris GL. Gabapentin. Epilepsia 1999; 40(suppl 5):S63–S70.
95. Taylor CP, Gee NS, Su TZ, et al. A summary of mechanistic hypotheses of gabapentin pharmacology. Epilepsy Res 1998; 29(3):233–249.
96. Honmou O, Oyelese AA, Kocsis JD. The anticonvulsant gabapentin enhances promoted release of GABA in hippocampus: a field potential analysis. Brain Res 1995; 692(1-2): 273–277.
97. Honmou O, Kocsis JD, Richerson GB. Gabapentin potentiates the conductance increase induced by nipecotic acid in CA1 pyramidal neurons in vitro. Epilepsy Res 1995; 20(3): 193–202.
98. Gee NS, Brown JP, Dissanayake VU, et al. The novel anticonvulsant drug, gabapentin (Neurontin): binds to the alpha2delta subunit of a calcium channel. J Biol Chem 1996; 271(10):5768–5776.
99. Sobieszek G, Borowicz KK, Kimber-Trojnar Z, et al. Zonisamide: a new antiepileptic drug. Pol J Pharmacol 2003; 55(5):683–689.
100. Schauf CL. Zonisamide enhances slow sodium inactivation in Myxicola. Brain Res 1987; 413(1):185–188.
101. Suzuki S, Kawakami K, Nishimura S, et al. Zonisamide blocks T-type calcium channel in cultured neurons of rat cerebral cortex. Epilepsy Res 1992; 12(1):21–27.
102. Masuda Y, Karasawa T. Inhibitory effect of zonisamide on human carbonic anhydrase in vitro. Arzneimittelforschung 1993; 43(4):416–418.
103. Kawata Y, Okada M, Murakami T, et al. Effects of zonisamide on K+ and Ca2+ evoked release of monamine as well as K+ evoked intracellular Ca2+ mobilization in rat hippocampus. Epilepsy Res 1999; 35(3):173–182.
104. Okada M, Kaneko S, Hirano T, et al. Effects of zonisamide on dopaminergic system. Epilepsy Res 1995; 22(3):193–205.

105. Okada M, Kawata Y, Mizuno K, et al. Interaction between Ca2+, K+, carbamazepine and zonisamide on hippocampal extracellular glutamate monitored with a microdialysis electrode. Br J Pharmacol 1998; 124(6):1277–1285.
106. Mori A, Noda Y, Packer L. The anticonvulsant zonisamide scavenges free radicals. Epilepsy Res 1998; 30(2):153–158.
107. Reynolds EH, Chanarin I, Milner G, et al. Anticonvulsant therapy, folic acid and vitamin B12 metabolism and mental symptoms. Epilepsia 1966; 7(4):261–270.
108. Cheung H, Kamp D, Harris E. An in vitro investigation of the action of lamotrigine on neuronal voltage-activated sodium channels. Epilepsy Res 1992; 13(2):107–112.
109. Zona C, Avoli M. Lamotrigine reduces voltage-gated sodium currents in rat central neurons in culture. Epilepsia 1997; 38(5):522–525.
110. Leach MJ, Marden CM, Miller AA. Pharmacological studies on lamotrigine, a novel potential antiepileptic drug: II. Neurochemical studies on the mechanism of action. Epilepsia 1986; 27(5):490–497.
111. Stefani A, Spadoni F, Siniscalchi A, et al. Lamotrigine inhibits Ca2+ currents in cortical neurons: functional implications. Eur J Pharmacol 1996; 307(1):113–116.
112. Wang SJ, Huang CC, Hsu KS, et al. Inhibition of N-type calcium currents by lamotrigine in rat amygdalar neurones. Neuroreport 1996; 7(18):3037–3040.
113. Hovinga CA. Levetiracetam: a novel antiepileptic drug. Pharmacotherapy 2001; 21 (11):1375–1388.
114. Noyer M, Gillard M, Matagne A, et al. The novel antiepileptic drug levetiracetam (ucb L059) appears to act via a specific binding site in CNS membranes. Eur J Pharmacol 1995; 286(2):137–146.
115. Lynch BA, Lambeng N, Nocka K, et al. The synaptic vesicle protein SV2A is the binding site for the antiepileptic drug levetiracetam. Proc Natl Acad Sci U S A 2004; 101 (26):9861–9866.
116. McLean MJ, Schmutz M, Wamil AW, et al. Oxcarbazepine: mechanisms of action. Epilepsia 1994; 35(suppl 3):S5–S9.
117. Stefani A, Pisani A, De Murtas M, et al. Action of GP 47779, the active metabolite of oxcarbazepine, on the corticostriatal system. II. Modulation of high-voltage-activated calcium currents. Epilepsia 1995; 36(10):997–1002.
118. Calabresi P, de Murtas M, Stefani A, et al. Action of GP 47779, the active metabolite of oxcarbazepine, on the cotricostriatal system. I. Modulation of corticostraital synaptic transmission. Epilepsia 1995; 36(10):990–996.
119. Warner G, Figgitt DP. Pregabalin: as adjunctive treatment of partial seizures. CNS Drugs 2005; 19(3):265–272 (discussion 273–274).
120. Taylor CP, Angelotti T, Fauman E. Pharmacology and mechanism of action of pre-gabalin: the calcium channel alpha2-delta (alpha2-delta) subunit as a target for anti-epileptic drug discovery. Epilepsy Res 2007; 73(2):137–150.
121. Borden LA, Murali Dhar TG, Smith KE, et al. Tiagabine, SK&F 89976-A, CI-966, and NNC-711 are selective for the cloned GABA transporter GAT-1. Eur J Pharmacol 1994; 269(2):219–224.
122. Roepstorff A, Lambert JD. Comparison of the effect of the GABA uptake blockers, tiagabine and nipecotic acid, on inhibitory synaptic efficacy in hippocampal CA1 neurones. Neurosci Lett 1992; 146(2):131–134.
123. Leach JP, Brodie MJ. Tiagabine. Lancet 1998; 351(9097):203–207.
124. Mumford JP, Cannon DJ. Vigabatrin. Epilepsia 1994; 35(suppl 5):S25–S28.
125. Lippert B, Metcalf BW, Jung MJ, et al. 4-amino-hex-5-enoic acid, a selective catalytic inhibitor of 4-aminobutyric-acid aminotransferase in mammalian brain. Eur J Pharmacol 1977; 74(3):441–445.
126. Leach JP, Sills GJ, Majid A, et al. Effects of tiagabine and vigabatrin on GABA uptake into primary cultures of rat cortical astrocytes. Seizure 1996; 5(3):229–234.
127. Rogawski MA. Diverse mechanisms of antiepileptic drugs in the development pipeline. Epilepsy Res 2006; 69(3):273–294.

2 Treatment of Acute Manic and Mixed Episodes

Paul E. Keck, Jr., Susan L. McElroy, and Jeffrey R. Strawn
Lindner Center of HOPE, Mason, and Department of Psychiatry, University of Cincinnati College of Medicine, Cincinnati, Ohio, U.S.A.

INTRODUCTION

Antiepileptic agents have been used to treat bipolar manic and mixed episodes since early investigational pilot trials dating back to the 1960s (1). Research into the potential efficacy of antiepileptic agents in the treatment of bipolar disorder has been based on empirical observations of the efficacy of specific agents as well as heuristic models of the potential pathogenesis of bipolar disorder, such as the kindling hypothesis (2). Antiepileptic agents include a broad group of compounds with diverse pharmacological properties and differential efficacy in various forms of epilepsy. In this chapter, we review the evidence to date regarding the efficacy of antiepileptic agents in the treatment of bipolar manic and mixed episodes, with particular attention to agents studied in randomized, controlled trials.

VALPROIC ACID

Various formulations of valproic acid (valproate, divalproex sodium, valpromide) have been shown to be efficacious for the treatment of acute manic and mixed episodes in a number of randomized, controlled trials (Table 1). In three, three-week, placebo-controlled, monotherapy trials among hospitalized patients, divalproex (3,4) and divalproex extended release (ER) (5) were superior to placebo in reduction of manic symptoms. These large trials confirmed the findings of smaller, placebo-controlled, crossover pilot studies (6,7).

The efficacy of the divalproex formulation in acute bipolar mania has also been studied in direct comparator trials against olanzapine (8,9) and lithium (10,11) in adults and against quetiapine in adolescents (12). Most of these latter, comparator trials were not powered sufficiently to detect potential differences in efficacy among agents and generally yielded comparable efficacy results. However, one of the olanzapine comparator trials included a sufficiently large sample of patients to detect a potential difference in efficacy between agents and found a slight difference in favor of olanzapine over divalproex (8). In both olanzapine comparator trials, divalproex had better overall tolerability (8,9).

A number of studies have specifically examined the efficacy, safety, and tolerability of divalproex oral loading, which has been administered either as 20 mg/kg/day (13–15), 25 mg/kg/day (ER formulation) (5), or 30 mg/kg/day for two days, followed by 20 mg/kg/day (9,11).

Although none of these trials was adequately powered to detect a significant difference in efficacy of the oral loading strategy, this approach was nevertheless found to be well tolerated. In addition, in a study comparing this strategy with haloperidol specifically in patients with psychotic mania, divalproex-treated patients had comparable reductions in psychotic as well as manic symptoms (15).

Divalproex has also been used as a comparator in adjunctive treatment trials (16–23). All but one of such studies (16) compared the acute efficacy of placebo added

TABLE 1   Randomized, Controlled Trials of Divalproex in Bipolar Manic and Mixed Episodes

Study	Diagnostic criteria	Design	Results
Bowden et al., 2006	Bipolar I, manic or mixed episode (DSM-IV)	DBPC, LOCF (3-wk), DVPX ER 25 mg/kg, increased by 500 mg on day 3, and adjusted to serum concentrations of 85–125 μg/mL	DVPX ER > placebo, mean MRS[3] DVPX ER (48%) > placebo (34%), response
DelBello et al., 2006	Bipolar I, manic or mixed episode (DSM-IV)	DBC, LOCF (4-wk), DVPX vs. QTP in adolescents	QTP = DVPX
Sachs et al., 2004	Bipolar I, manic episode (DSM-IV)	DBPC (3-wk), QTP + Li or DVPX vs. Li or DVPX monotherapy Lithium target levels: 0.7–1.0 mEq/L; valproic acid serum concentrations 50–100 μg/mL. QTP dosed 100 mg (day 1) and increased 100 mg/day until day 4 and optimized to between 200 and 800 mg/day by day 21	QTP + Li (56%) or + DVPX (53%) > Li (27%) or DVPX (36%) monotherapy, YMRS response
Yatham et al., 2004	Bipolar I, manic episode (DSM-IV)	DBPC (3 or 6 wk), QTP + Li or DVPX. Li and DVPX dosed to serum levels of 0.7–1.0 mEq/L and 50–100 μg/mL, respectively. QTP flexibly dosed to 800 mg/day	QTP + DVPX/Li (15.9) > Li/DVPX alone (12.2), improvement in YMRS score
Muller-Oerlinghausen et al., 2003	Acute manic episode (ICD-10 criteria)	DBPC (3-wk) of adjunctive VPA (20 mg/kg, fixed-dose) in patients treated with neuroleptic therapy	VPA > placebo, neuroleptic dose (primary outcome measure) DVPX (70%) > placebo (46%), YMRS[4] 50% reduction.
Tohen et al., 2002	Bipolar I, manic or mixed episode (DSM-IV)	DBC of flexable-dose OLZ (5–20 mg/day) and DVPX (500–2500 mg/day).	OLZ (54%) > DVPX (42%), YMRS[4] 50% reduction
Zajecka et al., 2002	Bipolar I, manic episode (DSM-IV)	DBC (3-wk) of flexable-dose olanzapine and DVPX with 12 week follow-up	No difference between DVPX and OLZ, MRS[3] score.
Bowden et al., 1994	Research Diagnostic Criteria for manic disorder	DBPC, LOCF (3-wk), Li (adjusted to 1.5 mmol/L) vs. DVPX	DVPX 48%, Li 49%, placebo 25%, MRS[3] 50% reduction
Freeman et al., 1992	Bipolar I, manic episode or "mixed state" (DSM-IIIR)	DBPC (3-wk). Li vs. VPA	Li = DVPX, on MRS, GAS, BPRS
Pope et al., 1991	Bipolar I, manic or mixed (DSM-IIIR)	DBPC (3-wk), Li nonresponders. DVPX dose adjusted to serum concentration of 50–125 μg/mL	DVPX (54%) > placebo (5%), YMRS score DVPX (20 point improvement) > placebo (0 point improvement), GAS

Abbreviations: ICD, International Classification of Diseases; DSM, Diagnostic And Statistical Manual Of Mental Disorders; DBPC, double-blind, placebo-controlled trial; DBC, double-blind, controlled trial; DVPX, divalproex; LCOF, last observation carried forward; MRS, Mania Rating Scale; YMRS, Young Mania Rating Scale; ER, extended release; QTP, quetiapine; Li, lithium; OLZ, olanzapine; GAS, Global Assessment Scale; BPRS, Brief Psychiatric Rating Scale.

to divalproex or lithium with a second-generation (atypical) antipsychotic (SGA) added to divalproex or lithium in patients with bipolar mania with or without psychotic symptoms. SGAs, either begun in combination with divalproex or lithium or added adjunctively to pre-existing and usually only partially successful mono-therapy with divalproex or lithium, were superior to placebo in these trials. One study addressed whether the addition of valproate was superior to placebo in patients receiving first-generation antipsychotics for patients with acute mania (16). Significantly, more valproate-treated patients displayed a decrease in the need for concomitant antipsychotic medication by the three-week study end point.

A number of post hoc analyses have been conducted to examine potential predictors of response to valproate in patients with acute mania (24,25). These anal-yses indicated that patients with manic and mixed episodes had comparable response rates to valproate and that the number of prior mood episodes did not adversely affect valproate response. In addition, the presence or absence of psychosis did not appear to affect response either (9,11). A post hoc analysis of pooled intent-to-treat data from three randomized, placebo-controlled studies of divalproex studies in patients with acute mania found a linear relationship between serum valproate concentration and response and that the target serum concentration of valproate for optimal response was above 94 mg/L (26). In summary, data from the controlled trials reviewed above indicate that valproate has a broad spectrum of efficacy in both acute manic and mixed episodes, with or without psychosis, and appears to be comparable to lithium and antipsychotics in overall acute antimanic efficacy.

CARBAMAZEPINE

Although 14 double-blind, controlled trials provided preliminary evidence of carbamazepine's efficacy in the treatment of acute mania (27), these findings were only recently replicated in two large, multicenter, randomized, placebo-controlled, parallel-group trials (Table 2) (28,29). In the first of these two trials (28), there was no significant difference in mean reduction of manic symptoms in patients with

TABLE 2 Selected Randomized Controlled Trials of Carbamazepine in Bipolar Manic and Mixed Episodes

Study	Diagnostic criteria	Design	Results
Zhang et al., 2007	Bipolar I, mixed or manic episode (DSM-IV)	DBPC (12-wk), LOCF. CBZ+ FEWP vs. CBZ or placebo	CBZ (93%) > placebo (57%), YMRS 50% reduction No efficacy difference between CBZ+ FEWP and CBZ
Weisler et al., 2005	Bipolar I, mixed or Manic episode (DSM-IV)	DBPC (3-wk) LOCF, CBZ beaded-extended release) 200 mg BID increased (as necessary, tolerated) by 200 mg/day to 1600 mg/day	CBZ > placebo, YMRS total score reduction and CGI score
Weisler et al., 2004	Bipolar I, mixed or manic episode (DSM-IV)	DBPC (3-wk) LOCF, CBZ (beaded-extended release) 400 mg/day increased to 1600 mg/day	CBZ (42%) > placebo (22%), YMRS 50% reduction

Abbreviations: BID, twice a day; CBZ, carbamazepine; DBPC, double-blind, placebo-controlled trial; DBC, double-blind, controlled trial; LOCF, last observation carried forward; YMRS, Young Mania Rating Scale; FEWP, Free and Easy Wanderer Plus (Jia-wey Shiau-Yau San, Chinese herbal remedy).

mixed episodes treated with carbamazepine compared with placebo, due in part to a high placebo response in the subgroup. However, in the second trial (29), response rates were significantly higher in both manic and mixed patients receiving carbamazepine compared with placebo. Aside from the subgroup analyses in these two trials, there are no consistent data regarding clinical predictors of acute response to carbamazepine.

Carbamazepine had previously been compared with lithium (30,31) and chlorpromazine (32,33) in head-to-head studies without a placebo group. These studies, although individually limited by small sample sizes, in aggregate found comparable antimanic efficacy among patients receiving carbamazepine, lithium, or chlorpromazine.

There are few controlled studies involving carbamazepine as adjunctive or combination treatment in patients with acute bipolar mania. In an eight-week, double-blind comparison trial of carbamazepine with lithium versus haloperidol with lithium involving 33 patients with acute mania, both treatment groups had comparable mean reductions in both manic and psychotic symptoms as well as similar response rates at end point (34). Risperidone was compared with placebo in combination with carbamazepine, lithium, or divalproex in patients with acute mania in another trial (35). Interestingly, risperidone was superior to placebo in combination with lithium of divalproex, but not with carbamazepine. This may have been due to induction of risperidone metabolism in the carbamazepine group, leading to subtherapeutic risperidone serum concentrations. Finally, carbamazepine was utilized as the principal antimanic agent in a study comparing a Chinese herbal medicine formulation with placebo in patients with acute mania (36). In this trial, the herbal medicine in combination with carbamazepine was no more efficacious than placebo with carbamazepine.

OXCARBAZEPINE

Oxcarbazepine, the 10-keto analogue of carbamazepine, has been studied in five controlled trials as monotherapy for patients with acute bipolar mania (37–41). The first double-blind study was a small pilot trial involving six patients in an A-B-A crossover design (37). The improvement seen during the oxcarbazepine component of this trial led to two double-blind comparison trials versus haloperidol and lithium, respectively (38,39).

In both studies, oxcarbazepine and the respective comparator agent were of similar efficacy. However, both studies were limited by small samples, the use of chlorpromazine as an as-needed adjunctive medication, and the absence of a placebo control group (42). In more recent controlled trials, the efficacy of oxcarbazepine in the treatment of acute bipolar mania has not yet been convincingly established. For example, in an open-label on-off-on study, four (33%) of 12 patients were classified as responders to oxcarbazepine, and antimanic effects were evident primarily in patients with mild-to-moderate symptoms (40). In the only large, randomized, double-blind, placebo-controlled, parallel-group trial of oxcarbazepine reported to date, a seven-week study conducted in children and adolescents with acute bipolar manic or mixed episodes, oxcarbazepine was not superior to placebo in reduction of manic symptoms (41).

PHENYTOIN

Two small controlled trials of phenytoin in the treatment of manic symptoms have recently been reported (43,44). The first trial compared the combination of phenytoin and haloperidol with placebo and haloperidol in a five-week study of patients with bipolar or schizoaffective disorder with manic symptoms (43). Significantly, more improvement in manic symptoms was evident in patients receiving the combination of phenytoin and haloperidol. The second trial examined the use of phenytoin in the prevention of manic symptoms in patients with allergies, pulmonary, or rheumatological illnesses receiving corticosteroid treatment (44). Thus, this trial was designed to prevent the occurrence of manic symptoms due to corticosteroids and not in patients with bipolar disorder per se.

The phenytoin-treated group displayed significantly smaller increases on patient self-report measures of manic symptoms compared with patients receiving placebo. Taken together, these findings are intriguing and suggest that phenytoin may have antimanic properties. However, these initial findings require confirmation in placebo-controlled studies of phenytoin monotherapy in patients with acute bipolar manic and mixed episodes.

TOPIRAMATE

In four randomized, placebo-controlled, parallel-group, three-week trials in adult patients with bipolar mania, two of which also included a lithium comparison group, topiramate was not found to have significant antimanic efficacy compared with placebo (45). These results could not be explained by a high placebo response. Moreover, the lithium groups were superior to placebo in the two trials utilizing a lithium control group. A placebo-controlled trial of topiramate monotherapy in children and adolescents with acute bipolar mania was discontinued upon analysis of the adult trial data described above (46). Thus, the results of this study, which was limited by a small sample, were inconclusive. Lastly, topiramate was also compared with placebo as an adjunct to lithium or valproate in patients with acute bipolar I mania (47). As in the monotherapy trials, there was no significant reduction in manic symptoms in patients receiving topiramate compared with placebo. Of note, topiramate treatment was associated with a significant reduction in body weight compared with placebo. This secondary finding is consistent with observations of topiramate's weight loss effects in other studies in patients with bipolar disorder (48,49), epilepsy (50), migraine (51), diabetic neuropathy (52), obesity (53), and binge-eating disorder associated with obesity (54).

GABAPENTIN

Two placebo-controlled trials of gabapentin in the treatment of acute bipolar mania failed to find significant efficacy of gabapentin over placebo (55,56). These included a large, multicenter, parallel-group trial of gabapentin as adjunctive therapy in patients with bipolar I manic or mixed episodes (55) and a small crossover trial in patients with rapid cycling bipolar disorders refractory to previous trials of mood stabilizing agents (56). In an interesting analysis of a sample of 43 patients with bipolar disorder who were treatment refractory to mood stabilizers and who received gabapentin in an open-label trial, significant improvement was observed in a subgroup of patients with comorbid anxiety and/or alcohol abuse (57). These preliminary observations suggest that gabapentin may have utility in the treatment of patients with bipolar disorder with comorbid anxiety or alcohol-use disorders.

LAMOTRIGINE

In three randomized, controlled trials, lamotrigine was not found to be significantly superior to placebo in the treatment of bipolar manic symptoms (56,58,59). In the first of these studies, a series of six-week crossover trials comparing lamotrigine, gabapentin, and placebo in patients with treatment-refractory rapid-cycling bipolar disorders, there was no significant difference in reduction of manic symptoms during the lamotrigine trials compared with the placebo trials (56). However, manic symptoms were low at baseline in this study, raising the possibility that treatment effects may have been obscured among the treatment groups in this pole of the illness. In the second lamotrigine bipolar mania trial, lamotrigine or placebo was added to ongoing lithium treatment in patients who were inadequately responsive to lithium or was administered as monotherapy in patients who could not tolerate lithium side effects (58). Again, there were no significant differences in reduction of manic symptoms among the patients receiving lamotrigine or placebo.

The third lamotrigine study in patients with bipolar mania was a small comparison trial with lithium in which both treatments produced significant reductions in manic symptoms (59). However, the small sample size ($N = 30$), low mean lithium levels (0.7 mEq/L), and absence of a placebo group limit interpretation of these results. Thus, although lamotrigine has demonstrated efficacy as a maintenance treatment for patients with bipolar I disorder (60,61), there are no compelling data to indicate that it exerts acute antimanic efficacy.

SUMMARY

Although a number of antiepileptic agents have been studied in the treatment of bipolar manic and mixed episodes, only two, valproic acid and carbamazepine, have established efficacy in rigorous randomized, placebo-controlled, parallel-group trials. Topiramate, lamotrigine, and gabapentin have not been shown to be superior to placebo in controlled trials. Phenytoin and oxcarbazepine have not been studied adequately in definitive trials and thus must be regarded as unproven in their efficacy in manic and mixed episodes.

REFERENCES

1. Bowden CL. Anticonvulsants in bipolar disorder. Aust N Z J Psychiatry 2006; 40: 386–393.
2. Post RM, Weiss SR. Convergences in course of illness and treatments of the epilepsies and recurrent affective disorders. Clin EEG Neurosci 2004; 35:14–24.
3. Pope HG Jr., McElroy SL, Keck PE Jr. Valproate treatment of acute mania: a placebo-controlled study. Arch Gen Psychiatry 1991; 48:62–68.
4. Bowden CL, Brugger AM, Swann AC, et al. Efficacy of divalproex versus lithium and placebo in the treatment of mania. JAMA 1994; 271:918–924.
5. Bowden CL, Swann AC, Calabrese JR, et al. A randomized, placebo-controlled, multi-center study of divalproex extended release in the treatment of acute mania. J Clin Psychiatry 2006; 67:1501–1510.

6. Emrich HM, Von Zerssen D, Kissling W. On a possible role of GABA in mania: therapeutic efficacy of sodium valproate. In: Costa E, Dicharia G, Gessa GL, eds. GABA and Benzodiazepine Receptors. New York, NY: Raven Press, 1981:287–296.
7. Brennan MIW, Sandyk R, Borsook D. Use of sodium valproate in the management of affective disorders: basic and clinical aspects. In: Emrich HM, Okuma T, Muller AA, eds. Anticonvulsants in Affective Disorders. Amsterdam, The Netherlands: Exerpta Medica, 1984:56–65.
8. Tohen M, Baker RW, Altshuler LL, et al. Olanzapine versus divalproex in the treatment of acute mania. Am J Psychiatry 2002; 159:1011–1017.
9. Zajecka JM, Weisler R, Sachs G, et al. A comparison of the efficacy, safety, and tolerability of divalproex sodium and olanzapine in the treatment of bipolar disorder. J Clin Psychiatry 2002; 63:1148–1155.
10. Freeman TW, Clothier JL, Pazzaglia P, et al. A double-blind comparison of valproic acid and lithium in the treatment of acute mania. Am J Psychiatry 1992; 149:247–250.
11. Hirschfeld RM, Allen MH, McEvoy J, et al. Safety and tolerability of oral loading of divalproex in acutely manic bipolar patients. J Clin Psychiatry 1999; 60:815–818.
12. DelBello MP, Kowatch RA, Adler CM, et al. A double-blind randomized pilot study comparing quetiapine and divalproex for adolescent mania. J Am Acad Child Adolesc Psychiatry 2006; 45:305–313.
13. Keck PE Jr., McElroy SL, Tugrul KC, et al. Valproate oral loading in the treatment of acute mania. J Clin Psychiatry 1993; 54:305–308.
14. McElroy SL, Keck PE Jr., Tugrul KC, et al. Valproate as a loading treatment in acute mania. Neuropsychobiol 1993; 27:146–149.
15. McElroy SL, Keck PE Jr., Stanton SP, et al. A randomized comparison of divalproex oral loading versus haloperidol in the initial treatment of acute psychotic mania. J Clin Psychiatry 1998; 59:142–146.
16. Müller-Oerlinghausen B, Retzow A, Henn FA, et al. Valproate as an adjunct medication for the treatment of acute mania: a prospective, randomized, double-blind, placebo-controlled trial. European Valproate Mania Study Group. J Clin Psychopharmacol 2000; 20:195–203.
17. Yatham LN, Paulsson B, Mullen J, et al. Quetiapine versus placebo in combination with lithium or divalproex for the treatment of bipolar mania. J Clin Psychopharmacol 2004; 24:599–606.
18. Sachs G, Chengappa KNR, Suppes T, et al. Quetiapine with lithium or divalproex for the treatment of bipolar mania: a randomized, double-blind, placebo-controlled study. Bipolar Disord 2004; 6:213–223.
19. Yatham LN, Binder C, Kusumaker V, et al. Risperidone plus lithium versus risperidone plus valproate in acute and continuation treatment of mania. Int Clin Psychopharmacol 2004; 19:103–109.
20. Sachs GS, Grossman F, Ghaemi SN, et al. Combination of a mood stabilizer with risperidone or haloperidol for the treatment of acute mania: a double-blind, placebo-controlled comparison of efficacy and safety. Am J Psychiatry 2002; 159:1146–1154.
21. Tohen M, Chengappa KNR, Suppes T, et al. Efficacy of olanzapine in combination with valproate or lithium in the treatment of mania in patients partially nonresponsive to valproate or lithium monotherapy. Arch Gen Psychiatry 2002; 59:62–69.
22. Bahk WM, Shin YC, Woo JM, et al. Topiramate and divalproex in combination with risperidone for acute mania: a randomized open-label study. Prog Neuropsychopharmacol Biol Psychiatry 2005; 29:115–121.
23. DelBello MP, Schweirs ML, Rosenberg HL, et al. A double-blind, randomized, placebo-controlled study of quetiapine as adjunctive treatment for adolescent mania. J Am Acad Child Adolesc Psychiatry 2002; 41:1216–1223.
24. Swann AC, Bowden CL, Calabrese JR, et al. Differential effects of number of previous episodes of affective disorder in response to lithium or divalproex in acute mania. Am J Psychiatry 1999; 156:1264–1266.
25. Swann AC, Bowden CL, Morris D, et al. Depression during mania: treatment response to lithium or divalproex. Arch Gen Psychiatry 1997; 54:37–42.

26. Allen MH, Hirschfeld RM, Wozniak PJ, et al. Linear relationship of valproate serum concentration to response and optimal serum levels for acute mania. Am J Psychiatry 2006; 163:272–275.
27. Keck PE Jr., McElroy SL, Nemeroff CB. Anticonvulsants in the treatment of bipolar disorder. J Neuropsychiatr Clin Neurosci 1992; 4:595–605.
28. Weisler RH, Kalali AH, Ketter TA, et al. A multicenter, randomized, double-blind, placebo-controlled trial of extended release carbamazepine capsules as monotherapy for bipolar patients with manic or mixed episodes. J Clin Psychiatry 2004; 65:478–484.
29. Weisler RH, Keck PE Jr., Swann AC, et al. Extended release carbamazepine capsules as monotherapy for acute mania in bipolar disorder: a multicenter, randomized, double-blind, placebo-controlled trial. J Clin Psychiatry 2005; 66:323–330.
30. Lerer B, Moore N, Meyendorff E, et al. Carbamazepine versus lithium in mania: a double-blind study. J Clin Psychiatry 1987; 48:89–93.
31. Small JG. Anticonvulsants in affective disorders. Psychopharmacol Bull 1990; 26:25–36.
32. Grossi E, Sacchetti E, Vita A. Carbamazepine vs. Chlorpromazine in mania: a double-blind trial. In: Emrich HM, Okuma T, Muller AA, eds. Anticonvulsants in Affective Disorders. Amsterdam, The Netherlands: Exerpta Medica, 1984:184–194.
33. Okuma T, Inanga K, Otsuki S, et al. Comparison of the antimanic efficacy of carbamazepine and chlorpromazine. Psychopharmacol 1979; 66:211–217.
34. Small JG, Klapper MH, Marhenke JD, et al. Lithium combined with carbamazepine or haloperidol in the treatment of mania. Psychopharmacol Bull 1995; 31:265–272.
35. Yatham LN, Grossman F, Augustyns I, et al. Mood stabilizers plus risperidone or placebo in the treatment of acute mania. Br J Psychiatry 2003; 182:141–147.
36. Zhang ZJ, Kang WH, Tan QR, et al. Adjunctive herbal medicine with carbamazepine for bipolar disorders: a double-blind, randomized, placebo-controlled study. J Psychiatr Res 2007; 41(3–4):360–369.
37. Emrich HM, Altmann H, Dose M, et al. Therapeutic effects of GABA-ergic drugs in affective disorders: a preliminary report. Pharmacol Biochem Behav 1983; 19:369–373.
38. Emrich HM. Studies with oxcarbazepine (Trileptal) in acute mania. Int Clin Psychopharmacol 1990; 5(suppl 1):83–88.
39. Muller AA, Stoll KD. Carbamazepine and oxcarbazepine in the treatment of manic syndromes: studies in Germany. In: Emrich HM, Okuma T, Muller AA, eds. Anticonvulsants in Affective Disorders. Amsterdam, The Netherlands: Experta Medica, 1984:222–229.
40. Hummel B, Walden J, Stampfer R, et al. Acute antimanic efficacy and safety of oxcarbazepine in an open trial with on-off-on design. Bipolar Disord 2002; 4:412–417.
41. Wagner KD, Kowatch RA, Emslie GJ, et al. A double-blind, randomized, placebo-controlled trial of oxcarbazepine in the treatment of bipolar disorder in children and adolescents. Am J Psychiatry 2006; 163:1179–1186.
42. Jefferson JW. Oxcarbazepine in bipolar disorder. J Clin Psychiatry 2001; 3:181.
43. Mishory A, Yaroslavsky Y, Bersudsky Y, et al. Phenytoin as an antimanic anticonvulsant. Am J Psychiatry 2000; 157:463–465.
44. Brown ES, Stuard G, Liggin JD, et al. Effect of phenytoin on mood and declarative memory during prescription corticosteroid therapy. Biol Psychiatry 2005; 57:543–548.
45. Kushner SF, Khan A, Lane R, et al. Topiramate monotherapy in the management of acute mania: results of four double-blind placebo-controlled trials. Bipolar Disord 2006; 8:15–27.
46. DelBello MP, Findling RL, Kushner S, et al. A pilot controlled trial for mania in children and adolescents with bipolar disorder. J Am Acad Child Adolesc Psychiatry 2005; 44:539–547.
47. Chengappa KNR, Schwarzman LK, Hulihan JF, et al. Adjunctive topiramate therapy in patients receiving a mood stabilizer for bipolar I disorder: a randomized, placebo-controlled trial. J Clin Psychiatry 2006; 67:1698–1706.
48. McElroy SL, Suppes T, Keck PE Jr., et al. Open-label adjunctive topiramate in the treatment of bipolar disorders. Biol Psychiatry 2000; 47:1025–1033.

49. Chengappa KNR, Levine J, Rathore D, et al. Long-term effects of topiramate on bipolar mood instability, weight change and glycemic control: a case-series. Eur Psychiatry 2001; 16:186–190.
50. Biton V. Effect of antiepileptic drugs on bodyweight: overview and clinical implications for the treatment of epilepsy. CNS Drugs 2003; 17:781–791.
51. Brandes JL, Saper JR, Diamond M, et al. Topiramate for migraine prevention: a randomized controlled trial. JAMA 2004; 291:965–973.
52. Raskin P, Donofrio PD, Vinik AI, et al. Efficacy, safety, and metabolic effects of topiramate in a multicenter, controlled trial of painful diabetic neuropathy. Neurol 2004; 63:865–873.
53. Wilding J, Van Gaal L, Rissanen A, et al. A randomized double-blind placebo-controlled study of the long-term efficacy and safety of topiramate in the treatment of obese subjects. Int J Obesity 2004; 28:1399–1410.
54. McElroy SL, Arnold LM, Shapira NA, et al. Topiramate in the treatment of binge eating disorder associated with obesity: a randomized, placebo-controlled trial. Am J Psychiatry 2003; 160:255–261.
55. Pande AC, Crockatt JG, Janney CA, et al. Gabapentin in bipolar disorder: a placebo-controlled trial of adjunctive therapy. Bipolar Disord 2000; 2:249–255.
56. Frye MA, Ketter TA, Kimbrell TA, et al. A placebo-controlled study of lamotrigine and gabapentin monotherapy in refractory mood disorders. J Clin Psychopharmacol 2000; 20:607–614.
57. Perugi G, Toni C, Frare F, et al. Effectiveness of adjunctive gabapentin in resistant bipolar disorder: is it due to anxious-alcohol abuse comorbidity? J Clin Psychopharmacol 2002; 22:584–591.
58. Anand A, Oren DA, Berman RM, et al. Lamotrigine treatment of lithium failure in oupatient mania: a double-blind, placebo-controlled trial. Third International Conference on Bipolar Disorder, Pittsburgh, Pennsylvania, June 16, 1999 (abstr).
59. Ichim L, Berk M, Brook S. Lamotrigine compared with lithium in mania: a double-blind, placebo-controlled trial. J Affect Disord 2000; 12:5–10.
60. Bowden CL, Calabrese JR, Sachs GS, et al. A placebo-controlled 18-month trial of lamotrigine and lithium maintenance treatment in recently manic or hypomanic patients with bipolar I disorder. Arch Gen Psychiatry 2003; 60:392–400.
61. Calabrese JR, Bowden CL, Sachs GS, et al. A placebo-controlled 18-month trial of lamotrigine and lithium maintenance treatment in recently depressed patients with bipolar I disorder. J Clin Psychiatry 2003; 64:1013–1024.

3 The Role of Antiepileptic Drugs in Long-Term Treatment of Bipolar Disorder

Charles L. Bowden and Vivek Singh
Department of Psychiatry, University of Texas Health Science Center at San Antonio, San Antonio, Texas, U.S.A.

INTRODUCTION

Long-term management of bipolar disorder is complex and challenging, largely because of the inherent complexity of the disorder and the multitude of interacting psychosocial stressors and supports that interweave over time. Bipolar disorder comprises four to six behavioral/symptomatic domains, and each requires unique attention psychopharmacologically when present. Studies consistently report factors for depression, mania, irritability, anxiety, and psychosis. Impulsivity and affective/mood instability are the closest to a universal symptom complex in bipolar disorder, appearing to some degree in all phases of the illness and even in patients recovered with continuing care (1,2). No drug, neither a single lifestyle modification nor a form of psychotherapy effectively eliminates all symptoms. Because of the persisting expression of symptomatology of bipolar illness in even the best functioning individuals, treatment needs to be continued over the lifetime and periodically modified to target symptoms that may emerge during the course of long-term treatment. Tolerability and consequently adherence, factors that translate efficacious into effective treatments, should drive drug selection and continuation in maintenance treatment of bipolar disorder.

Mood stabilizers are considered the foundation of treatment of bipolar disorder. Although definitions of the phrase mood stabilizer vary, all of the definitions emphasize that the drug must benefit one or more primary mood states of bipolar illness, be effective in acute and maintenance phase treatment and not worsen any aspect of the illness (3,4).

Antiepileptic drugs (AEDs), also called anticonvulsants, are mainstays of long-term treatment of bipolar disorder. A paradigm shift in long-term management of bipolar disorder has been an increased focus on the aggressive management of interepisode symptomatology and related psychosocial dysfunction, with less but certainly still important attention to syndromal mood states.

We present the evidence for efficacy, safety, and practical guidelines for long-term use in bipolar disorder of all approved AEDs, including those AEDs for which clear evidence indicates that they have no primary roles in treatment of bipolar disorder. Although the emphasis is on long-term treatment since acute episodes occur in the course of illness, this aspect of AED use is also addressed.

VALPROATE

Divalproex, a stable formulation of sodium valproate and valproic acid with delayed release properties, was approved by the United States Food and Drug Administration (FDA) in 1995 for the treatment of acute mania following a large randomized, double blind, parallel-group clinical trial of divalproex versus lithium versus placebo published in 1994 (5). Although the mechanism of action of valproate in bipolar disorder is unclear, more is known about its and lithium's central nervous system (CNS) related actions than any other treatments employed in bipolar disorder. Principally from animal studies, but in some cases human investigations, it is known to reduce protein kinase C (PKC) activity in manic patients (6), inhibit glycogen synthase kinase 3 (GSK-3), activate the extracellular signal-regulated kinase (ERK) pathway (7), increase the expression of the cyto-protective protein B-cell lymphoma/leukemia-2 gene (bcl-2) (8), reduce inositol biosynthesis, lengthen the period of circadian rhythms and increase arrhythmicity in *Drosophila*, and reverse early DNA damage caused by amphetamine in an animal model of mania (9). The impact on circadian rhythms is of particular interest given in recent data, implicating sets of genes associated with circadian rhyth-micity in bipolar disorder (10). For most of the above-summarized effects, similar results have been observed with both valproate and lithium. Each of the above systems has been associated with manic states and animal models for mania (11). However, valproate's mechanisms of action are unique, resulting from decreased myo-inositol 1-phosphate synthase inhibition (12) and inhibition of histone deacetylase (13).

Profile of Actions

In short-term studies, both divalproex and lithium significantly decreased impul-sivity and hyperactivity, whereas divalproex, but not lithium, improved irritability (1). Neither drug was superior to placebo in alleviating anxiety components. In a recent study indicating efficacy of a sustained release formulation of divalproex in mania, the specific areas of superiority of divalproex over placebo were for racing thoughts, decreased need for sleep, and items reflecting hyperactivity (14). Of interest in the study, extended release divalproex showed greater benefits in more seriously ill manic patients (14). In other monotherapy studies in acute mania, valproate was equivalent in efficacy to haloperidol in patients with psy-chotic mania (15), to olanzapine in two studies (16,17), and superior to carba-mazepine (18).

The efficacy of valproate in combination with other agents with proven efficacy as monotherapy in the treatment of mania has been demonstrated by several randomized, double-blind, placebo controlled studies. These studies also indicate that when antipsychotics are used in combination with lithium or valproate, patients receiving combination therapy regimens can be effectively treated with lower doses than are used for antipsychotic drug monotherapy (19–21). Analysis of the data from the Sachs et al. study did not demonstrate any advantage of the combination treatment in the cotherapy group (patients in a manic state without any treatment in whom risperidone and either lithium or valproate were initiated concomitantly), whereas in the add-on therapy group (patients nonresponsive to monotherapy with lithium or valproate at an adequate dose for two weeks or more in whom risperidone was then added), there was a distinct advantage to the addition of risperidone. Each of the other studies required some degree of failure with monotherapy prior to initiation of combi-nation treatment. In another study, the addition of valproate to a typical anti-psychotic (haloperidol) led to greater improvement in manic symptomatology than using haloperidol alone (21). These findings suggest that combination therapy should be initiated in patients who have either failed to respond or have responded partially to a monotherapeutic approach at an adequate dosage for an adequate duration of time.

Maintenance Efficacy

In patients with bipolar I disorder who were randomized to one year of maintenance treatment with divalproex, lithium, or placebo following meeting recovery criteria within three months of an index manic episode, divalproex showed a trend for superiority over lithium ($P = 0.06$) on the primary efficacy measure, time to a full mood episode, with neither drug significantly superior to placebo, due to a lower than expected rate of relapse among placebo-treated subjects (22). On most secondary measures, divalproex was superior to placebo. These included rate of early discontinuation for onset of any mood episode, onset of a depressive episode, and dropout for any reason (23,24). Divalproex was superior to lithium in prolonging the duration of successful prophylaxis in the study and improvement in global assessment function (GAF) scores. Similar results were reported in an earlier randomized, open study comparing valpromide with lithium (25). Divalproex also appeared better than lithium with regard to depressive outcomes. Compared with those randomized to lithium, patients randomized to divalproex had lesser worsening of depressive symptomatology, a lower probability of relapse into depression (particularly if they had demonstrated a response to divalproex when manic), and better response if a selective serotonin reuptake inhibitor (SSRI) was added following the development of a depressive episode (23).

Maintenance Outcome Comparisons with Placebo

Smith et al. recently conducted a thorough meta-analysis of all randomized control trials in the maintenance phase of bipolar disorder. The rate of study withdrawal for any reason was 18% [95% confidence interval (CI) 4–30%] less with valproate than with placebo (24,26). The rate of relapse to any mood episode was 18% less with valproate than with placebo with the rate of relapse to a manic episode being 27% less with valproate than with placebo. The relapse rate to a depressive episode was 60% less (CI 18–80%) in the valproate group than with placebo. The risk ratio for withdrawal for adverse effects was higher with valproate than with placebo (4.19, 95% CI 1.3–13.5%).

Maintenance Outcome Comparisons with Lithium

In comparisons with lithium, the withdrawal rate was 48% higher with lithium than with valproate (27). Combining the Bowden et al. and Calabrese et al. studies, the risk ratio withdrawal rate was 21% higher for lithium than for valproate (4,26). The relapse rates for any mood episode were 34% greater for lithium than for valproate. The relapse rates due to a manic episode did not differ significantly between the two agents (3% more for lithium than valproate) but the rate of relapse due to a depressive episode was 50% higher for lithium than for valproate. The withdrawal rate due to an adverse event was 81% higher for lithium than for valproate. Taken in the aggregate, these analyses indicate a broader spectrum of efficacy for valproate compared with both placebo and lithium, substantially better tolerability for valproate than for lithium, and evidence of at least as much benefit on depressive as for manic recurrences.

Maintenance Effectiveness in Adjunct Therapy

One small study with 99 subjects compared adjunctive olanzapine with mood stabilizer monotherapy, either valproate or lithium (28). The only outcome reported for all randomized subjects was time to relapse for any mood episode. There were nonsignificantly fewer relapses in the monotherapy group than in the adjunctive olanzapine group (13%, CI 45% fewer to 131% more). An even smaller subgroup of the acutely enrolled patients who were defined post hoc as in both symptomatic and syndromal remission had significantly longer time to mania relapse, but not depression relapse, with mood stabilizer monotherapy than with adjunctive olanzapine.

A second small study of 12 participants compared valproate plus lithium with lithium alone (29). Although the difference was reported as significantly favoring valproate plus lithium over lithium alone, the possibility of no benefit of the combination was not excluded. In the aggregate, the two studies suggest that adjunctive regimens including valproate may be more effective than monotherapy regimens with either lithium or other mood stabilizers, but more systematic, adequately designed studies are needed for this aspect.

A 47-week maintenance study comparing divalproex and olanzapine (17) in bipolar patients with an index episode of acute mania did not meet criteria for inclusion in the Smith et al. meta-analysis (26), because patients were randomized during the acute episode and not following achievement of mood stability. Rates of completion were low for both treatments (15% vs. 16%), and though symptomatic remission occurred earlier with olanzapine, efficacy was equivalent for the two drugs over the latter portion of the study. The two drugs did not differ in the rates of manic relapse and the median time to a manic relapse (19). Patients who attained remission at the end of acute treatment were more likely to complete the 47-week trial than those who did not (divalproex 26% vs. 11%; olanzapine 20% vs. 11%, $P = 0.001$), indicating that acute treatment response, while manic, for both valproate and olanzapine, is predictive of more effective treatment with the same drug during maintenance therapy. In addition, long-term treatment with divalproex was associated with significant reductions in both total and low-density cholesterol, compared with increases with olanzapine. Weight gain was greater with olanzapine than with divalproex (17).

In a 20-month, randomized, double-blind maintenance study of valproate or lithium monotherapy in bipolar patients with rapid cycling, only one quarter of patients enrolled, met criteria for an acute bimodal response to either drug and less than 25% of those randomized maintained benefits without relapse (27). These findings indicate that monotherapy regimens have limited efficacy in the treatment of rapid-cycling patients.

Efficacy in the Young and the Elderly

Open studies of valproate have demonstrated moderate to marked sustained improvement in over half of manic youth aged 8 through 18 years (30–33). An open-label, randomized 6-week study ($N = 42$) assessing the efficacy of divalproex, lithium, and carbamazepine in bipolar I and II patients experiencing manic or mixed manic episodes did not show any significant difference in rates of response between the three treatment groups, though the effect size for improvement was largest with divalproex (divalproex 1.63, lithium 1.06, carbamazepine 1.00) (34).

A randomized, placebo-controlled study ($N = 56$) reported significant benefits for valproate on irritability and agitation associated with dementia (35). These findings were consistent with open studies that have demonstrated benefit on some aspects of irritability and agitation in elderly patients with varying symptomatology (36–38). More systematic, controlled studies are needed to draw conclusions on valproate's effectiveness in these age groups.

Dosage and Serum Level Monitoring

Placebo-controlled trials have shown that acutely manic patients with valproate serum levels ≥45 µg/mL are significantly more likely to have at least a 20% improvement in their manic symptomatology (24,39–41). During maintenance treatment, valproate levels between 75 and 99 µg/mL were more likely to maintain prophylaxis than serum levels above or below this range and provided significantly superior outcomes than those observed with placebo (Table 1) (42).

Tolerability

Valproate is generally well tolerated as evidenced in the largest maintenance trial of divalproex in bipolar disorder, in which weight gain and tremors were the only adverse events more common with divalproex than placebo (22). Common dose/serum level related side effects seen with valproate include tremors, nausea, and related gastrointestinal distress, sedation, and reduction in platelets and white blood cell count (43,44). Alopecia can occur, in part consequent to chelation of trace elements, such as selenium and zinc, by valproic acid in the gut. Therefore the time of valproate dosing should be separated by several hours from that of taking a multivitamin preparation containing zinc and selenium. Low rates of hepatotoxicity (1/49,000) and pancreatitis (<1%) have been reported with valproate. Hepatic impairment, almost limited to children less than two years of age treated for epilepsy, may be a consequence of the interference of valproate with rapidly dividing cells in the immature liver. A similar mechanism is plausibly linked to neural tube defects and hair loss. In long-term studies, including the 12-month maintenance study of divalproex, valproate has not been associated with worsening of any hepatic indices by laboratory assessments, and in some instances, small but significant improvements in indices occurred (24). Routine monitoring of hepatic function and amylase levels is not indicated, unless active hepatic or pancreatic dysfunction is present (Table 1). Weight gain (about 3–24 pounds) is seen in 3% to 20% of patients on valproate. Valproate serum levels greater than 125 µg/mL are more likely to cause weight gain than levels below 125 mg/mL (24).

Valproate is an FDA Pregnancy Category D drug and has been associated with neural tube defects (1–4%) (24). The risk of CNS abnormalities is dose and serum level dependent, with the higher doses customarily employed in treating epilepsy associated with higher rates than those clinically utilized for bipolar disorder.

LAMOTRIGINE

Lamotrigine is FDA approved and recommended for the maintenance treatment of bipolar disorder, principally for the depressive manifestations of the illness. Although the specific mechanisms by which lamotrigine prevents recurrent depressive episodes in bipolar disorder are unknown, lamotrigine has several recognized mechanisms that distinguish it from other mood-stabilizing as well as antiepileptic drugs. Lamotrigine inhibits use-dependent voltage-sensitive sodium

TABLE 1 Characteristics of Antiepileptics Evaluated in Bipolar Disorder[a]

	VPA	CBZ	OXC	LAM	GBP	TMP	ZON	LEV	PHT
Time to steady state (days)	1–3	21–28[b]	2	3–15	1–2	4–5	5–15	2	7–28
Half-life (hr)	9–16	12–17[c]	2–9[d]	25–30	5–7	19–23	63	6–8	7–22
Bioavailability (%)	>95	85	100	98	60–27[e]	80	100	100	100[f]
Protein binding (%)	90–95	40–90	40	40–50	0–3	13–17	40	<10	93–98
Metabolism	Liver	Liver	Liver/biliary	Liver	None	Minimal	Liver	Liver	Liver
Clinically relevant metabolite	2-propyl-4-pentenoic acid (may cause toxicity)	10,11-epoxide (clinically active and may cause toxicity)	10-hydroxy carbazepine (clinically active)	None	None	None	None	None	None
Dosage range (mg/day)	200–2500	200–1200	300–2400	50–400	600–3600	100–600	100–600	1000–3000	100–400
Target blood levels (μg/mL)	50–125	6–12	10–35	N	N	N	10–40	N	10–20
Monitoring of drug levels	RB	R	NR	NR	NR	NR	NR	NR	NR
Monitoring of liver functions	R	R	NR	NR	NR	NR	NR	NR	NR
Monitoring of renal functions	NR	NR	NR	NR	NR	R[g]	NR	NR	NR
Monitoring of blood counts	R	R	NR	NR	NR	NR	NR	NR	NR
Monitoring of lipids	NR	NR	NR	NR	NR	NR	NR	NR	NR
Monitoring of blood sugar	NR	NR	NR	NR	NR	NR	NR	NR	NR
US-FDA pregnancy category	D	D	C	C	C	C	C	C	D

[a]Ref. 52.
[b]After completion of autoinduction.
[c]Due to autoinduction.
[d]Two hours for parent compound, nine hours for active metabolite.
[e]60% at 900 mg/day in divided doses and progressively decreases to 27% at 4800 mg/day in divided doses.
[f]Ref. 70.
[g]Ref. 71.

Abbreviations: VPA, valproate or divalproex; CBZ, carbamazepine; OXC, oxcarbazepine; LAM, lamotrigine; GBP, gabapentin; TMP, topiramate; ZON, zonisamide; LEV, levetiracetam; PHT, phenytoin or fosphenytoin; NR, not required; RB, required at baseline; R, required; N, not defined.

channel activity. It also modulates presynaptic release of excitatory amino acid neurotransmitters such as glutamate. These effects reduce rates of repetitive neuronal after-discharges.

Maintenance Efficacy

Lamotrigine was the second agent after lithium to be approved by the FDA for maintenance treatment of bipolar disorder. This approval was based on findings from two paired, randomized, parallel-group, placebo-controlled, multicenter studies that demonstrated its prophylactic efficacy in patients with bipolar I disorder (45,46). These studies were designed to assess the safety and efficacy of lamotrigine and lithium for preventing relapse or recurrence of any mood episode in patients with bipolar I disorder. Both studies consisted of a screening of up to 2 weeks: an open-label phase of up to 8 to 16 weeks during which lamotrigine (dosage range of 100–200 mg/day) was started as monotherapy or as adjunctive treatment to ongoing treatment and an 18-month, double-blind phase wherein patients were randomized to receive lamotrigine (100–400 mg/day), lithium (flexibly dosed to achieve blood levels of 0.8–1.1 mEq/L), or placebo. Since all subjects received and adequately tolerated lamotrigine, and met randomization criteria while receiving lamotrigine alone, these studies qualified as enriched design trials (i.e., both selected for patients who benefited acutely from lamotrigine). The first study ($n = 175$) consisted of patients who were in the midst of or had experienced a recent episode of mania/hypomania (45), while the second study included patients who were experiencing or had recently experienced a major depressive episode ($n = 463$) (46). On the primary efficacy measure, time to intervention for any mood episode, lamotrigine and lithium were each superior to placebo in both studies. Lamotrigine, but not lithium, in both studies demonstrated superiority over placebo in delaying time to intervention for depression, whereas lithium, but not lamotrigine, was superior to placebo in time to delaying mania. In a pooled combined analysis of the two studies, both lamotrigine and lithium demonstrated superior efficacy than placebo on the primary efficacy measure, time to intervention for any mood episode. While lamotrigine, but not lithium, demonstrated superiority to placebo in prolonging time to intervention for a depressive episode, both lamotrigine and lithium were more efficacious than placebo in prolonging time to intervention for a manic, hypomanic, or mixed episode. Patients on lamotrigine were more likely to experience a recurrence or relapse to an episode of the same polarity than of an opposite one (47). The risk of switching to mania, hypomania, or a mixed state was similar between lamotrigine and lithium (5% vs. 7%).

In a large, 26-week, placebo-controlled study in 182 patients with rapid cycling bipolar disorder, lamotrigine (dosage range 100–500 mg/day) did not demonstrate superiority to placebo on the primary efficacy measure, time to intervention with additional pharmacotherapy for any mood episode, in the general cohort of patients and those with bipolar I disorder, but did show a trend toward superiority in patients with bipolar II disorder (48). Moreover, survival analysis (time to dropout for any reason) showed lamotrigine's superiority over placebo in the general group of patients and those with bipolar II disorder, but showed no significant separation from placebo in bipolar I patients.

The Smith et al. meta-analysis provides an important comparative data from these three studies (26).

Maintenance Outcome Comparisons with Placebo
Participants were 29% less likely to withdraw for any reason with lamotrigine than with placebo (26). The rate of relapse due to any mood episode was 32% lower with lamotrigine than with placebo (CI 15–45%). The rate of relapse due to a manic episode was nonsignificantly lower with lamotrigine (25%) but did not exclude the possibility of an increased risk (95% CI 51% fewer to 11% more). The relapse rate due to a depressive episode was 35% lower (CI 9–54%) with lamotrigine than with placebo. There were 5% fewer withdrawals due to an adverse event with lamotrigine than with placebo, although the upper confidence interval did not exclude an increased risk.

Maintenance Outcome Comparisons with Lithium
Hazard rate estimates indicated 9% more withdrawals for any reason with lithium than lamotrigine (26). Rates of relapse due to any mood episode were 7% lower with lithium than with lamotrigine (CI 30% fewer to 25% more). Relapse rates due to mania were 44% lower with lithium than with lamotrigine while relapse rates due to depression were 22% higher for lithium than for lamotrigine. Withdrawal rates due to an adverse event were 120% higher for lithium than for lamotrigine (CI 31–270%). In the aggregate, these results indicate that lamotrigine has marked efficacy compared with both placebo and lithium for prophylaxis of depression, but not mania. They also indicate superior tolerability to lithium.

Dosing
Lamotrigine should be titrated gradually to minimize the emergence of adverse events, particularly serious rash. Clinicians should initiate lamotrigine at 25 mg/day for the first two weeks, titrate to 50 mg/day for weeks 3 and 4, and then increase the dosage by 50 to 100 mg/wk to a target dose of 200 mg/day or as clinically indicated (Table 2) (49). If lamotrigine is part of a combination regimen involving carbamazepine, a powerful inducer of lamotrigine's clearance, the initiating dose of lamotrigine should be doubled and lamotrigine titration accelerated. When lamotrigine is added to ongoing treatment with valproate, an inhibitor of lamotrigine's clearance, lamotrigine should be initiated at 12.5 mg/day or 25 mg every other day for weeks 1 and 2 and the rate of titration should be slower.

Tolerability
Lamotrigine has a high tolerability profile and, in placebo controlled studies, did not appear to cause the switching or cycle acceleration associated with antidepressants (47). The most commonly reported adverse events in these studies included headache, ataxia, dizziness, tremors, nausea, somnolence, diplopia, and blurred vision (50–53). Lamotrigine is not associated with weight gain or sexual

TABLE 2 Initial Dosing Regimens of Lamotrigine

	Lamotrigine alone	Lamotrigine + valproate	Lamotrigine + carbamazepine
Weeks 1 and 2	25 mg q.d.	25 mg q.o.d. or 12.5 mg/day	25 mg b.i.d.
Weeks 3 and 4	50 mg q.d.	25 mg q.d.	50 mg b.i.d.
Week 5	100 mg q.d.	50 mg q.d.	100 mg b.i.d.
Week 6	200 mg q.d.	100 mg q.d.	150 mg b.i.d.
Week 7	—	—	200 mg b.i.d.

dysfunction and does not negatively impact cognitive functioning (47,54). In a published analysis of the rates of rash in 12 multicenter clinical trials involving 3,153 patients exposed to lamotrigine, 11.6% developed a benign rash while less than 0.1% developed a serious rash (47). The risk of developing a rash is increased with a dosage titration rate that is more rapid than recommended. In a recent study, there was no evidence that the risk of rash, either benign or serious, was increased when lamotrigine was added to ongoing valproate treatment, or when valproate was added to ongoing lamotrigine treatment if patients had been taking a steady dose of lamotrigine for at least two weeks prior to valproate addition (55). Oral contraceptives (e.g., ethinylestradiol and levonorgestrel) cause a significant decrease in serum trough levels of lamotrigine via estrogenic induction of glu-curonidation (AUC by 52%, C_{max} by 39%) during the 21 days that the oral contraceptives are administered. The serum trough concentration of lamotrigine increases rapidly by twofold by the end of the "pill free" period (56). Consequently, the prophylactic efficacy of lamotrigine may be compromised when oral contraceptives are initiated in patients on a steady dose of lamotrigine. In addition, the risk of rash may be increased during the "pill free" period."

The FDA lists lamotrigine as a Pregnancy Category C drug. Category C refers to drugs that have not been studied. The 2005 Interim Report of the International Lamotrigine Pregnancy Registry reported data on the teratogenic potential of lamotrigine based on the frequency of birth defects seen in patients who were exposed to lamotrigine monotherapy during the first trimester of pregnancy (2.6%, 95% CI 1.7–3.8%) compared with a background rate estimated at 2% to 3% for patients with epilepsy (57). There was a significant increase in the rate of birth defects (11.9%, 95% CI 6.6–20.2%) among patients who were exposed to a combination regimen of lamotrigine and valproate. However, in those exposed to lamotrigine polytherapy that did not include valproate, the rate was 2.6% (05% CI 1.2–6.5%). These preliminary data indicate that lamotrigine exposure during the first trimester of pregnancy does not increase teratogenicity beyond 2% to 3% baseline rate seen in patients with epilepsy (2–3%). Since most data on teratogenicity for AEDs are derived from patients with epilepsy where AEDs dosages tend to be higher compared with dosages used in patients with bipolar disorder, extrapolations to the latter should be interpreted with caution (57).

CARBAMAZEPINE

Carbamazepine is a trycyclic compound with a broad spectrum of efficacy in epilepsy. Similar to valproate, its antimanic properties were noted through serendipitous observation. Less is known about its mechanisms of action, which do not appear to encompass most of those of lithium or valproate. Carbamazepine enhances GABAergic transmission and possesses antiglutamatergic properties (58). Two recent large randomized, placebo-controlled studies have established its efficacy in mania, though neither study included an active comparator (59,60). In addition, in the first study, carbamazepine was superior to placebo on change in mania score at day 21 only. No acute data beyond three weeks are available from randomized studies. One small, randomized, blind study provides comparative data. Valproate yielded significantly greater and earlier improvement than carbamazepine and proved superior to carbamazepine on four mania scale items— elevated mood, irritability, speech disturbance, and thought disturbance (18). Carbamazepine did not prove superior to valproate on any of the manic items and more carbamazepine-treated patients required rescue medications. Rates of adverse events were four times higher for carbamazepine than those for valproate.

Maintenance Treatment

One maintenance study enrolled 94 bipolar patients who were randomized to carbamazepine or lithium either during an acute mood episode ("acutely randomized," $N = 41$) or at entry into the maintenance phase of the study ("prophylactically randomized," $N = 53$). Lithium was significantly superior to carbamazepine in delaying time to treatment for a new episode in both patient groups (61). In an open randomized study, time to a new episode or discontinuation for other reasons was significantly longer for lithium than for carbamazepine (62). Among patients with bipolar II disorder, with small samples of 28 and 29 subjects treated with lithium and carbamazepine respectively, there was no significant differences in time to discontinuation for any protocol defined reason (63). One small study of 22 subjects compared carbamazepine with placebo. No differences in rates of efficacy between carbamazepine and placebo were found (64). One study compared rates of withdrawal for any reason for carbamazepine or lithium-treated patients, and found 32% fewer withdrawals for any reason with lithium than with carbamazepine (65). Taken in the aggregate, there are insufficient data to recommend carbamazepine for maintenance treatment of bipolar disorder unless other treatments with more robust evidence have failed. Additionally, although the studies are of limited methodological clarity, the available data suggest that carbamazepine is inferior to lithium and valproate.

Dosage and Serum Level Monitoring

Dosing of carbamazepine is essentially empirical, based on patient tolerability and response. Carbamazepine's induction of its own metabolism and its adverse effects on the CNS, particularly in the early course of treatment, warrants that it be started at low doses, in the treatment of both bipolar disorder and epilepsy, and increased gradually until response or adverse events ensue. Initial dosing is generally started at 100 to 200 mg b.i.d. and increased as needed to a dosage up to 1200 mg/day, usually given in divided dosages (Table 1). The recent availability of extended release formulations (e.g., Equetro) offers the advantages of less frequent dosing and fewer side effects (e.g., psychomotor disturbances), which are partially linked to peak serum levels. No studies specifically focused on dosing or correlating serum level and response in the maintenance treatment of bipolar disorder, however, have been published.

Tolerability

Carbamazepine's role, both in the acute and maintenance treatment phases of bipolar disorder, is significantly limited by its adverse event profile. The side effects associated with carbamazepine are attributed to its major metabolite, carbamazepine-epoxide (16,66). The discontinuation rate due to adverse events in a randomized, double-blind, crossover maintenance study was higher in the carbamazepine group (22%) than in the lithium group (4%) (67). Dose related side effects with carbamazepine include dizziness, sedation, ataxia, diplopia, and nystagmus (68). Agranulocytosis and aplastic anemia, both idiosyncratic in nature, are seen in 1 per 10,000 to 100,000 patients treated with carbamazepine. Benign and transient leucopenia are observed in 10% of patients; thrombocytopenia and sustained leucopenia are both seen in 2% of patients. Mild hyponatremia caused by carbamazepine may manifest more seriously in the geriatric or medically ill patient subgroups. Carbamazepine is associated with a benign rash in 10% of patients, which may be the harbinger of a life threatening Stevens-Johnson syndrome. By inducing the cytochrome P450 enzymes, particularly P450-3A4, carbamazepine lowers the plasma levels of other drugs, including other AEDs (valproate, lamotrigine, zonisamide, topiramate, phenytoin, and oxcarbazepine), antipsychotics (aripiprazole, clozapine, haloperidol, olanzapine, risperidone, and ziprasidone), antidepressants (bupropion, citalopram, and tricyclic antidepressants), anxiolytics/ sedatives (buspirone, clonazepam, and alprazolam), stimulants (methylphenidate, modafinil), and oral contraceptives (68,69). As a result, higher doses of some medications, such as oral contraceptives, need to be administered when they are taken concomitantly with carbamazepine to maintain continued efficacy.

Other AEDs with Reported use in Bipolar Disorder

Several other AEDs have had case reports and/or small open-label studies suggesting long-term effectiveness in bipolar disorder. These include phenytoin, oxcarbazepine, topiramate, levetiracetam, gabapentin, vigabatrin, and zonisamide. Unless future evidence of long-term efficacy and tolerability in bipolar disorder are published, the use of any of these agents for maintenance treatment of bipolar disorder is not recommended.

CONCLUSION

In recent years, several AEDs have been investigated for their potential mood-stabilizing properties. These drugs are characterized by heterogeneity, both in regards to mechanisms of action and possessing differential efficacy in the various mood states of bipolar disorder. Among the AEDs, only valproate, lamotrigine, and carbamazepine have been rigorously studied for prophylaxis in bipolar disorder. Evidence from well-controlled studies support the role of valproate and lamotrigine for specific, but not necessarily broad, use in maintenance treatment of bipolar disorder. Importantly, both drugs show better tolerability than lithium in randomized blind studies.

The last decade has seen significant improvement in our understanding of bipolar disorder. A wider therapeutic armamentarium is needed as a large proportion of bipolar patients have frequent relapses and recurrences during long-term treatment. As additional AEDs become available, rigorously designed studies examining the safety and efficacy of monotherapeutic and combination strategies of these agents in the long-term treatment of bipolar disorder should be employed to better guide the practicing clinician in providing evidence-based treatments for patients with this disabling illness.

REFERENCES

1. Swann AC, Bowden CL, Calabrese JR, et al. Pattern of response to divalproex, lithium, or placebo in four naturalistic subtypes of mania. Neuropsychopharmacology 2002; 26(4): 530–536.
2. Janowsky DS, Morter S, Hong L, et al. Myers Briggs Type Indicator and tridimensional personality questionnaire differences between bipolar patients and unipolar depressed patients. Bipolar Disord 1999; 1(2):98–108.

3. Sachs GS. Bipolar mood disorder: practical strategies for acute and maintenance phase treatment. J Clin Psychopharmacol 1996; 16(suppl 1):32S–47S.
4. Bowden CL, Swann AC, Calabrese JR, et al. Maintenance clinical trials in bipolar disorder: design implications of the divalproex-lithium-placebo study. Psychopharmacol Bull 1997; 33(4):693–699.
5. Bowden CL, Brugger AM, Swann AC, et al. Efficacy of divalproex vs. lithium and placebo in the treatment of mania. JAMA 1994; 271:918–924.
6. Hahn CG, Umapathy, Wang HY, Koneru R, et al. Lithium and valproic acid treatments reduce PKC activation and receptor-G protein coupling in platelets of bipolar manic patients. J Psychiatr Res 2005; 39(4):355–363.
7. Einat H, Yuan P, Gould TD, et al. The role of the extracellular signal-regulated kinase signaling pathway in mood modulation. J Neurosci 2003; 23(19):7311–7316.
8. Gray NA, Zhou R, Du J, et al. The use of mood stabilizers as plasticity enhancers in the treatment of neuropsychiatric disorders. J Clin Psychiatry 2003; 64(suppl 5):3–17.
9. Andreazza AC, Frey BN, Stertz L, et al. Effects of lithium and valproate on DNA damage and oxidative stress markers in an animal model of mania. Bipolar Disord 2007; 9(S1):16.
10. Dokucu ME, Yu L, Taghert PH. Lithium- and valproate-induced alterations in circadian locomotor behavior in Drosophila. Neuropsychopharmacology 2005; 30(12):2216–2224.
11. Einat H, Manji HK. Cellular plasticity cascades: genes-to-behavior pathways in animal models of bipolar disorder. Biol Psychiatry 2006; 59(12):1160–1171.
12. Shaltiel G, Shamir A, Shapior J, et al. Valproate decreases inositol biosynthesis. Biol Psychiatry 2004; 56:868–874.
13. Harwood AJ, Agam G. Search for a common mechanism of mood stabilizers. Biochem Pharmacol 2003; 66(2):179–189.
14. Bowden CL. Valproate in mania: from Pierre Lambert to New Delhi Study. Neuropsychopharmacology 2006; 16(S4):S587.
15. McElroy SL, Keck PE, Stanton SP, et al. A randomized comparison of divalproex oral loading versus haloperidol in the initial treatment of acute psychotic mania. J Clin Psychiatry 1996; 57:142–146.
16. Zajecka JM, Weisler R, Sachs G, et al. A comparison of the efficacy, safety, and tolerability of divalproex sodium and olanzapine in the treatment of bipolar disorder. J Clin Psychiatry 2002; 63:1148–1155.
17. Tohen M, Ketter TA, Zarate CA. Olanzapine versus divalproex sodium for the treatment of acute mania and maintenance of remission: a 47-week study. Am J Psychiatry 2003; 160:1263–1271.
18. Vasudev K, Goswami U, Kohli K. Carbamazepine and valproate monotherapy: feasibility, relative safety and efficacy, and therapeutic drug monitoring in manic disorder. Psychopharmacology 2000; 150:15–23.
19. Sachs G, Grossman F, Okamoto A, et al. Risperidone plus mood stabilizer versus. placebo plus mood stabilizer for acute mania of bipolar disorder: a double-blind comparison of efficacy and safety. Am J Psychiatry 2002; 159:1146–1156.
20. Yatham LN, Grossman F, Augustyns I, et al. Mood stabilisers plus risperidone or placebo in the treatment of acute mania. International, double-blind, randomised controlled trial. Br J Psychiatry 2003; 182:141–147.
21. Muller-Oerlinghausen B, Retzow A, Henn FA, et al. Valproate as an adjunct to neuroleptic medication for the treatment of acute episodes of mania: a prospective, randomized, double-blind, placebo-controlled, multicenter study. J Clin Psychopharmacol 2000; 20(2):195–203.
22. Bowden CL, Calabrese JR, McElroy SL, et al. A randomized, placebo-controlled 12-month trial of divalproex and lithium in treatment of outpatients with bipolar I disorder. Arch Gen Psychiatry 2000; 57:481–489.
23. Gyulai L, Bowden CL, McElroy SL, et al. Maintenance efficacy of divalproex in the prevention of bipolar depression. Neuropsychopharmacology 2003; 28(7):1374–1382.
24. Bowden CL. Valproate. Bipolar Disord 2003; 5:189–202.

25. Lambert PA, Venaud G. Comparative study of valpromide versus. lithium as prophylactic treatment in affective disorders. Nervure 1992; 5(2):57–65.
26. Smith LA, Cornelius V, Warnock A, et al. Effectiveness of mood stabilizers and anti-psychotics in the maintenance phase of bipolar disorder: a systematic review of randomized controlled trials. Bipolar Disord 2007; 9(4):394–412.
27. Calabrese JR, Shelton MD, Rapport DJ, et al. A 20-month, double-blind, maintenance trial of lithium versus divalproex in rapid-cycling bipolar disorder. Am J Psychiatry 2005; 162(11):2152–2161.
28. Tohen M, Chengappa KN, Suppes T, et al. Relapse prevention in bipolar I disorder: 18-month comparison of olanzapine plus mood stabiliser vs mood stabiliser alone. Br J Psychiatry 2004; 184(4):337–345.
29. Solomon DA, Ryan CE, Keitner GI, et al. A pilot study of lithium carbonate plus divalproex sodium for the continuation and maintenance treatment of patients with bipolar I disorder. J Clin Psychiatry 1997; 58(3):95–99.
30. Deltito JA, Levitan J, Damore J, et al. Naturalistic experience with the use of divalproex sodium on an in-patient unit for adolescent psychiatric patients. Acta Psychiatr Scand 1998; 97(3):236–240.
31. Mandoki MW. Valproate-lithium combination and verapamil as treatments of bipolar disorder in children and adolescents. Neuropsychopharmacology 1993; 9(suppl):183S.
32. Papatheodorou G, Kutcher SP. Divalproex sodium treatment in late adolescent and young adult acute mania. Psychopharmacol Bull 1993; 29:213–219 (abstr).
33. Wagner KD, Weller E, Carlson G, et al. An open-label trial of divalproex in children and adolescents with bipolar disorder. J Am Acad Child Adolesc Psychiatry 2002; 41(10): 1224–1230.
34. Kowatch RA, Suppes T, Carmody TJ, et al. Effect size of lithium, divalproex sodium, and carbamazepine in children and adolescents with bipolar disorder. J Am Acad Child Adolesc Psychiatry 2000; 39(6):713–720.
35. Porsteinsson AP, Tariot PN, Erb R, et al. Placebo-controlled study of divalproex sodium for agitation in dementia. Am J Geriatr Psychiatry 2001; 9(1):58–66.
36. McFarland BH, Miller MR, Straumfjord AA. Valproate use in the older manic patient. J Clin Psychiatry 1990; 51:479–481.
37. Narayan N, Nelson J. Treatment of dementia with behavioral disturbance using dival-proex or a combination of divalproex and a neuroleptic. J Clin Psychiatry 1997; 58(8): 351–354.
38. Niedermier JA, Nasrallah HA. Clinical correlates of response to valproate in geriatric inpatients. Ann Clin Psychiatry 1998; 10(4):165–168.
39. Bowden CL, Janicak PG, Orsulak P, et al. Relation of serum valproate concentration to response in mania. Am J Psychiatry 1996; 153(6):765–770.
40. Petty F, Davis LL, Nugent AL, et al. Valproate therapy for chronic, combat-induced postraumatic stress disorder. J Clin Psychopharmacol 2002; 22(1):100–101.
41. Pope HG Jr., McElroy SL, Keck PE Jr., et al. Valproate in the treatment of acute mania: a placebo-controlled study. Arch Gen Psychiatry 1991; 48:62–68.
42. Keck PE Jr., Bowden CL, Meinhold JM, et al. Relationship between serum valproate and lithium levels and efficacy and tolerability in bipolar maintenance therapy. Int J Psychiatry Clin Pract 2005; 9(4):271–277.
43. DeVane CL. Pharmacokinetics, drug interactions, and tolerability of valproate. Psycho-pharmacol Bull 2003; 37(S2):25–42.
44. Acharya S, Bussel JB. Hematologic toxicity of sodium valproate. J Pediatr Hematol Oncol 2000; 22(1):62–65.
45. Bowden CL, Calabrese JR, Sachs G, et al. A placebo-controlled 18-month trial of lamotrigine and lithium maintenance treatment in recently manic or hypomanic patients with bipolar I disorder. Arch Gen Psychiatry 2003; 60:392–400.
46. Calabrese JR, Bowden CL, Sachs G, et al. A placebo-controlled 18-month trial of lamotrigine and lithium maintenance treatment in recently depressed patients with bipolar I disorder. J Clin Psychiatry 2003; 64:1013–1024.

47. Calabrese JR, Vieta E, Shelton MD. Latest maintenance data on lamotrigine in bipolar disorder. Eur Neuropsychopharmacol 2003; 13:S57–S66.
48. Calabrese JR, Suppes T, Bowden CL, et al. A double-blind placebo-controlled prophylaxis study of lamotrigine in rapid cycling bipolar disorder. J Clin Psychiatry 2000; 61: 841–850.
49. GlaxoSmithKline. 2001. GlaxoSmithKline, Five Moore Drive, RTP, North Carolina 27709.
50. Wang PW, Ketter TA, Becker OV, et al. New anticonvulsant medication uses in bipolar disorder. CNS Spectr 2003; (12):941–947.
51. Muzina DJ, El-Sayegh S, Calabrese JR. Antiepileptic drugs in psychiatry-focus on randomized controlled trial. Epilepsy Res 2002; 50(1–2):195–202.
52. Physicians' Desk Reference. 59th ed. Montvale, NJ: Thomson PDR, 2005.
53. Van Parys JA, Meinardi H. Survey of 260 epileptic patients treated with oxcarbazepine (Trileptal) on a named-patient basis. Epilepsy Res 1994; 19(1):79–85.
54. Bowden CL, Calabrese JR, Ketter TA, et al. Impact of lamotrigine and lithium on weight in obese and nonobese patients with bipolar I disorder. Am J Psychiatry 2006; 163(7): 1199–1201.
55. Singh V, Bowden C. Mixed states (MS) as predictors of polarity of relapse in bipolar disorder (BD). Presented at the American College of Neuropsychology in Hollywood, Florida, 2006 (abstr).
56. Johannessen SI, Battino D, Berry DJ, et al. Therapeutic drug monitoring of the newer antiepileptic drugs. Ther Drug Monit 2003; 25(3):347–363.
57. GlaxoSmithKline. 2007. Lamotrigine Pregnancy Registry. Interim Report. 1 September 1992 through 31 March 2007, issued July 2007. Available at: http://pregnancyregistry .gsk.com/index.html.
58. Bowden CL. Carbamazepine in bipolar disorder. In: Goodnick PJ, ed. Predictors of Treatment Response in Mood Disorders. Washington, DC: American Psychiatric Press, 1996:119–132.
59. Weisler RH, Keck PE Jr., Swann AC, et al. Extended-release carbamazepine capsules as monotherapy for acute mania in bipolar disorder: a multicenter, randomized, double-blind, placebo-controlled trial. J Clin Psychiatry 2005; 66(3):323–330.
60. Weisler RH, Kalali AH, Ketter TA, and SPD417 Study Group. A Multicenter, Randomized, Double-Blind, Placebo-Controlled Trial of extended-release carbamazepine capsules as monotherapy for bipolar disorder patients with manic or mixed episodes. J Clin Psychiatry 2004; 65:478–484.
61. Hartong EG, Moleman P, Hoogduin CA, et al. Prophylactic efficacy of lithium versus carbamazepine in treatment-naive bipolar patients. J Clin Psychiatry 2003; 64(2):144–151.
62. Greil W, Kleindienst N. The comparative prophylactic efficacy of lithium and carbamazepine in patients with bipolar I disorder. Int Clin Psychopharmacol 1999; 14(5):277–281.
63. Greil W, Kleindienst N. Lithium versus carbamazepine in the maintenance treatment of bipolar II disorder and bipolar disorder not otherwise specified. Int Clin Psychopharmacol 1999; 14(5):283–285.
64. Okuma T, Inanage K, Otsuki S, et al. A preliminary double-blind study on the efficacy of carbamazepine in prophylaxis of manic-depressive illness. Psychopharmacology 1981; 73: 95–96.
65. Greil W, Ludwig-Mayerhofer W, Erazo N, et al. Lithium versus carbamazepine in the maintenance treatment of bipolar disorders—a randomised study. J Affect Disord 2007; 43(2):151–161.
66. Freeman TW, Clothier JL, Pazzaglia P, et al. A double-blind comparison of valproate and lithium in the treatment of acute mania. Am J Psychiatry 1992; 149:108–111.
67. Denicoff KD, Smith-Jackson EE, Disney ER, et al. Preliminary evidence of the reliability and validity of the prospective life-chart methodology (LCM-p). J Clin Psychiatry 1997; 58: 470–478.
68. Ketter TA, Wang PW, Post RM. Carbamazepine and oxcarbazepine. In: Schatzberg AF, Nemeroff CB, eds. The American Psychiatric Publishing Textbook of Psychopharmacology 3rd ed. Washington, DC, London, England: American Psychiatric Publishing, Inc., 2004:581–606.

69. Hellewell JS. Oxcarbazepine (Trileptal) in the treatment of bipolar disorders: review of efficacy and tolerability. J Affect Disord 2002; 72(S1):S23–S34.
70. Fischer JH, Patel TV, Fischer PA. Fosphenytoin: clinical pharmacokinetics and comparative advantages in the acute treatment of seizures. Clin Pharmacokinet 2003; 42(1): 33–58.
71. Chengappa KN, Gerhson S, Levine J. The evolving role of topiramate among other mood stabilizers in the management of bipolar disorder. Bipolar Disord 2001; 3(5):215–232.

4 Antiepileptic Drugs in the Treatment of Rapid-Cycling Bipolar Disorder and Bipolar Depression

David E. Kemp, Keming Gao, and Joseph R. Calabrese
*Bipolar Disorders Center for Intervention and Services Research,
Case Western Reserve University, Cleveland, Ohio, U.S.A.*

David J. Muzina
Cleveland Clinic Psychiatry and Psychology, Cleveland, Ohio, U.S.A.

INTRODUCTION

In 1974, Dunner and Fieve described a variant of bipolar disorder marked by extensive mood fluctuations, giving rise to the concept of rapid cycling (1). Now incorporated into our current diagnostic nomenclature, rapid cycling is defined by the DSM-IV (Diagnostic and Statistical Manual of Mental Disorders, 4th Edition) as the occurrence of four or more mood episodes during a 12-month period, inclusive of mixed episodes, mania, hypomania, or major depression. Over the past 30 years, rapid cycling as a modifier of the course of bipolar disorder has been substantiated by differences in gender, bipolar subtype, propensity for thyroid dysfunction, and prospectively defined outcomes (2–6). It is now recognized that patients with rapid cycling must contend with an earlier age of mood disorder onset, a higher lifetime number of mood episodes, and greater mood episode severity (2). In fact, compared with their non-rapid-cycling counterparts, patients with rapid-cycling experience eight times more depressive and nine times more hypomanic/manic episodes over a 12-month period (4).

Given the increased affective morbidity associated with rapid cycling, at-risk patients should be identified and treated with interventions intended to stabilize mood from both the manic and depressive poles. Considered the hallmark of rapid cycling, major depressive episodes are the most prevalent, persistent, and difficult-to-treat illness dimension (7). Although antiepileptic drugs (AEDs) have traditionally been regarded as "mood stabilizers," the rationale to support their use in bipolar disorder has primarily been derived from the treatment of mania. However, there is growing evidence to support the use of certain AEDs in the acute and long-term treatment of bipolar depression. This chapter will review both rapid-cycling bipolar disorder and bipolar depression, highlighting their often-coupled clinical presentation and more treatment refractory course. The results of randomized clinical trials involving AEDs will be reviewed in order to translate research findings into clinically meaningful approaches to patient care.

RAPID-CYCLING BIPOLAR DISORDER

The occurrence of rapid cycling is neither rare nor inconsequential. Approximately one in five patients presents with a rapid-cycling pattern, and its prevalence is estimated to range from 13% to 56% (8). Historically, females and individuals with bipolar II disorder were believed to account for the majority of rapid-cycling cases

(3,5,7–9), though recent studies have begun to question the higher association with bipolar II disorder (2,4). A Systematic Treatment Enhancement Program for Bipolar Disorder (STEP-BD) report found equal rates of rapid cycling occurring among patients diagnosed with either bipolar subtype (4), while a prospective study of 539 outpatients found a higher occurrence of rapid cycling in patients with bipolar I (41.3%) as compared with bipolar II (27.9%) disorder (2). Regardless of subtype predominance, the continuous mood cycling uniformly suggests greater illness severity, including a heightened risk for attempted suicide. Data from our prospectively collected cohort of 564 patients with rapid-cycling bipolar disorder demonstrate that 41% have attempted suicide, with the highest prevalence among those with comorbid substance use disorders (10). Although there is no direct evidence to substantiate higher rates of completed suicide in rapid-cycling patients, longitudinal data from the National Institute of Mental Health Collaborative Depression Study indicate that patients with rapid-cycling bipolar disorder are more than twice as likely as non-rapid-cycling patients to attempt suicide (11).

Antiepileptic Drugs in the Treatment of Rapid Cycling
Lithium and Carbamazepine
In 1980, Kukopulos et al. (12) identified one of the earliest disease features to be associated with rapid cycling, namely, a poor response to lithium prophylaxis. In this report, inadequate lithium response occurred in 84% (42/50) of patients who received treatment for more than one year. Likewise, a five-year prospective study of patients with bipolar I disorder found an absence of rapid cycling in good responders to lithium but a 26% incidence among nonresponders (13). Over time, accumulating reports revealed that more than 70% of patients respond poorly or only partially to lithium (14), and a need was realized for pharmacologic agents more effective at managing the rapid-cycling variant.

To meet this need, investigators shifted from the study of lithium and began to explore agents in the anticonvulsant drug class. Endeavoring to find more effective treatments, carbamazepine was selected as the first anticonvulsant to be specifically studied in rapid cycling. One early report suggested carbamazepine possessed antimanic properties (15). However, a year later, results from an open-label study showed that while carbamazepine was effective for a select group of rapid-cycling patients, the majority did not demonstrate a robust response (16). Furthermore, a retrospective study of 215 bipolar patients identified that a history of rapid cycling or circular continuous cycling was a predictor of poor response not only to lithium but to carbamazepine as well (17).

In contrast, to use in monotherapy, carbamazepine may be better suited for the treatment of rapid cycling when used in conjunction with another mood stabilizer. When used alone, carbamazepine has demonstrated a 19% rate of response, but when combined with lithium, the response rate rose to 56% (18). In this same study, lithium monotherapy was associated with a disappointing 28% rate of response. Despite the added improvement when using carbamazepine in combination with lithium, this drug regimen remains limited in its ability to achieve mood stabilization for nearly half of all subjects.

Valproate
On the basis of preliminary open data, Calabrese et al. hypothesized that the AED valproate may be efficacious for the treatment of rapid cycling. In order to test this

theory, a homogenous cohort of 101, prospectively defined rapid-cycling bipolar outpatients were administered valproate either as monotherapy or adjunctive therapy for up to 17.2 months (14,19). Seventy-seven percent of patients were found to demonstrate a marked antimanic response with valproate. However, only 38% showed a prophylactic effect against new depressive episodes. In total, marked prophylactic responses were seen in 72% of manic, 94% of mixed-state, and 33% of depressed patients. These results suggest that valproate is better suited to treat mania and mixed states in rapid cycling and offers only minimal to moderate efficacy in treating depression.

For the next 12 years, the belief that valproate and other AEDs were superior to lithium at treating rapid cycling was commonplace, but it was not until 2005 that a head-to-head, randomized, double-blind, parallel-group trial of lithium and valproate (as divalproex) was conducted to objectively compare outcomes (20). In this trial, patients were eligible for enrollment if they were diagnosed with rapid-cycling bipolar I or II disorder and had a history of at least one episode of mania, hypomania, or a mixed state within the past three months. Patients were first stabilized for up to six months with the open-label combination of lithium and divalproex, and any additional psychotropic medications were slowly weaned over a three-month period. Subjects were then eligible for randomization into the double-blind, maintenance phase upon meeting the following criteria: a 24-item Hamilton Depression Rating Scale (HAM-D) score less than or equal to 20, a Global Assessment Scale score greater than of equal to 51, a Young Mania Rating Scale (YMRS) score less than or equal to 12, lithium levels greater than or equal to 0.8 mEq/L, and valproate levels greater than or equal to 50 μg/mL for a minimum of four consecutive weeks. This trial design ensured that patients tolerated both treatments and were experiencing only mild-to-moderate symptoms of hypomania and/or depression prior to entering the maintenance phase; by definition, they were in partial remission. Upon meeting these eligibility criteria, patients were randomly assigned to treatment with either lithium or divalproex monotherapy and were followed for up to 20 months.

Of the 254 patients entering the initial stabilization phase of the trial, 65 (26%) did not respond to the combination of lithium and divalproex, with the majority exhibiting symptoms of refractory depression. Sixty patients (24%) completed the stabilization phase and underwent randomization to double-blind maintenance monotherapy (lithium: $N = 32$, divalproex: $N = 28$). For these patients, the mean lithium level was 0.92 mEq/L (dose range 900–2100 mg/day) and the mean valproate level was 77 μg/mL (dose range 750–2750 mg/day), respectively.

No significant difference between the lithium and divalproex groups was found on the primary outcome measure of time to treatment for emerging symptoms of relapse (Fig. 1). Likewise, no significant difference was observed in time to premature discontinuation for any reason, time to treatment for depression, or time to treatment for a manic/hypomanic/mixed episode.

Divalproex-treated patients experienced lower rates of tremors and polyuria/polydipsia, but no difference in discontinuations due to adverse events was found between treatment groups. Overall survival in the study was low, with only 16% of lithium-treated and 29% of divalproex-treated patients completing the 20-month maintenance phase. For a monotherapy study conducted over 20 months' duration, the low completion rates were surprising but consistent with a 12-month maintenance study comparing divalproex and lithium monotherapy, where 38% of divalproex-treated and 24% of lithium-treated patients completed the trial (21).

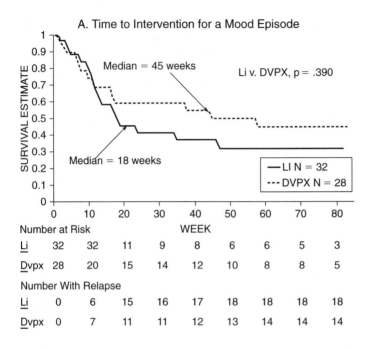

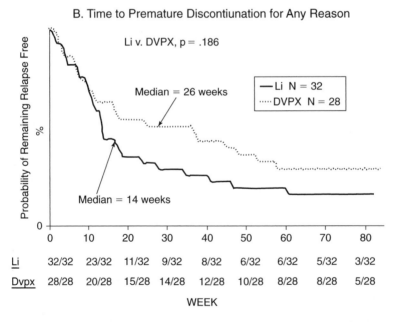

FIGURE 1 (**A**) and (**B**) Time to treatment intervention for any mood episode and time to study discontinuation among stabilized rapid-cycling bipolar disorder patients randomly assigned to double-blind maintenance monotherapy with lithium or divalproex. *Source*: From Ref. 20.

The results of this study did not confirm prior notions that valproate would be more effective than lithium in rapid-cycling bipolar disorder. As the observed treatment effect between valproate and lithium was small, the study was underpowered to detect a significant difference between agents. The estimated hazard ratio of 0.74 (95% CI = 0.36 to 1.49) reflected a need for 364 patients per study arm, substantially higher than the cumulative enrollment of 60 patients in the actual study.

Despite this limitation, the results pertain to treatment with two commonly used mood stabilizers and are generalizable to clinical practice. The up to six-month stabilization period and requirement that patients demonstrate continued improvement over four consecutive weeks prior to maintenance-phase randomization ensured that results would represent a true prophylactic effect of lithium or valproate monotherapy, as opposed to the effect of discontinuation of prestudy medications or relapse back into the index mood episode. The 20-month maintenance phase is the longest duration ever studied in a population of rapid cyclers and allowed for the assessment of recurrence over a meaningful time period. Perhaps of greatest relevance to clinicians is the realization that the combination of valproate and lithium will not be adequate for the majority of rapid-cycling patients. Most cases of mood episode nonresponse were due to refractory depressive symptoms. This reinforces observations that depression is the most common presentation of rapid-cycling bipolar disorder and raises awareness that novel compounds to treat and prevent rapid-cycling depressive states continue to be urgently needed.

With the results of this trial in hand, it becomes more apparent that the early studies of lithium suffered a design flaw by comparing lithium only to placebo. In order to truly gauge lithium's efficacy in the treatment of rapid cycling, it would need to be contrasted with an active comparator as accomplished in the Calabrese et al. study (20). Thus, the early lithium trials were accurate in detecting that rapid cycling is an indicator of difficult-to-treat illness, but lacked adequate assay sensitivity by not comparing lithium to agents within the anticonvulsant drug class (17,22). In support of this conclusion, a post hoc analysis of a 47-week maintenance study comparing the atypical antipsychotic olanzapine to divalproex in manic or mixed rapid-cycling patients found no difference in efficacy between treatments (23). Among the divalproex-treated patients, improvement in YMRS scores were initially better in rapid- than non-rapid-cycling patients, but this difference was only maintained during the first two study weeks.

Lamotrigine

During its clinical development for epilepsy, the AED lamotrigine was shown to exert positive effects on mood (24). Reports of efficacy in treatment-resistant bipolar disorder (25), bipolar depression (26), and open-label data suggesting benefit in rapid cycling (27) led to the evaluation of lamotrigine monotherapy for the long-term prophylaxis of mood episodes in patients with rapid-cycling bipolar disorder (28). This study was the first placebo-controlled assessment of any medication in a prospectively defined group of patients with rapid-cycling bipolar disorder.

The trial consisted of two phases: a preliminary, open-label stabilization phase and a randomized, double-blind continuation phase. Initially, patients received the addition of lamotrigine (titrated to between 100 and 300 mg/day) to their current psychotropic medication regimen. After four to eight weeks of lamotrigine exposure, all concomitant medications were tapered and discontinued. Subjects tolerating open-label lamotrigine with a HAM-D score less than or equal to 14 and a Mania Rating Scale (MRS) score less than or equal to 12 over a two-week period were randomized to lamotrigine or placebo for up to 26 weeks. Of 342 patients entering the preliminary phase, 182 patients were randomized to the continuation phase.

Time to additional pharmacotherapy to treat an emerging mood episode, the primary outcome measure, did not differ between groups. Median survival times were 18 weeks for lamotrigine-treated and 12 weeks for placebo-treated subjects (Fig. 2). However, when overall survival in the study was examined, lamotrigine-treated subjects remained in treatment significantly longer than those taking placebo (lamotrigine = 14 weeks vs. placebo = 8 weeks; $p = 0.036$). For patients requiring additional pharmacotherapy, 80% necessitated treatment for depressive symptoms. A comparison between patients with bipolar I and II disorder found that the bipolar II subgroup treated with lamotrigine survived significantly longer; namely 17 weeks, in contrast to 7 weeks for placebo-treated patients ($p = 0.015$). No drug-placebo difference in survival was detected for patients with bipolar I disorder. When assessing patients who remained stable without relapse for six months, a greater percentage were treated with lamotrigine (41%, 37/90) compared with placebo (26%, 23/87; $p = 0.04$). Once again, a statistical difference was observed among the bipolar II (46% vs. 18%; $p = 0.04$), but not the bipolar I, cohort.

A statistical difference favoring lamotrigine over placebo in both study survival and prevention of relapse suggests a differential effectiveness in patients with bipolar II compared to bipolar I disorder. The finding is intriguing, given that a controlled trial found lamotrigine to be superior to placebo for treating depressive symptoms in bipolar I disorder (26). Part of the difference may be attributable to the high placebo response observed in the patients with bipolar I disorder. Another explanation is that the lack of strong prophylactic antimanic effects with lamotrigine undermines its usefulness as a monotherapy in patients with rapid cycling. Overall, the results of this study support the use of lamotrigine as monotherapy for the treatment of rapid-cycling bipolar disorder, but primarily for patients with the bipolar II subtype.

Lamotrigine has also been evaluated in a double-blind, randomized, placebo-controlled, crossover study with the AED gabapentin (29). The sample consisted of 31 patients with refractory mood disorders treated successively with lamotrigine, gabapentin, or placebo for six weeks. Rapid-cycling patients composed 92% of the population, most of whom were diagnosed with bipolar I (11/31) or bipolar II (14/31) disorder. A significantly greater percentage of patients responded to lamotrigine compared to gabapentin or placebo as indicated by a Clinical Global Impressions Scale modified for bipolar disorder (CGI-BP) score of much or very much improved. Fifty-two percent (16/31) of lamotrigine-treated patients met

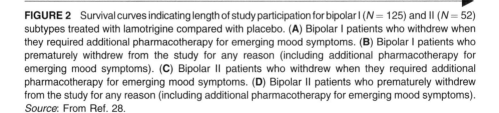

FIGURE 2 Survival curves indicating length of study participation for bipolar I ($N = 125$) and II ($N = 52$) subtypes treated with lamotrigine compared with placebo. (**A**) Bipolar I patients who withdrew when they required additional pharmacotherapy for emerging mood symptoms. (**B**) Bipolar I patients who prematurely withdrew from the study for any reason (including additional pharmacotherapy for emerging mood symptoms). (**C**) Bipolar II patients who withdrew when they required additional pharmacotherapy for emerging mood symptoms. (**D**) Bipolar II patients who prematurely withdrew from the study for any reason (including additional pharmacotherapy for emerging mood symptoms). *Source*: From Ref. 28.

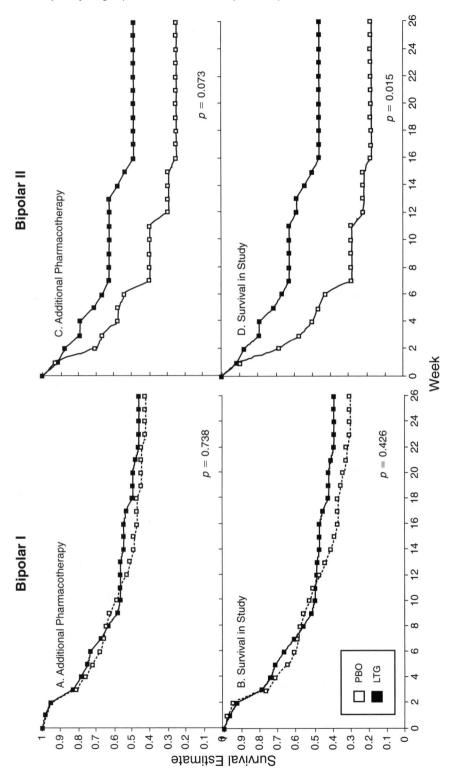

response criteria, compared with 26% (8/31) treated with gabapentin and 23% (7/31) treated with placebo.

Newer AEDs in the Treatment of Rapid Cycling

Less commonly used AEDs in the treatment of rapid-cycling bipolar disorder include tiagabine (30–32), levetiracetam (33,34), and topiramate (35,36). Topiramate has been evaluated in a study of 27 female rapid-cycling outpatients as an adjunctive treatment to lithium or divalproex (36). Fifteen patients achieved a significant improvement in mood as assessed by the 21-item HAM-D and YMRS, reaching a state of euthymia by 10 weeks of treatment. Eight (53%) of these 15 patients completed 40 weeks of treatment and remained euthymic. Weight loss of greater than or equal to 5% was experienced by nine (33%) patients; other side effects included ataxia, confusion, drowsiness, and the re-emergence of psychosis. A case report exists of a 38-year old woman with a 22-year history of rapid-cycling bipolar I disorder refractory to multiple treatments. The patient demonstrated a remarkable improvement with the combination of clozapine and topiramate, experiencing sustained remission for a period of three years (35). Despite these favorable reports, four separate placebo-controlled trials of topiramate mono-therapy in bipolar I mania or mixed states have failed to demonstrate efficacy. The lack of randomized, double-blind evidence for the use of topiramate in bipolar depression or rapid cycling speaks for restraint in its routine use as a mood stabilizer (37).

Levetiracetam has been reported to disrupt the sequence of rapid cycling in two cases, improving symptoms of depression and mania/mixed mania (33) One patient with a history of rapid-cycling bipolar disorder and comorbid substance abuse reportedly responded to levetiracetam monotherapy after failing 15 different psychotropic medications and remained well for one year (34).

Case studies suggest that some patients may benefit from the gamma-aminobutyric acid (GABA) reuptake inhibitor tiagabine as an add-on therapy during the long-term treatment of rapid-cycling bipolar disorder (31). However, other case series report tiagabine to be poorly tolerated and to offer little evidence of effectiveness in refractory bipolar illness (32). With rapid dose escalation, tia-gabine has been associated with possible seizure induction and should be used extremely cautiously (30).

Rapid-Cycling Bipolar Disorder and Comorbid Alcohol and Substance Use Disorders

A substantial area of unmet need involves the management of bipolar disorder and co-occurring substance use disorders (38). Perhaps not surprisingly, bipolar I and II disorder are the Axis I conditions observed to have the highest lifetime prevalence rates of alcohol abuse or dependence (46.2% and 39.2%, respectively) (39). Nega-tively influencing the course of bipolar disorder, comorbid alcoholism results in more frequent mood episodes and a shorter duration of remission between epi-sodes (40). Indeed, a lifetime history of drug abuse has been shown to be an independent predictor of rapid-cycling status (2).

To compare differences in treatment response among patients with active substance use disorders, our group recently completed enrollment in the first maintenance trial that compared lithium monotherapy with the combination of lithium plus divalproex in 149 rapid-cycling bipolar I or II patients with an alcohol or drug use disorder (41). In this trial, all patients met DSM-IV criteria for alcohol, cannabis, and/or cocaine abuse or dependence and were required to have had an episode of hypomania or mania within three months preceding study entry. Patients were also integrated into a 12-step-based intensive outpatient chemical dependency treatment program. Initially, patients were treated with a combination of lithium and divalproex ($N = 149$); responders were then randomized to double-blind treatment with lithium alone or lithium plus divalproex for up to six months. Thirty-eight subjects (25%) did not respond to open-label treatment with the combination of lithium and divalproex, and thus were not randomly assigned. Approximately equal numbers of these patients were experiencing refractory depressive or manic/hypomanic/mixed states. A total of 31 (21%) patients demonstrated a bimodal response to the treatment combination and were randomized to the maintenance phase.

On the primary outcome measure of time to treatment for a new mood episode, the median survival for combination-treated patients was 17.8 weeks compared with 15.9 weeks for lithium monotherapy-treated patients ($p = 0.6$). No significant difference in time to treatment intervention for a depressive or manic episode was evidenced between either group. Interestingly, among randomized subjects, more than half no longer met abuse criteria or had entered into early full remission of their respective substance use disorder. This suggests that in acutely symptomatic patients who are actively abusing alcohol or other substances, treatment with appropriate mood stabilizer therapy can treat not only the acute mood episode, but can also be beneficial in managing the co-occurring substance use disorder.

RAPID CYCLING AND DEPRESSION: A COMMON GROUND

Accumulating data suggest a distinct relationship between depression and rapid cycling. Nearly two decades ago, depression was identified as the index episode for the majority of patients with rapid cycling (42). Newer studies also report a high frequency of depression as the index episode, including the previously described placebo-controlled maintenance trial of lamotrigine (28) and the maintenance study comparing lithium with divalproex (20). Moreover, during the course of each of these trials, depression emerged as the most frequently recurring mood state. The spectrum of prophylactic efficacy of valproate, possessing substantial antimanic but only modest antidepressant activity, further supports the prominence of depression in rapid cycling (14,19). A meta-analysis of patients enrolled in the former Stanley Foundation Bipolar Network identified that rapid-cycling patients spend more days depressed than non-rapid-cycling patients (145 vs. 121 days) (2). Throughout the one-year assessment, patients experienced depression 35.6% of the time, considerably greater than the 12.6% of the time spent manic/hypomanic or the 3.3% of the time spent cycling or in a mixed state.

Depression is a substantial cause of morbidity and mortality in bipolar I and II disorders, and remains the primary clinical challenge in treating bipolar disorder in general and rapid cycling in particular. Patients with bipolar I disorder followed an average of 12.8 years spent 31.9% of the time depressed, in comparison with 8.9% of the time manic/hypomanic and 5.9% of the time cycling/mixed (43). Results indicate that depressive symptoms are even more predominant in patients with bipolar II disorder, occurring almost 40 times as frequently as hypomanic symptoms (44). The observation that depression is the primary morbidity in bipolar disorder has also been confirmed by a naturalistic, prospective study of outpatients followed daily for one year. Patients spent three times as many days depressed as manic, with depressive episodes lasting four times as long as manic episodes (45). Not surprisingly, the negative impact depression extols on psychosocial functioning leads to suicide in approximately 20% of patients (46). Nearly 30% of bipolar patients attempt suicide (47,48), a rate double than that observed in unipolar depression (47). Depression could also be considered as a marker of chronicity. At intake, patients presenting with a purely depressive episode are expected to have greater symptom persistence than patients presenting with a purely manic episode (43). Coryell et al. (49) noted that depressive symptoms occurring early in the course of bipolar disorder predicted depression at 15-year follow-up. No such relationship was identified for the persistence of manic symptoms.

Depression in bipolar disorder has not been studied as extensively as has mania. Lithium, divalproex, carbamazepine, and every second-generation antipsychotic with the exception of clozapine, is FDA approved for the treatment of mania. There are only two FDA approved treatments for bipolar depression, an olanzapine-fluoxetine combination and quetiapine. Additional research is needed to develop agents effective for all aspects of bipolar depression, including subsyndromal symptoms and phase-specific (acute, continuation, and maintenance) interventions. A summary of acute bipolar depression trials involving AEDs is provided in Table 1.

AEDs in the Treatment of Bipolar Depression
Carbamazepine
Developed in 1957, carbamazepine was one of the earliest anticonvulsants to be investigated for the relief of acute bipolar depression. Using a double-blind, placebo-controlled, off-on-off again design, carbamazepine was shown to result in response for 63% (15/24) of bipolar subjects at an average dose of 971 mg/day (50) Studies demonstrating the antidepressant properties of carbamazepine are limited by the use of heterogeneous samples, which combined patients with unipolar and bipolar disorder along with those suffering from treatment-refractory illness (51) Adding to carbamazepine's complexity of use is the requirement for routine monitoring of hematological and hepatic parameters. The incidence of agranulocytosis with carbamazepine use is around 1:100,000 (52). Although perhaps less likely to result in weight gain than valproate (53), patients receiving carbamazepine for the treatment of depression may be more susceptible to weight gain than those treated for mania (54). Given the limited study of carbamazepine in depressive states and the significant potential for adverse effects, it is not regarded as a first-line agent for the treatment of bipolar depression.

A related compound, oxcarbazepine, differs from carbamazepine by the addition of a ketone substitution. However, it does not require routine blood monitoring, does not cause induction of its own metabolism, and is associated with less prominent drug interactions (55). There are no published controlled trials of oxcarbazepine in bipolar depression. The only published controlled study of oxcarbazepine monotherapy in bipolar disorder involves the treatment of mania or mixed states in youths with bipolar I disorder. In this trial, no difference was evidenced between oxcarbazepine and placebo (56).

Valproate/Divalproex
Initial support for the use of valproate in the treatment of acute bipolar depression was noted by Winsberg et al. (57) in a 12-week open-label study of bipolar II

TABLE 1 Blinded, Controlled, Trials of Anticonvulsants in the Treatment of Acute Bipolar Depression

Agent	Design	Subjects	Number randomized	Duration	Primary outcome measure	Primary outcome results	Key findings
Divalproex Davis et al. (2005) 58	DB, PC	BP I	DVX (N = 13) PBO (N = 12)	8 wk	Percentage change from baseline to end point on HAMD	DVX Δ = 43.5% PBO Δ = 27.0% p < 0.001	DVX superior to PBO at reducing depression and anxiety
Divalproex extended release	DB, PC	BP I, II, NOS	DVP (N = 10)	6 wk	Change from baseline to end point on MADRS	DVX Δ = −13.6	DVX superior to PBO at reducing depression
Ghaemi et al. (2007) 60			PBO (N = 8)			PBO Δ = −1.4 p = 0.003	No difference in response[a] rates between DVX and PBO
Lamotrigine	DB, PC	BP I	LTG 50 mg/day (N = 66)	7 wk	Change from baseline to end point on MADRS[d]	LTG 200 mg/day	Greater rates of response[a] on LTG 50 and 200 mg/day than on PBO
Calabrese et al. (1999) 26			LTG 200 mg/day (N = 63) PBO (N = 66)			Δ = −13.3 LTG 50 mg/day Δ = −11.2 PBO Δ = −7.8 p < 0.05 for LTG 200 mg/day vs. PBO	LTG 200 mg/day showed greater efficacy than 50 mg/day
Lamotrigine/ Citalopram	Adjunctive, DB, CIT active comparator	BP I, II	LTG (N = 10)	12 wk	Change from baseline to end point on MADRS	LTG Δ = −13.3	LTG and CIT equally effective at reducing depression
Schaffer et al. (2006) 75			CIT (N = 10)			CIT Δ = −14.2 p = NS	Combined response[a] rose from 31.6% at wk 6 to 52.6% at wk 12

(Continued)

TABLE 1 Blinded, Controlled, Trials of Anticonvulsants in the Treatment of Acute Bipolar Depression (*Continued*)

Agent	Design	Subjects	Number randomized	Primary outcome measure	Duration	Primary outcome results	Key findings
Lamotrigine/ gabapentin Frye et al. (2000) 29	DB, PC, crossover	BPI, II MDD	LTG (N = 31) GBP (N = 31) PBO (N = 31)	Responder[b] analysis based on CGI-BP	6 wk	LTG = 52% GBP = 26% PBO = 23% $p = 0.031$	LTG superior to both GBP and PBO in the treatment of refractory mood disorders
Lamotrigine/ olanzapine-fluoxetine combination Brown et al. (2006) 86	DB, OFC active comparator	BP I	LTG (N = 205) OFC (N = 205)	Change from baseline to end point on CGI-S	7 wk	OFC showed greater improvement than LTG on CGI-S $p = 0.002$	OFC modestly superior to LTG in reducing depression OFC associated with greater weight gain and metabolic abnormalities
Topiramate/ bupropion SR McIntyre et al. (2002) 69	Adjunctive, SB, BUP active comparator	BP I, II	TOP (N = 18) BUP (N = 18)	Responder[c] analysis based on HAMD-17	8 wk	TOP = 56% BUP = 59% $p = $ NS	TOP and BUP equally effective at reducing depression as adjunctive therapy Most patients in both treatment groups experienced weight loss

[a] ≥50% reduction in MADRS score.
[b] Rated as much or very much improved.
[c] ≥50% reduction in Hamilton Depression Rating Scale (HAMD-17) score.
[d] Primary outcome measure not defined a priori.

Abbreviations: Δ, change; BP I, bipolar I disorder; BP II, bipolar II disorder; BP NOS, bipolar disorder not otherwise specified; BUP, bupropion SR; CIT, citalopram; CGI-BP, Clinical Global Impressions scale for Bipolar Illness; CGI-S, Clinical Global Impressions Severity of Illness Scale; DB, double-blind; DVX, divalproex sodium; GBP, gabapentin; HAMD, Hamilton Depression Scale; Li, lithium; LTG, lamotrigine; MADRS, Montgomery-Åsberg Depression Rating Scale; MDD, unipolar major depressive disorder; OFC, olanzapine-fluoxetine combination; PBO, placebo; PC, placebo-controlled; SB, single-blind; TOP, topiramate.

outpatients. A mean divalproex dose of 882 mg/day resulted in a 63% response rate (12/19) as assessed by the 17-item HAM-D. The highest rate of response tended to be in medication naïve (82%) compared with mood-stabilizer naïve (38%) patients, but this difference did not reach statistical significance ($p < 0.08$). One published trial by Davis et al. of 25 bipolar I–depressed patients randomized to double-blind treatment with divalproex or placebo found the rate of improvement in depressive symptoms over time to be twice as great with divalproex than placebo (58). In this study, a significant reduction in anxiety symptoms was also noted in divalproex-treated subjects. Divalproex was well tolerated, with only one patient withdrawing from the study because of adverse effects. An unpublished, multisite trial of divalproex in bipolar depression (I, II, or NOS) found no significant difference in the rate of response compared with placebo (43% vs. 27%) (59). Similar to the Davis et al. trial, this study enrolled a relatively small number of subjects ($N = 45$) and utilized the HAM-D as the primary outcome measure. However, the Davis et al. study was conducted at a single site, perhaps accounting for the detectable difference with divalproex as opposed to the negative multisite trial conducted by Sachs et al. A placebo-controlled study involving divalproex extended release (ER) in the treatment of bipolar depression was recently reported, enrolling 18 patients with bipolar I, II, or NOS disorders (60). Change from baseline to end point score on the Montgomery-Åsberg Depression Rating Scale (MADRS) was significant for a time by treatment interaction favoring divalproex ER over placebo ($p = 0.0078$). The absolute improvement in MADRS total score over time was 13.6 points with divalproex versus 1.4 points with placebo ($p = 0.003$).

A post hoc analysis to assess the efficacy of divalproex in the prevention of bipolar depression was carried out by Gyulai et al. in recently manic bipolar I patients ($N = 571$) enrolled in a 52-week maintenance trial (61). After completing an open-label stabilization phase, eligible patients were randomized to divalproex ($N = 187$), lithium ($N = 91$), or placebo ($N = 94$) in a 2:1:1 ratio. Divalproex-treated patients were less likely to discontinue early for depression than placebo-treated patients ($p < 0.05$). Divalproex was also more effective than lithium in delaying the time to depressive relapse among patients who responded to divalproex in the open-period and in those with a past history of psychiatric hospitalization.

In this trial, paroxetine or sertraline could be added for breakthrough depression. The combination of divalproex and a selective serotonin reuptake inhibitor (SSRI), but not lithium and an SSRI, was more effective than SSRI monotherapy in prophylaxing against depressive symptoms. Interestingly, this was the first time a randomized, controlled maintenance trial found antidepressant monotherapy to be inferior to an antidepressant plus a mood stabilizer in preventing breakthrough depression.

Lamotrigine

Treatment of acute bipolar depression. Lamotrigine was the first monotherapy agent to be investigated in a randomized, double-blind, parallel-group trial in bipolar I depression (26). A total of 195 subjects were enrolled in an equivalent fashion to lamotrigine 50 mg/day, lamotrigine 200 mg/day, or placebo for seven weeks. The sample was moderately ill; 50% of patients had prior hospitalizations and 30% had previously attempted suicide. Significant improvement from placebo began to emerge at week 3 when patients were taking lamotrigine 50 mg/day. At study end point, significant improvement was noted for lamotrigine 200 mg/day on the MADRS ($p < 0.05$) and approached significance for the 50 mg/day group $p = 0.058$). Significantly more patients in both groups demonstrated a response ($\geq 50\%$ improvement on MADRS total score), but only the lamotrigine 200 mg/day dose performed significantly better on the CGI-I. Neither dose of lamotrigine showed improvement over placebo on the HAM-D, perhaps reflecting the greater weighting toward somatic symptoms (e.g., insomnia, anxiety, and agitation) with this instrument. The low incidence of somnolence as a side effect may also have contributed to the limited improvement on HAM-D scores with lamotrigine in comparison with placebo.

A double-blind crossover study similarly found lamotrigine to be more effective than placebo in patients with refractory mood disorders, the majority of whom were diagnosed with bipolar disorder (29). However, four other double-blind, placebo-controlled trials of lamotrigine conducted in the acute treatment of bipolar depression failed to show drug-placebo separation on the primary outcome measures (62). In each of the four studies, the effect size was small on measures such as the MADRS and 31-item HAM-D, falling consistently below 0.2 (the lower limits of a small treatment effect). A large placebo response appeared to contribute to the inability of lamotrigine to demonstrate superiority over placebo in treating acute bipolar depression in these trials.

Prophylaxis against recurrent depression. In addition to the acute relief of depressive symptoms, the prevention of recurrence is of paramount concern in the longitudinal treatment of bipolar disorder. Over 90% of patients with bipolar disorder will experience a recurrence at some point in their lifetime (63). Even when following a guideline-based treatment algorithm, over the course of two years almost half of patients will suffer a recurrence, with most being depressive in nature (64).

To assess the prevention of relapse or recurrence of mood episodes in bipolar I disorder, a randomized, double-blind, placebo-controlled trial of lamotrigine was conducted in patients who recently experienced a manic or hypomanic episode (65). Lithium served as the active comparator arm, given its proven efficacy in the maintenance treatment of bipolar disorder. Patients who were currently or recently manic or hypomanic were enrolled into an initial 8- to –16-week open-label phase. During this period, lamotrigine was titrated to at least 100 mg/day and other psychotropic medications were gradually withdrawn. Patients demonstrating response entered into the double-blind, maintenance phase and were randomized to lamotrigine (100–400 mg/day, $N = 59$), lithium (serum level = 0.8–1.1 mEq/L, $N = 46$), or placebo ($N = 70$). Regarding the primary outcome measure, both lithium and lamotrigine were significantly superior to placebo on time to intervention for any mood episode. Lamotrigine, but not lithium, was superior to placebo at prolonging the time to treatment for a depressive episode (lamotrigine vs. placebo $p = 0.02$; lithium vs. placebo $p = 0.17$). Conversely, lithium, but not lamotrigine, was superior to placebo at prolonging the time to treatment for a manic, hypomanic, or mixed episode (lithium vs. placebo $p = 0.006$; lamotrigine vs. placebo $p = 0.28$). In this study, lamotrigine was well tolerated, with headache emerging as the only adverse event occurring more commonly than with lithium in the double-blind phase, while lithium was associated with a higher incidence of diarrhea.

In conjunction with the 18-month maintenance trial assessing lamotrigine in recently hypomanic or manic patients, an analogous trial was performed in recently depressed patients (66). Again, results showed that both lamotrigine and lithium monotherapy were superior to placebo at delaying the time to intervention for a mood episode. A complementary pattern of efficacy was also observed, with lithium significantly delaying the time to intervention for manic but not depressive episodes, and lamotrigine significantly delaying the time to intervention for depressive but not manic episodes. These trials employed moderately enriched designs, requiring patients to initially tolerate and respond to lamotrigine. Although this method will generally lead to decreased variance throughout the randomization phase, it may limit generalizability of results. The enriched design may also have led to exaggeration of the ineffectiveness of lithium in preventing recurrent episodes of depression. Collectively, however, the results of these two studies strongly support the use of lamotrigine for the prophylaxis of depressive episodes in bipolar disorder.

It has been proposed that in order to assess the true performance of a drug in preventing recurrence, relapses should be excluded by requiring patients to experience sustained relief of mood symptoms for at least two months prior to evaluating a drug's prophylactic efficacy (67). To assess whether lamotrigine exhibited pure maintenance efficacy, a post hoc analysis was performed on both of the lamotrigine 18-month maintenance studies (65,66) in which all potential relapses (mood episodes of same polarity as the index episode) that occurred within 90 and 180 days of randomization were excluded (68) Similar to results of the original analyses, lamotrigine was found to be superior to placebo in terms of overall study survival. Both lithium and lamotrigine were superior to placebo in delaying time to onset of a new mood episode, supporting the pure-maintenance effects of these agents.

Emerging Treatments for Bipolar Depression

In small, underpowered, preliminary studies, the mood stabilizers topiramate and zonisamide have demonstrated putative antidepressant properties. Topiramate was compared with bupropion slow release (SR) under single-blind conditions as an add-on treatment for bipolar I or II depression (69). After eight weeks of treatment, both agents resulted in comparable reductions in depressive symptoms, with 56% of topiramate-treated and 58% of bupropion SR-treated patients meeting response criteria ($\geq$50% reduction in HAM-D score). Weight loss was apparent in both treatment groups, but was statistically greater with topiramate. Zonisamide, one of the newest AEDs on the market, has been evaluated in small open-label studies for the treatment of mania (70) and bipolar depression (71,72). Mixed results were seen in a trial of 20 depressed patients who were administered open-label zonisamide as an adjunctive therapy (72). Twenty-five percent of patients (5/20) were deemed treatment responders based on a greater than or equal to 50% decline in MADRS score over eight weeks. However, 50% (10/20) of patients discontinued treatment mainly because of side effects. The most common adverse effects were sedation, nausea, dizziness, and cognitive dysfunction. It appears that zonisamide, similar to topiramate, may also be associated with weight loss in some patients. Zonisamide may prove promising as a treatment for bipolar disorder with mood stabilizing effects from below baseline, but until placebo-controlled trials are undertaken, evidence for its efficacy is limited at best and it should likely be considered for use only when patients have failed more established therapies.

Combination Therapy

For patients already taking a mood stabilizer but who continue to display depressive symptoms, it is unclear whether the next-step treatment should be to add an antidepressant or another mood stabilizer, such as an AED. Combining two or more mood stabilizing agents is becoming common practice and may be more efficacious than monotherapy (73,74). A small trial by Young et al. (74) found no difference in efficacy when a second mood stabilizer or an antidepressant was added to an existing mood stabilizer—both were equally useful in managing depressive symptoms. However, the addition of an antidepressant resulted in fewer dropouts. Likewise, in a separate trial evaluating the addition of lamotrigine or citalopram to depressed bipolar I or II patients taking divalproex, lithium, or carbamazepine, no significant difference in antidepressant efficacy was observed between study drugs (75). Both lamotrigine and citalopram resulted in similar reductions in depressive severity.

Lithium and divalproex are the most commonly prescribed drugs for bipolar disorder; yet when the two are used in combination they are ineffective at stabilizing mood in nearly 75% of rapid-cycling patients (18,19). Most of the refractory episodes are due to depression, or mood states "below baseline," as opposed to mania, hypomania, or subsyndromal mood elevation that would be characterized as episodes "above baseline." Ketter and Calabrese have offered that an agent effective at "stabilizing mood from below" would possess considerable antidepressant properties but would not worsen the course of illness by inducing (hypo) mania or cycle acceleration (76). Such treatment options are limited, and none of the AEDs have demonstrated consistently strong evidence to meet this definition. This suggests that future trials should aim at combining agents that work well at preventing episodes from above baseline with agents that prevent episodes from below baseline. Until such time, the current evidence base does not robustly support a front-line monotherapy role for any AED for acute bipolar depression, whether or not there is associated rapid cycling.

Treatment Guidelines for Bipolar Depression

A host of professional organizations and consensus panels have established guidelines for the treatment of bipolar depression, and there are considerable variations in their recommendations (see Table 2). Lithium is generally regarded as an acceptable monotherapy agent (77–81). The majority of guidelines also support the use of lamotrigine monotherapy for the depressed phase of bipolar disorder (77,79–82), primarily on the basis of positive results from one placebo-controlled acute depression trial (26) and two 18-month maintenance trials (65,66). With combination treatments becoming more common, several guidelines also recommend combined treatment with two mood stabilizers or a mood stabilizer plus an antidepressant as a first-line therapy (78,81–84). Although not an anticonvulsant, compelling evidence supports the use of quetiapine in bipolar depression. The most recent series of recommendations, published in 2006 by the Canadian Network for Mood and Anxiety Treatments, have newly included quetiapine monotherapy as an acceptable initial treatment and continue to recommend use of the antipsychotic olanzapine in combination with an SSRI (81).

TABLE 2 Summary of First-Line Recommended Treatments for Acute Bipolar Depression

Study	Monotherapy				Combination therapy					
	Li	LTG	QUE	VPA	Antimanic[a] + AD	Antimanic[a] + LTG	Li + LTG	Li + AD	LTG + AD	Li + VPA
APA (Hirschfeld et al. 2002) 77	Yes	Yes	No	No	No	No	No	No	No	No
World Federation of SBP (Grunze et al. 2002) 82	No	No	No	No	No	No	No	Yes	Yes	No
British Association for Psychopharmacology (Goodwin et al. 2003) 83	No	No	No	No	Yes	No	No	Yes	No	No
Expert Consensus Guidelines (Keck et al., 2004) 78	Yes	No	No	No	No	No	Yes	Yes	No	No
Australian and New Zealand Guidelines (Mitchell et al. 2004) 79	Yes	Yes	No	No	No	No	No	No	No	No
International Consensus Group (Calabrese et al. 2004) 80	Yes	Yes	No	No	No	No	No	No	No	No
Texas Medication Algorithms (Suppes et al. 2005) 84	No	Yes[b]	No	No	No	Yes	Yes	No	No	No
Canadian Network for Mood and Anxiety (Yatham et al. 2006) 81	Yes	Yes	Yes	No	Yes[c]	No	No	Yes	No	Yes

[a]An antimanic agent includes any medication that has evidence of being an effective treatment for mania.
[b]Only recommended if there is no history of severe or recent mania.
[c]Only Li, VPA, and Olanzapine are recommended as antimanic agents for use in combination with an AD.
Abbreviations: AD, antidepressant; APA, American Psychiatric Association; Li, lithium; LTG, lamotrigine; QUE, quetiapine; SBP, Societies of Biological Psychiatry; VPA, valproate.

CONCLUSIONS

AEDs have played an integral role in the management of rapid-cycling bipolar disorder and bipolar depression. Lamotrigine, the first agent ever studied in prospective, double-blind, placebo-controlled trials in both conditions, has established a rigorous standard of evidence for the maintenance treatment of bipolar disorder by which emerging therapies will be compared. The AEDs are not equivalent and clearly possess variant efficacy and tolerability profiles. For acute bipolar depression, despite some conflicting data, lamotrigine is the AED most supported by treatment guidelines and the extant literature; though for rapid cycling, lamotrigine's forte may be confined to patients with the bipolar II subtype. Valproate appears suited for the management of rapid cycling, and its modest antidepressant effects may make it most useful as an adjunctive therapy, perhaps in combination with an antidepressant or lamotrigine. There remains little evidence to recommend zonisamide, oxcarbazepine, gabapentin, levetiracetam, or topiramate in bipolar depression or rapid cycling, or, for that matter, any phase of bipolar disorder. However, these agents are not known to exacerbate manic switching and may be employed for the management of co-occurring anxiety (e.g., gabapentin) or substance use (e.g., topiramate) disorders or to offset weight loss associated with traditional mood stabilizer therapy (e.g., topiramate and zonisamide).

The AEDs have brought numerous benefits to the field, but their application has principally been evaluated in monotherapy studies. Long aware that monotherapy often falls short of improving symptom control and reducing relapse, clinicians often rely on multiple drug regimens. It is here that evidence is most limited to guide prescribing practices. On the horizon are trials aimed at assessing combination strategies to treat the most complex manifestations of bipolar disorder. Data collection in a group of rapid-cycling bipolar patients with comorbid substance use disorders is nearing completion and will compare the combination of divalproex and lithium with the triple therapy combination of divalproex, lithium, and lamotrigine. These results are highly anticipated and should help resolve whether exposure to multiple agents merely adds to the side-effect burden and treatment cost or rather provides greater efficacy and improved well-being for the estimated 169 million existing individuals worldwide that suffer from bipolar disorder (85).

Although not developed specifically to ease the burden of psychiatric illness, AEDs are a staple for patients with some of the most chronic and refractory variations of bipolar illness. Their expansion into the management of bipolar disorder will likely continue, and with that growth, bring promise for patients with rapid cycling, bipolar depression, and other states of unmet need.

REFERENCES

1. Dunner DL, Fieve RR. Clinical factors in lithium carbonate prophylaxis failure. Arch Gen Psychiatry 1974; 30(2):229–233.
2. Kupka RW, Luckenbaugh DA, Post RM, et al. Comparison of rapid-cycling and non-rapid-cycling bipolar disorder based on prospective mood ratings in 539 outpatients. Am J Psychiatry 2005; 162(7):1273–1280.
3. Bauer MS, Calabrese J, Dunner DL, et al. Multisite data reanalysis of the validity of rapid cycling as a course modifier for bipolar disorder in DSM-IV. Am J Psychiatry 1994; 151 (4):506–515.

4. Schneck CD, Miklowitz DJ, Calabrese JR, et al. Phenomenology of rapid-cycling bipolar disorder: data from the first 500 participants in the Systematic Treatment Enhancement Program. Am J Psychiatry 2004; 161(10):1902–1908.
5. Maj M, Magliano L, Pirozzi R, et al. Validity of rapid cycling as a course specifier for bipolar disorder. Am J Psychiatry 1994; 151(7):1015–1019.
6. Kupka RW, Luckenbaugh DA, Post RM, et al. Rapid and non-rapid cycling bipolar disorder: a meta-analysis of clinical studies. J Clin Psychiatry 2003; 64(12):1483–1494.
7. Calabrese JR, Shelton MD, Bowden CL, et al. Bipolar rapid cycling: focus on depression as its hallmark. J Clin Psychiatry 2001; 62(suppl 14):34–41.
8. Tondo L, Baldessarini RJ. Rapid cycling in women and men with bipolar manic-depressive disorders. Am J Psychiatry 1998; 155(10):1434–1436.
9. Coryell W, Solomon D, Turvey C, et al. The long-term course of rapid-cycling bipolar disorder. Arch Gen Psychiatry 2003; 60(9):914–920.
10. Gao K, Bilali S, Conroy C. Clinical impacts of comorbid anxiety disorder or substance use disorder on patients with rapid cycling bipolar disorder. Paper presented at: American Psychiatric Association Annual Meeting, May 20–25, 2006, Toronto, Canada.
11. Coryell W, Endicott J, Keller M. Rapidly cycling affective disorder. Demographics, diagnosis, family history, and course. Arch Gen Psychiatry 1992; 49(2):126–131.
12. Kukopulos A, Reginaldi D, Laddomada P, et al. Course of the manic-depressive cycle and changes caused by treatment. Pharmakopsychiatr Neuropsychopharmakol 1980; 13 (4):156–167.
13. Maj M, Pirozzi R, Magliano L, et al. Long-term outcome of lithium prophylaxis in bipolar disorder: a 5-year prospective study of 402 patients at a lithium clinic. Am J Psychiatry 1998; 155(1):30–35.
14. Calabrese JR, Woyshville MJ, Kimmel SE, et al. Predictors of valproate response in bipolar rapid cycling. J Clin Psychopharmacol 1993; 13(4):280–283.
15. Post RM, Uhde TW, Roy-Byrne PP, et al. Correlates of antimanic response to carba-mazepine. Psychiatry Res 1987; 21(1):71–83.
16. Joyce PR. Carbamazepine in rapid cycling bipolar affective disorder. Int Clin Psychopharmacol 1988; 3(2):123–129.
17. Okuma T. Effects of carbamazepine and lithium on affective disorders. Neuro-psychobiology 1993; 27(3):138–145.
18. Denicoff KD, Smith-Jackson EE, Disney ER, et al. Comparative prophylactic efficacy of lithium, carbamazepine, and the combination in bipolar disorder. J Clin Psychiatry 1997; 58(11):470–478.
19. Calabrese JR, Delucchi GA. Spectrum of efficacy of valproate in 55 patients with rapid-cycling bipolar disorder. Am J Psychiatry 1990; 147(4):431–434.
20. Calabrese JR, Shelton MD, Rapport DJ, et al. A 20-month, double-blind, maintenance trial of lithium versus divalproex in rapid-cycling bipolar disorder. Am J Psychiatry 2005; 162(11):2152–2161.
21. Bowden CL, Calabrese JR, McElroy SL, et al. A randomized, placebo-controlled 12-month trial of divalproex and lithium in treatment of outpatients with bipolar I disorder. Divalproex Maintenance Study Group. Arch Gen Psychiatry 2000; 57(5)481–489.
22. Di Costanzo E, Schifano F. Lithium alone or in combination with carbamazepine for the treatment of rapid-cycling bipolar affective disorder. Acta Psychiatr Scand 1991; 83 (6):456–459.
23. Suppes T, Brown E, Schuh LM, et al. Rapid versus non-rapid cycling as a predictor of response to olanzapine and divalproex sodium for bipolar mania and maintenance of remission: post hoc analyses of 47-week data. J Affect Disord 2005; 89(1–3):69–77.
24. Smith D, Chadwick D, Baker G, et al. Seizure severity and the quality of life. Epilepsia 1993; 34(suppl 5):S31–S35.
25. Calabrese JR, Bowden CL, McElroy SL, et al. Spectrum of activity of lamotrigine in treatment-refractory bipolar disorder. Am J Psychiatry 1999; 156(7):1019–1023.
26. Calabrese JR, Bowden CL, Sachs GS, et al. A double-blind placebo-controlled study of lamotrigine monotherapy in outpatients with bipolar I depression. Lamictal 602 Study Group. J Clin Psychiatry 1999; 60(2):79–88.

27. Calabrese JR, Fatemi SH, Woyshville MJ. Antidepressant effects of lamotrigine in rapid cycling bipolar disorder. Am J Psychiatry 1996; 153(9):1236.
28. Calabrese JR, Suppes T, Bowden CL, et al. A double-blind, placebo-controlled, prophylaxis study of lamotrigine in rapid-cycling bipolar disorder. Lamictal 614 Study Group. J Clin Psychiatry 2000; 61(11):841–850.
29. Frye MA, Ketter TA, Kimbrell TA, et al. A placebo-controlled study of lamotrigine and gabapentin monotherapy in refractory mood disorders. J Clin Psychopharmacol 2000; 20 (6):607–614.
30. Grunze H, Erfurth A, Marcuse A, et al. Tiagabine appears not to be efficacious in the treatment of acute mania. J Clin Psychiatry 1999; 60(11):759–762.
31. Schaffer LC, Schaffer CB, Howe J. An open case series on the utility of tiagabine as an augmentation in refractory bipolar outpatients. J Affect Disord 2002; 71(1–3):259–263.
32. Suppes T, Chisholm KA, Dhavale D, et al. Tiagabine in treatment refractory bipolar disorder: a clinical case series. Bipolar Disord 2002; 4(5):283–289.
33. Braunig P, Kruger S. Levetiracetam in the treatment of rapid cycling bipolar disorder. J Psychopharmacol 2003; 17(2):239–241.
34. Kaufman KR. Monotherapy treatment of bipolar disorder with levetiracetam. Epilepsy Behav 2004; 5(6):1017–1020.
35. Chen CK, Shiah IS, Yeh CB, et al. Combination treatment of clozapine and topiramate in resistant rapid-cycling bipolar disorder. Clin Neuropharmacol 2005; 28(3):136–138.
36. Kusumakar V, Yatham L, Kutcher S, et al. Preliminary, open-label study of topiramate in rapid-cycling bipolar women. Eur Neuropsychopharmacol 1999; 9:S357.
37. Kushner SF, Khan A, Lane R, et al. Topiramate monotherapy in the management of acute mania: results of four double-blind placebo-controlled trials. Bipolar Disord 2006; 8(1):15–27.
38. McElroy SL, Altshuler LL, Suppes T, et al. Axis I psychiatric comorbidity and its relationship to historical illness variables in 288 patients with bipolar disorder. Am J Psychiatry 2001; 158(3):420–426.
39. Regier DA, Farmer ME, Rae DS, et al. Comorbidity of mental disorders with alcohol and other drug abuse. Results from the Epidemiologic Catchment Area (ECA) Study. JAMA 1990; 264(19):2511–2518.
40. Brady KT, Lydiard RB. Bipolar affective disorder and substance abuse. J Clin Psychopharmacol 1992; 12(suppl 1):17S–22S.
41. Kemp DE, Gao K, Ganocy SJ, et al. Lithium monotherapy versus the combination of lithium and divalproex for rapid cycling bipolar disorder comorbid with substance abuse or dependence: a 6-month, double-blind, maintenance trial. Neuropsychopharmacology 2006; 31(suppl 1):S106.
42. Wehr TA, Sack DA, Rosenthal NE, et al. Rapid cycling affective disorder: contributing factors and treatment responses in 51 patients. Am J Psychiatry 1988; 145(2):179–184.
43. Judd LL, Akiskal HS, Schettler PJ, et al. The long-term natural history of the weekly symptomatic status of bipolar I disorder. Arch Gen Psychiatry 2002; 59(6):530–537.
44. Judd LL, Akiskal HS, Schettler PJ, et al. A prospective investigation of the natural history of the long-term weekly symptomatic status of bipolar II disorder. Arch Gen Psychiatry 2003; 60(3):261–269.
45. Post RM, Leverich GS, Nolen WA, et al. A re-evaluation of the role of antidepressants in the treatment of bipolar depression: data from the Stanley Foundation Bipolar Network. Bipolar Disord 2003; 5(6):396–406.
46. Goodwin FK, Jamison K. Manic-Depressive Illness. New York, NY: Oxford University Press, 1990.
47. Chen YW, Dilsaver SC. Lifetime rates of suicide attempts among subjects with bipolar and unipolar disorders relative to subjects with other Axis I disorders. Biol Psychiatry 1996; 39(10):896–899.
48. Fagiolini A, Kupfer DJ, Rucci P, et al. Suicide attempts and ideation in patients with bipolar I disorder. J Clin Psychiatry 2004; 65(4):509–514.
49. Coryell W, Turvey C, Endicott J, et al. Bipolar I affective disorder: predictors of outcome after 15 years. J Affect Disord 1998; 50(2–3):109–116.

50. Post RM, Uhde TW, Roy-Byrne PP, et al. Antidepressant effects of carbamazepine. Am J Psychiatry 1986; 143(1):29–34.
51. Ballenger JC, Post RM. Carbamazepine in manic-depressive illness: a new treatment. Am J Psychiatry 1980; 137(7):782–790.
52. Schatzberg AF, Cole JO, DeBattista C. Manual of Clinical Psychopharmacology. 4th ed. Washington, DC: American Psychiatric Publishing, Inc., 2003.
53. Mattson RH, Cramer JA, Collins JF. A comparison of valproate with carbamazepine for the treatment of complex partial seizures and secondarily generalized tonic-clonic seizures in adults. The Department of Veterans Affairs Epilepsy Cooperative Study No. 264 Group. N Engl J Med 1992; 327(11):765–771.
54. Joffe RT, Post RM, Uhde TW. Effect of carbamazepine on body weight in affectively ill patients. J Clin Psychiatry 1986; 47(6):313–314.
55. Baruzzi A, Albani F, Riva R. Oxcarbazepine: pharmacokinetic interactions and their clinical relevance. Epilepsia 1994; 35(suppl 3):S14–S19.
56. Wagner KD, Kowatch RA, Emslie GJ, et al. A double-blind, randomized, placebo-controlled trial of oxcarbazepine in the treatment of bipolar disorder in children and adolescents. Am J Psychiatry 2006; 163(7):1179–1186.
57. Winsberg ME, DeGolia SG, Strong CM, et al. Divalproex therapy in medication-naive and mood-stabilizer-naive bipolar II depression. J Affect Disord 2001; 67(1–3):207–212.
58. Davis LL, Bartolucci A, Petty F. Divalproex in the treatment of bipolar depression: a placebo-controlled study. J Affect Disord 2005; 85(3):259–266.
59. Sachs GS, Altshuler LL, Ketter T, et al. Divalproex versus placebo for the treatment of bipolar depression. Poster session presented at: The American College of Neuropsychopharmacology 40th Meeting, December 9–13, 2001, Waikoloa, Hawaii.
60. Ghaemi SN, Gilmer WS, Goldberg JF, et al. Divalproex in the treatment of acute bipolar depression: a preliminary double-blind, placebo-controlled pilot study. J Clin Psychiatry 2007; 68(12):1840–1844.
61. Gyulai L, Bowden CL, McElroy SL, et al. Maintenance efficacy of divalproex in the prevention of bipolar depression. Neuropsychopharmacology 2003; 28(7):1374–1382.
62. Calabrese JR, Huffman RF, White RL, et al. Lamotrigine in the acute treatment of bipolar depression: results of five double-blind, placebo-controlled clinical trials. Bipolar Disord 2008; 10(2):323–333.
63. Solomon DA, Keitner GI, Miller IW, et al. Course of illness and maintenance treatments for patients with bipolar disorder. J Clin Psychiatry 1995; 56(1):5–13.
64. Perlis RH, Ostacher MJ, Patel JK, et al. Predictors of recurrence in bipolar disorder: primary outcomes from the Systematic Treatment Enhancement Program for Bipolar Disorder (STEP-BD). Am J Psychiatry 2006; 163(2):217–224.
65. Bowden CL, Calabrese JR, Sachs G, et al. A placebo-controlled 18-month trial of lamotrigine and lithium maintenance treatment in recently manic or hypomanic patients with bipolar I disorder. Arch Gen Psychiatry 2003; 60(4):392–400.
66. Calabrese JR, Bowden CL, Sachs G, et al. A placebo-controlled 18-month trial of lamotrigine and lithium maintenance treatment in recently depressed patients with bipolar I disorder. J Clin Psychiatry 2003; 64(9):1013–1024.
67. Prien RF, Caffey EM Jr., Klett CJ. Prophylactic efficacy of lithium carbonate in manic-depressive illness. Report of the Veterans Administration and National Institute of Mental Health collaborative study group. Arch Gen Psychiatry 1973; 28(3):337–341.
68. Calabrese JR, Goldberg JF, Ketter TA, et al. Recurrence in bipolar I disorder: a post hoc analysis excluding relapses in two double-blind maintenance studies. Biol Psychiatry 2006; 59(11):1061–1064.
69. McIntyre RS, Mancini DA, McCann S, et al. Topiramate versus bupropion SR when added to mood stabilizer therapy for the depressive phase of bipolar disorder: a preliminary single-blind study. Bipolar Disord 2002; 4(3):207–213.
70. Kanba S, Yagi G, Kamijima K, et al. The first open study of zonisamide, a novel anticonvulsant, shows efficacy in mania. Prog Neuropsychopharmacol Biol Psychiatry 1994; 18(4): 707–715.
71. Anand A, Bukhari L, Jennings SA, et al. A preliminary open-label study of zonisamide treatment for bipolar depression in 10 patients. J Clin Psychiatry 2005; 66(2):195–198.

72. Ghaemi SN, Zablotsky B, Filkowski MM, et al. An open prospective study of zonisamide in acute bipolar depression. J Clin Psychopharmacol 2006; 26(4):385–388.
73. Solomon DA, Ryan CE, Keitner GI, et al. A pilot study of lithium carbonate plus divalproex sodium for the continuation and maintenance treatment of patients with bipolar I disorder. J Clin Psychiatry 1997; 58(3):95–99.
74. Young LT, Joffe RT, Robb JC, et al. Double-blind comparison of addition of a second mood stabilizer versus an antidepressant to an initial mood stabilizer for treatment of patients with bipolar depression. Am J Psychiatry 2000; 157(1):124–126.
75. Schaffer A, Zuker P, Levitt A. Randomized, double-blind pilot trial comparing lamotrigine versus citalopram for the treatment of bipolar depression. J Affect Disord 2006; 96(1–2):95–99.
76. Ketter TA, Calabrese JR. Stabilization of mood from below versus above baseline in bipolar disorder: a new nomenclature. J Clin Psychiatry 2002; 63(2):146–151.
77. Practice guideline for the treatment of patients with bipolar disorder (revision). Am J Psychiatry 2002; 159(suppl 4):1–50.
78. Keck PE, Perlis RH, Otto MW, et al. The expert consensus guideline series: treatment of bipolar disorder 2004. Postgraduate Med 2004; 1–19.
79. Australian and New Zealand clinical practice guidelines for the treatment of bipolar disorder. Aust N Z J Psychiatry 2004; 38(5):280–305.
80. Calabrese JR, Kasper S, Johnson G, et al. International consensus group on bipolar I depression treatment guidelines. J Clin Psychiatry 2004; 65(4):571–579.
81. Yatham LN, Kennedy SH, O'Donovan C, et al. Canadian Network for Mood and Anxiety Treatments (CANMAT) guidelines for the management of patients with bipolar disorder: update 2007. Bipolar Disord 2006; 8(6):721–739.
82. Grunze H, Kasper S, Goodwin G, et al. World Federation of Societies of Biological Psychiatry (WFSBP) guidelines for biological treatment of bipolar disorders. Part I: Treatment of bipolar depression. World J Biol Psychiatry 2002; 3(3):115–124.
83. Goodwin GM, Young AH. The British Association for Psychopharmacology guidelines for treatment of bipolar disorder: a summary. J Psychopharmacol 2003; 17(4 suppl):3–6.
84. Suppes T, Dennehy EB, Hirschfeld RM, et al. The Texas implementation of medication algorithms: update to the algorithms for treatment of bipolar I disorder. J Clin Psychiatry 2005; 66(7):870–886.
85. Kessler RC, Berglund P, Demler O, et al. Lifetime prevalence and age-of-onset distributions of DSM-IV disorders in the National Comorbidity Survey Replication. Arch Gen Psychiatry 2005; 62(6):593–602.
86. Brown EB, McElroy SL, Keck PE, et al. A 7-week, randomized, double-blind trial of olanzapine/fluoxetine combination versus lamotrigine in the treatment of bipolar I depression. J Clin Psychiatry 2006; 67(7):1025–1033.

5 Role of Antiepileptic Drugs in the Treatment of Major Depressive Disorder

Erik Nelson
Department of Psychiatry, University of Cincinnati Medical Center, Cincinnati, Ohio, U.S.A.

ANTIEPILEPTICS IN THE TREATMENT OF MAJOR DEPRESSIVE DISORDER

The effectiveness of antiepileptic drugs (AEDs), particularly valproate, carbamazepine, and lamotrigine, as mood stabilizers in bipolar disorder has been thoroughly documented over the past 30 years (1). However, the value of these agents in unipolar major depression is less well established and no AED is currently approved for this indication. Moreover, very few rigorous controlled trials have been conducted with these agents in samples of patients with unipolar depression (2). Nevertheless, the results of a number of studies suggest that some AEDs, including carbamazepine, valproate, phenytoin, lamotrigine, topiramate, gabapentin, and tiagabine, may have antidepressant effects in unipolar patients.

Carbamazepine

Carbamazepine is one of the three AEDs approved for the treatment of bipolar disorder. Its anticonvulsant effects appear to be, in part, mediated by a reduction in glutamate release due to the inhibition of voltage-gated sodium channels, although mood stabilization may depend on other mechanisms that occur with chronic administration, such as modulation of monoamine and gamma-aminobutryric acid (GABA) neurotransmission (1). Evidence that carbamazepine decreases the frequency of depressive episodes in bipolar disorder sparked interest in the possibility that it may have acute antidepressant effects in both bipolar and unipolar mood disorders (3). There is, however, only a single double-blind, placebo-controlled study of carbamazepine published to date that included a significant number of patients with unipolar depression (3). In this crossover study, 5 (45%) of 11 treatment-resistant unipolar depressed inpatients responded to carbamazepine monotherapy as indicated by an improvement of one point or more ("mild response") on the Bunney-Hamburg scale. Only two patients (18%) met the more stringent response criterion of improvement by two points or more on this 15-point scale ("good response"). In the bipolar depressed patients, 15 of 24 (63%) had a mild response and 10 (42%) had a good response. Although a greater percentage of bipolar patients responded to carbamazepine in this study, the difference in response rates between the diagnostic groups was not statistically significant. The difference between the mean depression rating score from the two weeks of placebo treatment and the rating from the four weeks of carbamazepine treatment, however, was significant only in the bipolar depressed group.

Nonetheless, several open-label studies suggest that carbamazepine may benefit patients with unipolar depression. In an open-label trial of carbamazepine monotherapy in patients with chronic depression, 11 out of 12 patients were described as "responders" to carbamazepine 400 to 600 mg/day, although the criterion for determining response was not given (4). Moreover, there was a significant improvement in the mean score on the Montgomery-Åsberg Depression Rating Scale (MADRS) (from 36.3 to 22.1) after carbamazepine therapy. Other studies report benefits with carbamazepine when used to augment the effects of antidepressants. Rybakowski et al. (5) randomized 59 patients with treatment-resistant depression, 18 of whom had unipolar depression, to either lithium or carbamazepine augmentation of ongoing antidepressant therapy. There was no significant difference between the two treatments; 16 (57.1%) of the 28 patients who received carbamazepine responded, with 9 (32.1%) reaching full remission. Although the response of the unipolar patients was not analyzed separately, there was no significant effect of unipolar/bipolar diagnosis on the response to either drug. In a series of patients with unipolar depression who had failed to respond to open-label venlafaxine, four out of six treated with carbamazepine augmentation were considered responders (6). Another study investigated the effects of carbamazepine augmentation in six patients who had failed to respond to four weeks of treatment with citalopram (7). In this open-label trial, there was a significant reduction in MADRS score after four weeks of adjunctive carbamazepine. The authors, however, warned that a reduction in the mean citalopram plasma concentration was observed after the addition of carbamazepine.

A retrospective chart review of 16 treatment-resistant depressed patients (13 of whom were unipolar) treated with carbamazepine also reported benefits with this agent (8). Seven patients out of the total sample had a moderate or marked response to the medication, despite the fact that only two patients in this group received concomitant antidepressant therapy. The authors noted that the rate of adverse effects in this study was rather high, which may have been related to the relatively older age of the patient sample (mean age 63.9 ± 10.5 years). Several case reports also describe antidepressant effects with carbamazepine when used as an adjunct to treatment with an antidepressant (9,10) or lithium (11). Moreover, two case reports point to potential benefits of carbamazepine therapy in the treatment of major depression with psychotic features. In one case, a patient with psychotic depression who was refractory to numerous medication trials responded to carbamazepine monotherapy (12). In the other case, a patient with "rapid cycling" psychotic depression benefited from a combination of carbamazepine and lithium (13).

Another potential role for carbamazepine therapy in the management of patients with unipolar depression is the prophylaxis of depressive episodes. Stuppaeck et al. (14,15) reported on a group of unipolar depressed patients treated with carbamazepine at two and five years of therapy. At the two-year time point, 17 out of the 24 patients described were diagnosed with unipolar depression, and all but four received carbamazepine monotherapy. Eleven of these patients were completely free of depressive episodes while on carbamazepine; two of these were taking concomitant lithium. An additional two patients were noted as having a decrease in episode frequency, while four patients had no change with carbamazepine prophylaxis. The mean number of depressive episodes per year decreased from 2.45 to 0.77 with carbamazepine treatment, a statistically significant change. In the report on longer-term carbamazepine prophylaxis, Stuppaeck et al. (15) describe the treatment of 17 patients with "major depression with melancholia" using 200 to 600 mg/day. Fifteen of these patients were treated with carbamazepine monotherapy, while two patients were treated with lithium as well. Five patients stopped taking carbamazepine during the five-year study, three because of lack of efficacy and two because of patient preference despite a good response to the drug. Seven of the fifteen patients were completely free of depression during the observation period. Of the remaining patients, five demonstrated a moderate decrease in episode frequency, two had no change in episode frequency, and one had an increase in episode frequency. As in the shorter prophylaxis study, there was a significant decrease in the mean number of episodes with prophylactic carbamazepine treatment, from 2.11 to 0.7 episodes per year. The mean prophylactic dose in this study was 480 mg and the mean carbamazepine plasma concentration was 6.2 μg/mL.

Lamotrigine

Like carbamazepine, lamotrigine appears to reduce excitatory glutamate release through its actions on voltage-gated sodium channels. Also, like carbamazepine, lamotrigine was first identified as having potential antidepressant effects when it was noted that patients taking it for epilepsy experienced an improvement in mood symptoms (16). It is currently approved for maintenance treatment of bipolar disorder, and the results of one double-blind, placebo-controlled study suggest that it has antidepressant properties in patients with bipolar I disorder (17). However, there are currently no published studies of lamotrigine as monotherapy for unipolar depression. Several studies have investigated the effects of lamotrigine as an adjunct to antidepressants in patients with major depression. Two randomized, placebo-controlled studies evaluated lamotrigine augmentation of antidepressants in samples predominantly consisting of unipolar depressed patients. In one study, 40 patients (33 of whom were unipolar) received lamotrigine or placebo added to ongoing paroxetine treatment (18). Although there was no significant difference compared with placebo in the change in Hamilton Depression Rating Scale (HAM-D) score, a significantly greater decrease in the Clinical Global Impression-Severity (CGI-S) score was reported in lamotrigine-treated patients. Moreover, the lamotrigine group demonstrated greater improvement compared with placebo-treated patients on the following HAM-D items: depressed mood, guilt, work nonproductivity, and lack of interest. In the other placebo-controlled augmentation study, patients who had failed at least one prior antidepressant trial were treated concurrently with fluoxetine 20 mg and either lamotrigine or placebo for six weeks (19). Again, there was no significant difference in the change in depression scores between patients treated with lamotrigine or placebo. However, there was a significantly greater improvement in the lamotrigine-treated group on the CGI-S and Clinical Global Impression-Improvement (CGI-I) scales.

Open-label studies also suggest potential benefits of the addition of lamotrigine to antidepressant therapy. Schindler et al. (20) conducted an eight-week, open-label comparison of lamotrigine and lithium augmentation of antidepressant therapy in 34 treatment-resistant unipolar patients. Both drugs produced a statistically significant improvement in symptom ratings, and the degree of change in scores was not significantly different between the two treatment groups. Specifically, 23% of the lamotrigine-treated patients met criteria for remission of the depressive episode, while 53% were considered responders on the basis of at least a 50% reduction in HAM-D score from baseline. In contrast, 18% of lithium-treated patients remitted, and 47% were considered responders. The mean dose of lamotrigine in this study was 153 mg. A smaller six-month trial also evaluated the effectiveness of lamotrigine added to antidepressants in 14 treatment-resistant unipolar patients (21). The addition of lamotrigine (dose range 50–200 mg) produced a significant improvement in depressive symptoms at both eight weeks and six months of therapy. At the end of the trial, four patients were rated as very much improved and seven much improved on the CGI-I scale. Furthermore, retrospective chart reviews (22–24) and case reports (25) also support the benefits of adjunctive lamotrigine in patients with treatment-resistant unipolar depression.

Valproate

Valproate, a broad spectrum AED that has effects on voltage-gated sodium channels and GABA neurotransmission, was the first anticonvulsant to be FDA approved for use in bipolar disorder. A few studies suggest that valproate therapy has acute and maintenance antidepressant effects in bipolar patients, (26,27), although its effects on depressive symptoms may be less robust than its antimanic properties. However, a dearth of studies has assessed the effectiveness of valproate in patients with unipolar depression. In fact, there are currently no published placebo-controlled trials of valproate monotherapy or valproate augmentation of antidepressants in nonbipolar depressed patients. Davis et al. (28) conducted the only prospective study of valproate monotherapy in unipolar patients, an eight-week open-label trial. At the end of the trial, 19 of the 22 study completers demonstrated a clinically significant response to the drug. The intent-to-treat analysis, which included 32 patients, demonstrated a statistically signficant improvement in overall depressive symptoms from baseline, which corresponded to an 11.9 point decrease in the mean HAM-D score (a decrease of 55%) from baseline. Debattista et al. (29) conducted an open-label study of valproate augmentation of antidepressants in 12 patients with major depression who were experiencing agitation as a symptom of their depressive episode. At the end of this four-week trial, patients displayed a statistically significant decrease in HAM-D scores (baseline 23.7 ± 5.9, end point 18.1 ± 8.1). Patients also exhibited a significant reduction in agitation during the trial that was independent of the overall antidepressant response. The authors commented that the antidepressant response observed was only modest compared with the effects on agitation, although it is important to note that the observation period of valproate therapy in this study was only four weeks, with up to two weeks for titration to the final dose. Although two to three weeks on a therapeutic dose of valproate may be sufficient for agitation effects to be optimized, this is generally not enough time for a complete antidepressant response to evolve.

Hayes et al. (30) conducted a retrospective chart review of long-term valproate use in psychiatric illness that included nine patients with major depression. Seven of these patients demonstrated improvement in Global Assessment of Functioning (GAF) scale scores after at least one year of treatment. The mean increase in GAF score was 27.7 ± 21.7 points for the depressed group (baseline GAF = 41.7 ± 14.7), which approximated that of the mixed bipolar group and resulted in the majority of the patients reaching the "mild symptom range or the virtually asymptomatic state." A few individual case reports also support the hypothesis that valproate has antidepressant properties in patients with unipolar major depression (31–33).

Phenytoin

Like lamotrigine and carbamazepine, phenytoin's anticonvulsant effects appear to be mediated by decreased glutamate release secondary to inhibition of voltage-gated sodium channels. Unlike these other AEDs, phenytoin is not approved for use in bipolar disorder, and there are relatively few studies investigating its therapeutic potential in bipolar patients. However, two controlled studies of phenytoin have been conducted in unipolar depression, one assessing its potential as monotherapy and the other evaluating its efficacy in augmenting SSRI antidepressants. The former study was a six-week trial comparing fluoxetine 20 mg and phenytoin 200 to 400 mg in patients with major depression (there was no placebo arm) (34). Twelve of fourteen patients in the phenytoin-treated group responded on the basis of a 50% or greater reduction in HAM-D score. There was no difference in the mean change in HAM-D score from baseline between the groups (−18.6 points for the fluoxetine group; −18.2 points for phenytoin). The mean blood level of phenytoin was 10.9 ± 2.0 µg/mL at week 6. It should be noted that a relatively low dose of fluoxetine was used, raising the concern that both treatments might have failed to demonstrate superiority over a placebo, had one been used in this study.

In the second controlled study, phenytoin was compared with placebo in patients who had received at least three weeks of treatment with adequate doses of fluvoxamine, fluoxetine, or paroxetine, but still had a score of 18 or higher on the HAM-D, 24 item version (35). After four weeks of double-blind treatment, there was no difference in change on the HAM-D between the phenytoin- and placebo-treated groups. The authors point out that a relatively high placebo response was observed in this study, which may have obscured any potential benefit of phenytoin augmentation. However, only 2 of 11 patients demonstrated a 30% or greater improvement in HAM-D score in the phenytoin group compared with seven of nine in the placebo group, making it unlikely that there was any clinically significant benefit of phenytoin augmentation in this trial.

Topiramate

Topiramate appears to modulate glutamatergic and GABA neurotransmission and is approved for the treatment of epilepsy and migraine headaches. Four double-blind, placebo-controlled studies have shown that topiramate is not efficacious for acute bipolar manic or mixed episodes (36). However, improvement in depressive symptoms after topiramate therapy has been reported in bipolar patients (37). There is currently one published double-blind, placebo-controlled study assessing topiramate as monotherapy for unipolar major depression (38). This trial compared the effects of 10 weeks of treatment with topiramate 200 mg or placebo in 64 women diagnosed with recurrent major depressive disorder. The change in mean depressive symptom scores from baseline to end point was significantly greater for the topiramate compared with the placebo group, though the total decrease in symptom scores was small for both groups (−3.9 points for topiramate, −1.1 for placebo). The authors also reported a decrease in expressed anger, improved attention, and increased health-related quality of life in the topiramate compared with the placebo group.

Several studies support the effectiveness of topiramate as a treatment for obesity and binge eating disorder (39). Accordingly, open-label studies and case reports have focused on the use of topiramate in depressed patients with comorbid obesity. Carpenter et al. (40) reviewed the charts of 16 women diagnosed with a major depressive episode (12 were unipolar) and mild-to-moderate obesity who received adjunctive topiramate. Although the response in unipolar patients was not analyzed separately, 4 of 11 (36%) patients were judged responders after treatment in the acute phase (4–8 weeks) and 7 of 16 (44%) responded at the end of extended treatment (mean duration 17.7 ± 13.4 weeks), according to the criterion of a CGI-I score at end point of much or very much improved. Despite a significant decrease in the Inventory of Depressive Symptoms-Self Rated Version score, only 2 of the 11 patients (18%) who completed this assessment demonstrated a decrease of 50% or more after acute-phase topiramate treatment, prompting the authors to qualify the antidepressant effect as "modest." Mean body weight decreased significantly with topiramate treatment in this trial (6.1 ± 8.2%), but interestingly, weight loss was not correlated with change in depressive symptoms. In addition to this larger retrospective study in depressed patients with obesity, there are two published case reports of successful topiramate augmentation in patients diagnosed with treatment-resistant depression and both comorbid binge eating disorder (41) and obesity (42).

Gabapentin
Gabapentin, a GABA-modulating drug that is approved for use in epilepsy and postherpetic neuralgia, was once thought to have significant potential as a mood-stabilizing agent. However, the results of controlled clinical trials suggest that it is not an effective monotherapy for bipolar disorder, although it may still have a role as an adjunct in treatment-resistant patients (43). There are no published placebo-controlled trials of gabapentin in either bipolar or unipolar depressed patients. However, a small number of open-label studies suggest that gabapentin may have antidepressant effects in bipolar patients (44,45). There are currently only two published studies, both retrospective chart reviews that addressed the response of unipolar depressed patients to adjunctive gabapentin therapy. In the first study, 2 of 10 patients were considered responders on the basis of a CGI-I score, reflecting moderate-to-marked improvement (46). The mean maximum dose of gabapentin in this review was 1699 ± 1237 mg/day. In the second study (47), 24 of the total 27 patients studied had a unipolar depressive disorder (20 with major depression). Although the response of the unipolar patients was not analyzed separately, there was a statistically significant improvement in CGI scores at study end point, and 10 (37%) patients met CGI-I response criteria after gabapentin augmentation. The mean final gabapentin dose was 904 ± 445 mg/day.

Oxcarbazepine
Oxcarbazepine is structurally similar to carbamazepine and appears to share its property of inhibiting voltage-gated sodium channels and subsequently reducing glutamate release. Unlike carbamazepine, it is not approved for use in bipolar disorder, although a number of smaller studies suggest that it is useful in this patient population, including patients who are in the depressed phase of the illness. To date, only two retrospective chart reviews have assessed the effectiveness of oxcarbazepine in unipolar depression by including a small number of such patients (48,49). Both studies reported significant improvement in patients who were depressed at the time of treatment but did not separately report the response of unipolar depressed patients. No other studies of oxcarbazepine in unipolar depression are available at this time.

Tiagabine
Tiagabine is a GABA reuptake inhibitor that is approved for adjunctive therapy in the treatment of partial seizures. A few studies have evaluated tiagabine in patients with bipolar disorder with mixed results (50,51), although no studies specifically

address its effectiveness in bipolar depression. Only one study of tiagabine has been conducted in unipolar depression, an eight-week, open-label prospective trial of tiagabine monotherapy in patients with depression and signficant anxiety symptoms (52). In this trial, there was a statistically significant change in HAM-D and Hamilton Anxiety Rating Scale scores (−14.9 points and −10.2 points, respectively). Seven out of 15 patients met the criteria for antidepressant response (CGI-I rating of much improved and ≥50% improvement in HAM-D score) at the study end point, while four met criteria for full remission of symptoms (score of ≤7 on the HAM-D).

ANTIEPILEPTICS AND SUICIDALITY

A higher rate of depression and suicidality has been reported in patients with epilepsy (53). This phenomenon has been attributed to various factors, including the pathophysiology of epilepsy (54), psychosocial factors related to this illness, and the effects of AEDs (55). Kalinin (56), in his review of AEDs and suicidality, concluded that some AEDs, particularly phenobarbital, appear to be associated with increased suicidality in patients with epilepsy, while others, such as valproate and carbamazepine, may be protective for some patients. The results regarding suicidal thoughts and behaviors for other AEDs are either mixed or inconclusive. Studies conducted in mood disorder patients confirm that certain AEDs, such as valproate and carbamazepine, may decrease the risk of suicidality (57). Some studies suggest that lithium offers greater protection against suicidality than AEDs (58,59), although not all studies have reported a greater benefit with lithium in this regard (57). There are currently no studies that specifically have addressed the effect of AEDs on suicidal behavior in unipolar depressed patients.

Importantly, a recent FDA analysis of 199 placebo-controlled trials of 11 AEDs found that patients receiving AEDs had approximately twice the risk of suicidal behavior or ideation (0.43%) compared with patients receiving placebo (0.22%) (60). The AEDs assessed were carbamazepine, felbamate, gabapentin, lamotrigine, levetiracetam, oxcarbazepine, pregabalin, tiagabine, topiramate, valproate, and zonisamide. The studies examined the effectiveness of these drugs in epilepsy, psychiatric disorders (e.g., bipolar disorder, depression, and anxiety), and other conditions (e.g., migraine and neuropathic pain syndromes). The increased risk of suicidal behavior and suicidal ideation was observed as early as one week after starting the AED and continued through 24 weeks. The results were generally consistent among the 11 drugs. Patients who were treated for epilepsy, psychiatric disorders, and other conditions were all at increased risk for suicidality when compared with placebo, and there did not appear to be a specific demographic subgroup of patients to which the increased risk could be attributed. However, the relative risk for suicidality was higher in patients with epilepsy (3.6) compared with patients with psychiatric (1.6) or other disorders (2.3) (60).

REFERENCES

1. Post RM, Ketter TA, Uhde T, et al. Thirty years of clinical experience with carbamazepine in the treatment of bipolar illness, principles and practice. CNS Drugs 2007; 21 (1):47–71.
2. Shelton RC. Mood-stabilizing drugs in depression. J Clin Psychiatry 1999; 60(suppl 5): 37–40.
3. Post RM, Uhde TW, Roy-Byrne PP, et al. Antidepressant effects of carbamazepine. Am J Psychiatry 1986; 143(1):29–34.

4. Prasad AJ. Efficacy of carbamazepine as an antidepressant in chronic resistant depressives. J Indian Med Assoc 1985; 83(7):235–237.
5. Rybakowski JK, Suwalska A, Chlopocka-Wozniak M. Potentiation of antidepressants with lithium or carbamazepine in treatment-resistant depression. Neuropsychobiology 1999; 40(3):134–139.
6. Ciusani E, Zullino DF, Eap CB, et al. Combination therapy with venlafaxine and carbamazepine in depressive patients not responding to venlafaxine, pharmacokinetic and clinical aspects. J Psychopharmacol 2004; 18(4):559–566.
7. Steinacher L, Vandel P, Zullino DF, et al. Carbamazepine augmentation in depressive patients non-responding to citalopram, a pharmacokinetic and clinical pilot study. Eur Neuropsychopharmacol 2002; 12(3):255–260.
8. Cullen M, Mitchell P, Brodaty H, et al. Carbamazepine for treatment-resistant melancholia. J Clin Psychiatry 1991; 52(11):472–476.
9. De la Fuente JM, Mendlewicz J. Carbamazepine addition in tricyclic antidepressant-resistant unipolar depression. Biol Psychiatry 1992; 32(4):369–374.
10. Otani K, Yasui N, Kaneko S, et al. Carbamazepine augmentation therapy in three patients with trazodone-resistant unipolar depression. Int Clin Psychopharmacol 1996; 11(1):55–57.
11. Kramlinger KG, Post RM. The addition of lithium to carbamazepine. Antidepressant efficacy in treatment-resistant depression. Arch Gen Psychiatry 1989; 46(9):794–800.
12. Schaffer CB, Mungas D, Rockwell E. Successful treatment of psychotic depression with carbamazepine. J Clin Psychopharmacol 1985; 5(4):233–235.
13. Arana GW, Santos AB, Knax EP, et al. Refractory rapid cycling unipolar depression responds to lithium and carbamazepine treatment. J Clin Psychiatry 1989; 50(9):356–357.
14. Stuppaeck C, Barnas C, Miller C, et al. Carbamazepine in the prophylaxis of mood disorders. J Clin Psychopharmacol 1990; 10(1):39–42.
15. Stuppaeck CH, Barnas C, Schwitzer J, et al. Carbamazepine in the prophylaxis of major depression, a 5-year follow-up. J Clin Psychiatry 1994; 55(4):146–150.
16. Edwards KR, Sackellares JC, Vuong A, et al. Lamotrigine monotherapy improves depressive symptoms in epilepsy, a double-blind comparison with valproate. Epilepsy Behav 2001; 2(1):28–36.
17. Calabrese JR, Bowden CL, Sachs GS, et al. A double-blind placebo-controlled study of lamotrigine monotherapy in outpatients with bipolar I depression. Lamictal 602 Study Group. J Clin Psychiatry 1999; 60(2):79–88.
18. Normann C, Hummel B, Scharer LO, et al. Lamotrigine as adjunct to paroxetine in acute depression, a placebo-controlled, double-blind study. J Clin Psychiatry 2002; 63(4):337–344.
19. Barbosa L, Berk M, Vorster M. A double-blind, randomized, placebo-controlled trial of augmentation with lamotrigine or placebo in patients concomitantly treated with fluoxetine for resistant major depressive episodes. J Clin Psychiatry 2003; 64(4):403–407.
20. Schindler F, Anghelescu IG. Lithium versus lamotrigine augmentation in treatment resistant unipolar depression, a randomized, open-label study. Int Clin Psychopharmacol 2007; 22(3):179–182.
21. Gabriel A. Lamotrigine adjunctive treatment in resistant unipolar depression, an open, descriptive study. Depress Anxiety 2006; 23(8):485–488.
22. Barbee JG, Jamhour NJ. Lamotrigine as an augmentation agent in treatment-resistant depression. J Clin Psychiatry 2002; 63(8):737–741.
23. Rocha FL, Hara C. Lamotrigine augmentation in unipolar depression. Int Clin Psychopharmacol 2003; 18(2):97–99.
24. Gutierrez RL, McKercher RM, Galea J, et al. Lamotrigine augmentation strategy for patients with treatment-resistant depression. CNS Spectr 2005; 10(10):800–805.
25. Maltese TM. Adjunctive lamotrigine treatment for major depression. Am J Psychiatry 1999; 156(11):1833.
26. Davis LL, Bartolucci A, Petty F. Divalproex in the treatment of bipolar depression, a placebo-controlled study. J Affect Disord 2005; 85(3):259–266.
27. Gyulai L, Bowden CL, McElroy SL, et al. Maintenance efficacy of divalproex in the prevention of bipolar depression. Neuropsychopharmacology 2003; 28(7):1374–1382.

28. Davis LL, Kabel D, Patel D, et al. Valproate as an antidepressant in major depressive disorder. Psychopharmacol Bull 1996; 32(4):647–652.
29. Debattista C, Solomon A, Arnow B, et al. The efficacy of divalproex sodium in the treatment of agitation associated with major depression. J Clin Psychopharmacol 2005; 25(5):476–479.
30. Hayes SG. Long-term use of valproate in primary psychiatric disorders. J Clin Psychiatry 1989; 50(suppl):35–39.
31. Mitchell P, Cullen MJ. Valproate for rapid-cycling unipolar affective disorder. J Nerv Ment Dis 1991; 179(8):503–504.
32. Pies R, Adler DA, Ehrenberg BL. Sleep disorders and depression with atypical features, response to valproate. J Clin Psychopharmacol 1989; 9(5):352–357.
33. Sharma V. Lithium augmentation of valproic acid in treatment resistant depression. Lithium 1994; 5:99–103.
34. Nemets B, Bersudsky Y, Belmaker RH. Controlled double-blind trial of phenytoin vs. fluoxetine in major depressive disorder. J Clin Psychiatry 2005; 66(5):586–590.
35. Shapira B, Nemets B, Trachtenberg A, et al. Phenytoin as an augmentation for SSRI failures, a small controlled study. J Affect Disord 2006; 96(1–2):123–126.
36. Kushner SF, Khan A, Lane R, et al. Topiramate monotherapy in the management of acute mania: results of four double-blind placebo-controlled trials. Bipolar Disord 2006; 8(1):15–27.
37. McIntyre RS, Mancini DA, McCann S, et al. Topiramate versus bupropion SR when added to mood stabilizer therapy for the depressive phase of bipolar disorder, a preliminary single-blind study. Bipolar Disord 2002; 4(3):207–213.
38. Nickel C, Lahmann C, Tritt K, et al. Topiramate in treatment of depressive and anger symptoms in female depressive patients, a randomized, double-blind, placebo-controlled study. J Affect Disord 2005; 87(2–3):243–252.
39. McElroy SL, Hudson JI, Capece JA, et al. Topiramate for the treatment of binge eating disorder associated with obesity, a placebo-controlled study. Biol Psychiatry 2007; 61 (9):1039–1048.
40. Carpenter LL, Leon Z, Yasmin S, et al. Do obese depressed patients respond to topiramate? A retrospective chart review. J Affect Disord 2002; 69(1–3):51–255.
41. Schmidt do Prado-Lima PA, Bacaltchuck J. Topiramate in treatment-resistant depression and binge-eating disorder. Bipolar Disord 2002; 4(4):271–273.
42. Dursun SM, Devarajan S. Accelerated weight loss after treating refractory depression with fluoxetine plus topiramate, possible mechanisms of action? Can J Psychiatry 2001; 46(3):287–288.
43. Carta MG, Hardoy MC, Hardoy MJ, et al. The clinical use of gabapentin in bipolar spectrum disorders. J Affect Disord 2003; 75(1):83–91.
44. Wang PW, Santosa C, Schumacher M, et al. Gabapentin augmentation therapy in bipolar depression. Bipolar Disord 2002; 4(5):296–301.
45. Young LT, Robb JC, Patelis-Siotis I, et al. Acute treatment of bipolar depression with gabapentin. Biol Psychiatry 1997; 42(9):851–853.
46. Ghaemi SN, Katzow JJ, Desai SP, et al. Gabapentin treatment of mood disorders, a preliminary study. J Clin Psychiatry 1998; 59(8):426–429.
47. Yasmin S, Carpenter LL, Leon Z, et al. Adjunctive gabapentin in treatment-resistant depression, a retrospective chart review. J Affect Disord 2001; 63(1–3):243–247.
48. Centorrino F, Albert MJ, Berry JM, et al. Oxcarbazepine, clinical experience with hospitalized psychiatric patients. Bipolar Disord 2003; 5(5):370–374.
49. Raja M, Azzoni A. Oxcarbazepine vs. valproate in the treatment of mood and schizoaffective disorders. Int J Neuropsychopharmacol 2003; 6(4):409–414.
50. Suppes T, Chisholm KA, Dhavale D, et al. Tiagabine in treatment refractory bipolar disorder, a clinical case series. Bipolar Disord 2002; 4(5):283–289.
51. Schaffer LC, Schaffer CB, Howe J. An open case series on the utility of tiagabine as an augmentation in refractory bipolar outpatients. J Affect Disord 2002; 71(1–3): 259–263.
52. Carpenter LL, Schecter JM, Tyrka AR, et al. Open-label tiagabine monotherapy for major depressive disorder with anxiety. J Clin Psychiatry 2006; 67(1):66–71.

53. Hawton K, Fagg J, Marsack P. Association between epilepsy and attempted suicide. J Neurol Neurosurg Psychiatry 1980; 43(2):168–170.
54. Harden CL. The co-morbidity of depression and epilepsy, epidemiology, etiology, and treatment. Neurology 2002; 59(6 suppl 4):S48–S55.
55. Suicide and epilepsy (no author listed). Br Med J 1980; 281(6239):530.
56. Kalinin VV. Suicidality and antiepileptic drugs, is there a link? Drug Saf 2007; 30(2): 123–142.
57. Yerevanian BI, Koek RJ, Mintz J. Bipolar pharmacotherapy and suicidal behavior. Part I, Lithium, divalproex and carbamazepine. J Affect Disord 2007; 103(1–3):5–11.
58. Goodwin FK, Fireman B, Simon GE, et al. Suicide risk in bipolar disorder during treatment with lithium and divalproex. JAMA 2003; 290(11):1467–1473.
59. Collins JC, McFarland BH. Divalproex, lithium and suicide among Medicaid patients with bipolar disorder. J Affect Disord. 2007 (in press) (epub ahead of print).
60. U.S. Food and Drug Administration (FDA). Information for healthcare professionals suicidality and antiepileptic drugs. Available at: http://www.fda.gov/cder/drug/InfoSheets/HCP/antiepilepticsHCP.htm. Accessed January 5, 2008.

6 Antiepileptics in the Treatment of Schizophrenia

Leslie Citrome

New York University School of Medicine, New York, New York, and Clinical Research and Evaluation Facility, Nathan S. Kline Institute for Psychiatric Research, Orangeburg, New York, U.S.A.

INTRODUCTION

In the absence of knowledge about the precise pathophysiology of schizophrenia, pharmacological treatments have been limited to symptoms. Although the reduction of positive symptoms such as hallucinations or delusions are important, particularly when they intrude on self-care or interactions with other people, there is growing appreciation of the importance of treating other symptom domains such as negative symptomatology, cognitive function, and persistent aggressive behavior. In this context, clinicians routinely turn to augmentation strategies when faced with the observation that antipsychotic monotherapy can be inadequate for many patients with schizophrenia. Prime medication candidates for use in combination with antipsychotics are those agents with a different mechanism of action so that there is the possibility of pharmacodynamic synergy, perhaps leading to a faster, better, or more sustainable therapeutic response. Antiepileptic drugs (AEDs) and lithium, medications used for bipolar disorder, are also commonly used in combination with antipsychotics to treat schizophrenia.

The evidence base supporting the use of adjunctive AEDs for patients with schizophrenia is mixed. Initial positive case reports and open-label studies have not always been followed by successful randomized clinical trials (Table 1). This chapter will review the utilization patterns of AEDs in patients with schizophrenia, the evidence base supporting this use, and end with pragmatic advice for the clinician on when and how to consider augmentation with a specific AED for an individual patient.

EXTENT OF USE

The use of adjunctive AEDs in patients with schizophrenia is extensive, especially among inpatients in intermediate and long-term care settings. Within the inpatient facilities operated by the New York State Office of Mental Health (NYSOMH), the percentage of inpatients with schizophrenia receiving adjunctive AEDs or lithium has leveled off at approximately 50% during the last five years (Fig. 1, lithium not shown). Although valproate is the most commonly used adjunctive anticonvulsant, others appear to be increasing in their popularity, albeit more slowly (1–3). Some AEDs are being used less often over time, such as adjunctive gabapentin or adjunctive carbamazepine.

The mean dose of AEDs used is substantial. Data available from NYSOMH inpatient facilities in 2006 reveals that among 7154 patients receiving antipsychotics (76.5% of whom had a diagnosis of schizophrenia or schizoaffective disorder), the average daily dose of valproate was 1677 mg ($N = 2813$), gabapentin 1552 mg ($N = 363$), oxcarbazepine 1183 mg ($N = 306$), carbamazepine 781 mg ($N = 178$), topiramate 237 mg ($N = 357$), and lamotrigine 225 mg ($N = 528$) [unpublished data updated from (4)]. Moreover, combinations of mood stabilizers are also

TABLE 1 Evidence for Adjunctive Use of Antiepileptics for the Treatment of Schizophrenia

Agent	Year introduced in United States	Case reports and open studies	Controlled clinical trials[a] (number of reports)	Utility (benefit?)
Carbamazepine	1974	Yes	Yes (7)	Maybe
Valproate	1978	Yes	Yes (8)	Maybe
Gabapentin	1993	Yes (±)	None	Probably not
Lamotrigine	1994	Yes (±)	Yes (6)	Maybe
Topiramate	1997	Yes (±)	Yes (3)	Probably not
Oxcarbazepine	2000	Yes (±)	None	Too early to tell

Note: ±, both positive and negative results.
[a]English-language reports.

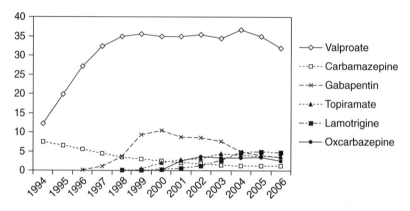

FIGURE 1 Percent inpatients with schizophrenia receiving adjunctive antiepileptics within the New York State Office of Mental Health from 1994 (*N* = 8405) to 2006 (*N* = 3132). *Source*: From unpublished data updated from Ref. 4.

used. Approximately half of all patients receiving a mood stabilizer received more than one, with the exception of patients receiving valproate where the rate of coprescribing of another AED or lithium was about 25% (4).

Somewhat lower utilization rates for adjunctive mood stabilizers are observed in other parts of the world. The overall trend over time, however, has been for increased use. In the treatment of acute episodes of schizophrenia in a German university hospital, adjunctive mood stabilizer use increased from 15% in 1998 to 26% in 2001 and 28% in 2004 (5). For all inpatients with schizophrenia at the same hospital, adjunctive use of AEDs specifically increased from approximately 3% in 1998 to 12% in 2003, while that for adjunctive lithium decreased from 13% to 4% (6). In the 10 hospitals participating in a drug surveillance program in Germany and Switzerland, among 745 patients with schizophrenia in 1995, 9.5% received AEDs, increasing to 15% of 1015 patients in 2001 (7).

Adjunctive AED use in outpatient populations has also been described. In a cross-sectional study of 456 outpatients with schizophrenia, in Rochester, New York (8), 39% of white patients and 25% of black patients received adjunctive lithium or AEDs in 2003 or 2004. The percentage is lower in China, where in a randomly selected sample of 250 stable outpatients with schizophrenia, 10% received a mood stabilizer (actual medications in this category were not defined) (9).

In an analysis of database data for both inpatient and outpatient encounters contained in the National Psychosis Registry of the U.S. Department of Veterans Affairs (10), among 77,243 patients with a diagnosis of schizophrenia or schizoaffective disorder in 1999 and 2000, concurrent treatment with a mood stabilizer was observed among 37% ($N = 2148$) of patients given prescriptions for antipsychotic polypharmacy and 27% ($N = 10,797$) of patients given prescriptions for antipsychotic monotherapy.

Thus, the use of adjunctive AEDs in both inpatients and outpatients with schizophrenia is extensive. There are international variations in practice, but overall use has increased with time.

EVIDENCE SUPPORTING AUGMENTATION WITH ANTIEPILEPTIC DRUGS

Table 1 outlines the variability in quality and quantity of the evidence supporting the use of adjunctive AEDs in the treatment of schizophrenia. Although uncontrolled case reports or case series provide relatively weak supporting evidence, they do provide a rationale for follow-up double-blind and/or randomized clinical trials. However, not all AEDs in use as adjunctive agents in the treatment of schizophrenia have been tested in controlled trials, and many of the published studies suffer from a variety of methodological flaws such as an inadequate number of subjects (insufficient statistical power to detect differences), lack of control of confounds such as affective symptomatology (seen when studies include patients with schizoaffective disorder), inadequate duration (usually too short), or inappropriate target populations (acute exacerbations of schizophrenia rather than treatment-refractory schizophrenia with persistent residual symptoms).

Carbamazepine

Carbamazepine was introduced in the United States in 1974 for the treatment of epilepsy. Initial reports from Finland on the possible use of carbamazepine in the treatment of violent patients with schizophrenia with and without EEG abnormalities (11) led to further investigations with carbamazepine in patients with schizophrenia with normal EEGs (12). The available controlled studies of adjunctive carbamazepine in the treatment of schizophrenia (double-blind and/or randomized) for which English-language reports are available are included in Table 2 (13–19). In the largest of these studies ($N = 162$) (15), a double-blind clinical trial of carbamazepine in patients with Diagnostic and Statistical Manual of Mental Disorders III (DSM-III) schizophrenia or schizoaffective disorder, there was a failure to detect significant improvement on the total Brief Psychiatric Rating Scale (BPRS) with adjunctive carbamazepine compared with adjunctive placebo. However, differences did emerge among the BPRS items of suspiciousness, uncooperativeness, and excitement. The other studies listed in Table 2 were substantially smaller in terms of sample size, and with the exception of an early crossover design study (13), they failed to detect any meaningful advantage for adjunctive carbamazepine use. Moreover, a recent comparison with a second-generation antipsychotic, olanzapine, demonstrated superiority of that agent over a combination of perazine and carbamazepine, particularly with positive symptoms (19). A comprehensive Cochrane Library Review meta-analysis (20) concluded on the basis of eight studies ($N = 182$), which compared adjunctive carbamazepine

TABLE 2 Controlled Studies of Adjunctive Carbamazepine in Schizophrenia

Author and year (reference)	N	Length (days)	Target daily dose of CBZ (mg)[a]	Design	Diagnosis	Outcome
Neppe 1983 (13)	11	42	600	AP + CBZ vs. AP + placebo (crossover)	Inpatients, 8 with schizophrenia (and EEG abnormalities)	Improvement in "overall clinical rating" with CBZ
Dose 1987 (14)	22	28	600–1200	HAL + CBZ vs. HAL + placebo	Inpatients with schizophrenia or schizoaffective disorder	No difference on BPRS
Okuma 1989 (15)	162	28	200–1200	AP + CBZ vs. AP + placebo (although double-blind, the study was not randomized)	Inpatients or outpatients with schizophrenia or schizoaffective disorder	No difference on BPRS; Possible improvement on suspiciousness, uncooperative-ness and excitement with CBZ
Nachshoni 1994 (16)	28	49	600	AP + CBZ vs. AP + placebo	Inpatients with "residual schizophrenia with negative symptoms"	No difference on BPRS or SANS
Simhandl 1996 (17)	42	42	15–42 μmol/L	AP + CBZ vs. AP + Li vs. AP + placebo	Schizophrenia (treatment-nonresponsive)	No difference on BPRS; within groups CBZ and Li improved on CGI from baseline
Hesslinger 1998 (18)	27	28	Mean 567	HAL vs. HAL + CBZ vs. HAL + VAL (although randomized, the study was not double-blind)	Inpatients with schizophrenia or schizoaffective disorder	CBZ was associated with significantly lower HAL plasma levels and with a worse clinical outcome compared with antipsychotic monotherapy
Ohlmeier 2007 (19)	33	21	Mean 404	Perazine + CBZ vs. olanzapine (although randomized, the study was not double-blind)	Inpatients with schizophrenia	Olanzapine monotherapy was superior to perazine plus CBZ on positive symptoms on PANSS and BPRS

[a]If unavailable mean daily dose or target plasma level is provided.
Abbreviations: HAL, Haloperidol; CBZ, Carbamazepine; Li, Lithium; VAL, Valproate; AP, Antipsychotic; BPRS, Brief Psychiatric Rating Scale; SANS, Scale for the Assessment of Negative Symptoms; CGI, Clinical Global Impression; PANSS, Positive and Negative Syndrome Scale.

with adjunctive placebo, that adding carbamazepine to antipsychotic treatment was as acceptable as adding placebo with no difference between the numbers leaving the study early from each group and that carbamazepine augmentation was superior compared with antipsychotics alone in terms of overall global improvement. However, there were no differences in the outcome of 50% reduction in BPRS scores. The authors concluded that carbamazepine cannot be recommended for routine clinical use for treatment or augmentation of antipsychotic treatment of schizophrenia, but that large, simple, well-designed, and reported trials are justified, especially if focusing on those populations for which data is especially scant: patients with schizophrenia with violent episodes and/or EEG abnormalities. Although the frequency of use of carbamazepine in psychiatric practice appears to have decreased in patients with bipolar disorder, schizophrenia, or schizoaffective disorder during the 1990s in the United States (2,21), this trend may reverse itself now that an extended-release formulation of carbamazepine received approval in December 2004 by the U.S. Food and Drug Administration (FDA) for the indication of bipolar mania (22). An important obstacle to the use of carbamazepine is that it induces its own metabolism (and that of other agents being administered), and hence dose adjustments are often needed for both carbamazepine and the antipsychotic being prescribed. For example, a recent study of the second-generation antipsychotic, aripiprazole, given with carbamazepine demonstrated substantially reduced plasma levels of the antipsychotic in the presence of carbamazepine cotherapy (23).

Valproate

Valproate is the active moiety of both valproic acid and divalproex sodium and is currently the most commonly used adjunctive AED in the treatment of schizophrenia. Valproic acid was introduced as a treatment for epilepsy in France in 1967 and was approved in the United States by the FDA in 1978 for the monotherapy and adjunctive therapy of complex partial seizures and simple or complex absence seizures. For patients with mental disorders, the pivotal year was 1995, when divalproex sodium was approved by the FDA for the indication of manic episodes associated with bipolar disorder. The first signals indicating the use of adjunctive valproate in the treatment of schizophrenia came from case reports and open-label studies. Early reports from 1976 (24) and 1979 (25) demonstrated reduced psychopathology in general, as measured by the BPRS, and improvement on emotional withdrawal, respectively. An open-label study of valproate and haloperidol in 30 patients with schizophrenia suggested that augmentation with valproate can result in improvements in suspiciousness, hallucinations, unusual thought content, and emotional withdrawal, as well as in fewer inpatient days (26). A report of the combination of valproate with the second-generation antipsychotic, risperidone, demonstrated clinical improvement in an otherwise treatment-resistant patient with schizophrenia (27).

The available controlled studies of adjunctive valproate in the treatment of schizophrenia (double-blind and/or randomized) for which English-language reports are available are included in Table 3 (18,28–34). Initial controlled studies of adjunctive valproate in patients with schizophrenia have been limited in terms of the number of subjects. In the first, Ko and colleagues (28) found no additional benefit with adjunctive valproate in a 28-day crossover study with six neuroleptic-resistant patients with chronic schizophrenia (not experiencing an exacerbation). In

TABLE 3 Controlled Studies of Adjunctive Valproate in Schizophrenia

Author and year (reference)	N	Length (days)	Target daily dose of VAL (mg)[a]	Design	Diagnosis	Outcome
Ko 1985 (28)	6	28	1600–2400	AP + VAL vs. AP + placebo (crossover)	Inpatients with neuroleptic-resistant chronic schizophrenia (not exacerbation)	No valproate effect noted
Fisk 1987 (29)	62	42	1200 or 1500	AP + VAL vs. AP + placebo	Inpatients with chronic psychosis and tardive dyskinesia	No differences in mental state and behavior as measured by the "Krawiecka scale" (85)[b]
Dose 1998 (30)	42	28	900–1200	HAL + VAL vs. HAL + placebo	Inpatients with acute, nonmanic schizophrenic or schizoaffective psychosis	No difference on BPRS; Possible effect on hostile belligerence
Hesslinger 1998 (18)	27	28	Mean 757	HAL vs. HAL + CBZ vs. HAL + VAL (although randomized, the study was not double-blind)	Inpatients with schizophrenia or schizoaffective	VAL had no significant effect on either plasma levels of HAL or on psychopathology
Wassef 2000 (31)	12	21	75–100 µg/mL	HAL + VAL vs. HAL + placebo	Inpatients with acute exacerbation of chronic schizophrenia	Significant Improvement in CGI and SANS but not BPRS
Casey 2003 (32)	249	28	Mean ~2300	RIS + VAL vs. OLZ + VAL vs. RIS + placebo vs. OLZ + placebo	Inpatients with acute schizophrenia	Improvement on PANSS
Abbott 2006 (33)	402	84	Mean ~2900	RIS + VAL vs. OLZ + VAL vs. RIS + placebo vs. OLZ + placebo	Inpatients with acute schizophrenia	No advantage for combination treatment with adjunctive VAL
Citrome 2007 (34)	33	56	50–100 µg/mL	RIS vs. RIS + VAL (although randomized, the study was not double-blind)	Inpatients with schizophrenia and hostile behavior	Although significantly fewer patients randomized to monotherapy completed the study, no significant differences between monotherapy and combination treatment were observed in change of the rating instruments used, including the PANSS

[a]If unavailable mean daily dose or target plasma level is provided.

Abbreviations: AP, antipsychotic; HAL, haloperidol; VAL, valproate; RIS, risperidone; OLZ, olanzapine; BPRS, Brief Psychiatric Rating Scale; SANS, Scale for the Assessment of Negative Symptoms; CGI, Clinical Global Impression; PANSS, Positive and Negative Syndrome Scale.

another study, this time among 42 patients with acute, nonmanic schizophrenic or schizoaffective psychosis comparing haloperidol and placebo versus haloperidol and valproate over 28 days, no difference on the BPRS was observed, but a possible effect on "hostile belligerence" was noted (30). In another study of acute patients with schizophrenia ($N = 12$) comparing adjunctive valproate with placebo in patients receiving haloperidol, a significant improvement was observed in the Clinical Global Impression (CGI) scale as well as on the Schedule for Assessment of Negative Symptoms (SANS) but not on the BPRS (31). Two other controlled studies found no meaningful advantage for adjunctive valproate (29,30). These initial randomized studies enrolled relatively small number of subjects, hence differences between the groups might have been difficult to detect because of lack of sufficient statistical power. They also included different types of patients—neuroleptic-resistant patients in one (28), chronic patients with tardive dyskinesia in another (29), and acute patients in the other three reports (18,30,31).

The published study with the largest number of subjects ($N = 249$) is that of a multicenter, randomized, double-blind, 28-day clinical trial of adjunctive divalproex in hospitalized patients with an acute exacerbation of schizophrenia conducted by the manufacturer of divalproex (32). Schizoaffective and treatment-refractory patients were specifically excluded, thus the study did answer the question whether or not adjunctive valproate has an effect on acute psychotic symptoms rather than on mood. However, this study did not answer the question whether or not adjunctive valproate would be useful in treatment-refractory patients with persistent symptoms of schizophrenia. The study design consisted of receiving one of four treatments for four weeks: olanzapine and divalproex, olanzapine and placebo, risperidone and divalproex, or risperidone and placebo. Doses of risperidone 6 mg/day or olanzapine 15 mg/day were reached by day 6. Divalproex was started at 15 mg/kg and titrated to a maximum of 30 mg/kg by day 14. The mean dose of divalproex achieved was approximately 2300 mg/day with a mean plasma level of approximately 100 µg/mL. The Positive and Negative Syndrome Scale (PANSS) was the primary outcome measure. Ratings were done at baseline, days 3, 5, 7, 10, 14, 21, and 28. PANSS total score significantly improved in the combination therapy group compared with the monotherapy group at specific time points (days 3, 5, 7, 10, 14, and 21) and throughout the study period [repeated measures analysis of variance (ANOVA), $P = 0.020$]. Significant treatment differences occurred as early as day 3. The major effect was on the positive symptoms of schizophrenia. No new safety concerns were observed; the combination therapy was as well tolerated as monotherapy. A post hoc analysis also revealed that patients receiving adjunctive divalproex had greater reductions in hostility on days 3 and 7 (as measured by the Hostility item in the Positive Subscale of the PANSS) compared with antipsychotic monotherapy and that this effect was independent of the effect on the positive symptoms of schizophrenia or sedation (35).

The above 28-day study provided the strongest evidence so far for a real effect of adjunctive AED treatment for schizophrenia and provided the impetus for the manufacturer to conduct a second study, this time with the extended-release preparation of divalproex with 402 patients with acute schizophrenia (33). The principal results of this 84-day multicenter, double-blind, randomized clinical trial have been publicly disclosed on the Web site clinicalstudyresults.org (www .clinicalstudyresults.org) and revealed that the study failed to demonstrate any benefit with combination treatment versus monotherapy with risperidone or olanzapine. This failure to replicate the earlier study (32) is consistent with the results of another recently reported clinical trial of adjunctive valproate in the treatment of patients with schizophrenia and hostility (34). This was an eight-week, open-label, rater-blinded, randomized, parallel-group clinical trial in hospitalized adults where patients were randomly assigned to receive risperidone alone ($N = 16$) or risperidone plus valproate ($N = 17$). Although significantly fewer patients randomized to monotherapy completed the study, no significant differences between monotherapy or combination treatment were observed in change of any of the rating instruments used, including the PANSS.

Evidence supporting the use of adjunctive valproate in the treatment of schizophrenia is thus limited. There remains active interest in this combination treatment, and small uncontrolled studies continue to be published showing advantages for combination treatment, such as the use of this strategy with older adults in a prospective, 12-week open-label study ($N = 20$) (36), a retrospective six-month study examining adjunctive divalproex ($N = 15$) or lithium ($N = 9$) added to clozapine and compared with clozapine monotherapy in treatment-resistant schizophrenia patients ($N = 25$) (37), and a four-week study of the effect of valproic acid on plasma levels of risperidone and its active metabolite ($N = 12$) (38). Pharmacoepidemiological evidence published includes the results of a large ($N = 10,262$) retrospective analysis of persistence of treatment with valproate augmentation versus switching antipsychotic medication (39). Diagnostic categories were not available. Valproate led to longer persistence of treatment than switching antipsychotics, but the average doses of valproate were small (<425 mg/day), as were the doses of the antipsychotics (risperidone < 1.7 mg/day, quetiapine < 120 mg/day, and olanzapine < 7.5 mg/day).

Although the use of an extended-release preparation may be particularly helpful when encouraging medication adherence for patients who are otherwise prescribed complicated medication regimens, different formulations of valproate may have different effects, as suggested by a prospective "quasi-experimental" clinical trial involving over 9000 psychiatric admissions over six years (40). Inpatients who initially received divalproex sodium had a 32.7% longer hospital stay and 3.8% higher readmission rate than did patients who initially received valproic acid. After other variables were controlled, the hospital stay of patients who continued the initial medication was 15.2% longer (2 days) for divalproex than valproic acid. Medication intolerance occurred in approximately 6.4% more patients taking valproic acid than divalproex. However, switching from valproic acid to divalproex did not significantly prolong length of stay over that for continuous divalproex or increase the rehospitalization rate. The authors concluded that lower peak valproate concentrations with divalproex sodium may have enhanced tolerability but may also explain the lower effectiveness, and that extended-release divalproex could lower effectiveness further and require higher doses. They suggested that inpatients should start with generic valproic acid and then change to delayed-release divalproex only if intolerance occurs. Switching to the extended-release preparation from the regular (delayed-release) preparation of divalproex does involve consideration of bioavailability differences; the average bioavailability of the extended-release preparation is 81% to 89% relative to delayed-release tablets given twice daily (41,42). The consequences of this difference were assessed in 30 patients with schizophrenia who were switched in a four-week open-label treatment trial (43). Patients were converted from divalproex delayed release to extended release on a 1.0:1.0 mg basis (rounded up to the nearest 500-mg increment), if baseline valproate plasma levels were at least 85 μg/mL; otherwise, the conversion rate was 1.0:1.2 mg (rounded up). Patients who converted on a 1:1 mg basis had lower end point valproate trough plasma levels than at baseline but did not experience deterioration in their psychopathology, presumably because they had a higher plasma level of valproate to begin with.

A comprehensive Cochrane Library Review meta-analysis (44) concluded on the basis of five studies ($N = 379$) that compared adjunctive valproate with adjunctive placebo that adding valproate did not demonstrate a significant effect on the participants' global state or general mental state at end point. The reviewers noted that subjects receiving valproate more frequently experienced sedation than those in the placebo group. Given this limited evidence, further large, simple, well-designed, and reported trials were thought necessary.

In reviewing all of the studies described above, larger and focused controlled trials examining the use of adjunctive valproate in specific subpopulations of patients with schizophrenia would be helpful, such as treatment-refractory patients and the more chronically ill.

Lamotrigine

Lamotrigine was commercialized in the United States as an AED in 1994, and the FDA approved it for the indication of maintenance treatment of bipolar I disorder in 2003. A report was published in 1999 of a case series of six patients with treatment-resistant schizophrenia who benefited from lamotrigine being added to their regimen of clozapine (45). In another open trial, patients receiving lamotrigine augmentation of clozapine had a significant decrease in BPRS scores after two weeks of treatment, but there was no significant improvement when lamotrigine was added to risperidone, haloperidol, olanzapine, or fluphenthixol (46). In contrast, others have found benefit in adding lamotrigine to regimens of antipsychotics other than clozapine, notably, zuclopenthixol, risperidone, and haloperidol in patients with treatment-resistant schizophrenia (47). These positive results are tempered by reports of other cases where a benefit of adjunctive lamotrigine with clozapine was not observed (48), a report of worsening of psychotic symptoms in a patient with schizophrenia when lamotrigine was added to quetiapine (49), and a case of remission of positive symptoms of schizophrenia when a regimen of lamotrigine and olanzapine was switched to carbamazepine and olanzapine in a patient with schizophrenia and EEG abnormalities (50). Additional case reports are available regarding the use of lamotrigine to augment clozapine in patients with both schizophrenia and alcohol dependence, where an anticraving effect may be observed (51).

The available controlled studies of adjunctive lamotrigine in the treatment of schizophrenia (double-blind and/or randomized) for which English-language reports are available are included in Table 4 (52–57). The first was conducted in Finland by Tiihonen and colleagues (52), where adjunctive lamotrigine was added to clozapine in patients with treatment-resistant schizophrenia in a small ($N = 34$), double-blind, placebo-controlled crossover trial. Patients who had failed clozapine monotherapy received lamotrigine (200 mg/day) for up to 12 weeks. Adjunctive lamotrigine resulted in the improvement of positive, but not negative, symptoms. Similarly, in a 10-week, double-blind, parallel-group clinical trial ($N = 38$) by Kremer and colleagues (53), administering adjunctive lamotrigine to treatment-resistant inpatients with schizophrenia resulted in improvement in the PANSS positive, general psychopathology, and total symptoms scores in completers ($N = 31$);

TABLE 4 Controlled Studies of Adjunctive Lamotrigine in Schizophrenia

Author and year (reference)	N	Length (days)	Target daily dose of LAM (mg)	Design	Diagnosis	Outcome
Tiihonen 2003 (52)	34	84	200	CLO + LAM vs. CLO + placebo (crossover)	Male inpatients with CLO-resistant chronic schizophrenia (not exacerbation)	Improvement in BPRS, PANSS positive, and PANSS general psychopathology; Most robust effect seen in the most ill patients ($N = 10$) (BPRS $\geq$ 45); No improvement in negative symptoms
Kremer 2004 (53)	38	70	400	AP + LAM vs. AP + placebo	Inpatients with treatment-resistant schizophrenia	Improvement in PANSS positive, general psychopathology, and total symptoms scores in completers; No difference in negative symptoms or total BPRS; No difference with intent-to-treat analyses
Akhondzadeh 2005 (54)	36	56	150	RIS + LAM vs. RIS + placebo	Inpatients with schizophrenia	Superiority over RIS alone in the treatment of negative symptoms, general psychopathology, and PANSS total scores; patients' attention improved on the Stroop color-naming subtest (time and error)
Zoccali 2007 (55)	60	168	200	CLO + LAM vs. CLO + placebo	Outpatients with treatment-resistant schizophrenia	Improvement on negative, positive, and general psychopathological symptomatology
Glaxo-Smith-Kline 2005 (56)	209	84	100–400	AP + LAM vs. AP + placebo	Inpatients or outpatients with schizophrenia and with stable, residual psychotic symptoms	SANS total score and CGI improved more with placebo than LAM
Glaxo-Smith-Kline 2006 (57)	210	84	100–400	AP + LAM vs. AP + placebo	Inpatients or outpatients with schizophrenia and with stable, residual psychotic symptoms	Cognitive composite score improved more with LAM than with placebo

Abbreviations: CLO, clozapine; LAM, lamotrigine; AP, antipsychotic; BPRS, Brief Psychiatric Rating Scale; SANS, Scale for the Assessment of Negative Symptoms; PANSS, Positive and Negative Syndrome Scale; CGI, Clinical Global Impression.

however, no differences were observed in negative symptoms or total BPRS scores, and no differences were found in the intent-to-treat (ITT) analysis. Response to lamotrigine did not differ between patients treated with first-generation compared with second-generation antipsychotics. In a third inpatient study conducted in Iran (54), 36 patients with schizophrenia were randomized to receive risperidone plus lamotrigine or risperidone plus placebo for eight weeks. Advantages for combination treatment were observed for negative symptoms, general psychopathology, and total PANSS but not for positive symptoms. Some additional cognitive effect was noted on a subtest assessing color naming. An outpatient study involving 60 patients with treatment-resistant schizophrenia assessed double-blind over a 24-week period (55) found improvement of positive and negative symptoms as well as improvement in measures of cognitive performance when lamotrigine was added to clozapine compared with placebo added to clozapine among the 51 completers.

The initial signals from the uncontrolled studies by Dursun (45,46) and the randomized clinical trial by Tiihonen (52) spurred the launch of two 12-week large-scale ($N = 209$ and $N = 210$) studies by the manufacturer of lamotrigine in patients with schizophrenia who had not responded adequately to second-generation antipsychotics alone (56–58). Patients were randomized to receive either adjunctive lamotrigine or adjunctive placebo. Results from these two trials did not support the effectiveness of lamotrigine as an add-on treatment for patients with residual psychotic symptoms of schizophrenia. Secondary objectives that evaluated additional measures of global response, negative symptoms, depressive symptoms, and quality of life also failed to support clinical effectiveness. The only indication of a possible therapeutic effect of lamotrigine was the improvement in the cognitive composite score in one study (57), but this effect was neither found in the other study (56) nor was it a primary hypothesis. These results are clearly at odds with the other published controlled trials (52–55). It is possible that the patients enrolled in the large multicenter studies conducted by the manufacturer were not as ill as the patients who participated in the other studies. In addition, placebo response in both of the manufacturer's studies was substantial, diminishing the ability to observe a therapeutic effect with lamotrigine.

A comprehensive Cochrane Library Review meta-analysis (59) concluded on the basis of five studies ($N = 537$) that compared adjunctive lamotrigine versus adjunctive placebo that the data are not robust and the effect sizes showing an advantage for combination therapy are small.

Topiramate

Topiramate was introduced in the United States in 1997 as an antiseizure medication. It does not have FDA approval for any psychiatric disorder per se. However, topiramate is one of the few medications that have been associated with weight loss. Thus this agent has attracted a great deal of interest among clinicians as an adjunct to second-generation antipsychotics to address the adverse event of weight gain. An early case report from 2000 described a patient with schizophrenia being treated with clozapine who lost 21 kg over five months when receiving adjunctive topiramate 125 mg/day (60). In a two-year retrospective case series analysis, weight loss was observed in 10 patients with schizophrenia and schizoaffective disorder with antipsychotic-induced weight gain and who received adjunctive topiramate at a mean daily dose of approximately 200 mg (61). Adjunctive topiramate limited the amount of weight gain observed among 60 male outpatients with schizophrenia receiving olanzapine in a 12-week, randomized, open-label, parallel-group trial conducted in Korea (62). The strongest evidence to date supporting the use of adjunctive topiramate for the treatment of excess weight in patients with schizophrenia is a 12-week, randomized, placebo-controlled prospective study of 66 hospitalized patients conducted in Korea (63). Patients were randomized to receive adjunctive topiramate at doses of 100 mg/day or 200 mg/day, or a placebo. Body weight, body mass index, waist measurement, and hip measurement decreased significantly in the 200-mg/day topiramate group compared with the 100-mg/day topiramate and placebo groups over 12 weeks. The waist-to-hip ratio did not change in any group.

The use of adjunctive topiramate in treating the symptoms of schizophrenia has also been studied. A case report from 2001 describes how adjunctive topiramate can attenuate the severity of negative symptoms of schizophrenia (64). However, negative reports also exist. In an open trial, no significant improvement was observed in nine patients receiving topiramate augmentation of clozapine, olanzapine, haloperidol, or fluphenthixol (46). Deterioration has also been described. For example, when using adjunctive topiramate up to the range of 200 to 300 mg/day to treat five patients with treatment-refractory schizophrenia (4 patients were taking clozapine), two patients deteriorated to the point that the investigators could not obtain reliable post-treatment PANSS scores, and for the remaining three patients, the PANSS total score deteriorated substantially (including both positive and negative symptoms) (65). In another case report, a patient with schizophrenia originally treated with clozapine and valproate experienced a worsening of psychosis in the context of replacing valproate with topiramate, which remitted when valproate was resumed (66). The cognitive side effects of topiramate have been suggested as one of the reasons patients with schizophrenia may deteriorate with adjunctive topiramate (67). Other case reports of adjunctive topiramate in treating schizophrenia have examined the potential role topiramate may play in reducing alcohol abuse (68).

The available controlled studies of adjunctive topiramate in the treatment of schizophrenia (double-blind and/or randomized) for which English-language reports are available are included in Table 5 (62,63,69). The sole extant study targeting psychopathology was conducted in Finland in 26 patients with treatment-resistant schizophrenia (69). The study was a randomized, double-blind, placebo-controlled trial in which 300 mg/day of topiramate was gradually added to the patient's ongoing treatment (clozapine, olanzapine, risperidone, or quetiapine) over two 12-week crossover treatment periods. In the ITT analysis, topiramate was more effective than placebo in reducing PANSS general psychopathological symptoms, but no significant improvement was observed in positive or negative symptoms.

Gabapentin

Although introduced in the United States in 1993, there is very limited published data on the use of adjunctive gabapentin for the treatment of schizophrenia. It does not have FDA approval for any psychiatric disorder per se. No controlled studies are available regarding adjunctive gabapentin for the treatment of schizophrenia. There is an early report of favorable long-term antianxiety and hypnotic effects of adjunctive gabapentin in patients with comorbid anxiety-related disorders (70). Among the 18 patients described in that naturalistic study, 10 were diagnosed with

TABLE 5 Controlled Studies of Adjunctive Topiramate in Schizophrenia

Author and year (reference)	N	Length (days)	Target daily dose of TOP (mg)	Design	Diagnosis	Outcome
Ko 2005 (63)	66	84	100 or 200	AP + TOP 100 mg vs. AP + TOP 200 mg vs. AP + placebo	Inpatients with schizophrenia and overweight	With TOP 200 mg, body weight, body mass index, waist measurement, and hip measurement decreased significantly compared with TOP 100-mg and placebo groups. Waist-to-hip ratio did not change in any group. BPRS decreased by 0.4%, 3.2%, and 2.9% in the placebo, TOP 100-mg, and TOP 200-mg groups, respectively
Tiihonen 2005 (69)	26	84	300	AP+TOP vs. AP + placebo (crossover)	Male inpatients with treatment-resistant chronic schizophrenia (on CLO, OLZ, or QUE)	Improvement in PANSS general; no difference in total PANSS, PANSS positive, or PANSS negative
Kim 2006 (62)	60	84	100	OLZ vs. OLZ + TOP (although randomized, the study was not double-blind)	Outpatients with schizophrenia	TOP was associated with less weight gain at weeks 4, 8, and end point. Improvement on the PANSS total were observed in both groups and not significantly different

Abbreviations: AP, antipsychotic; TOP, topiramate; CLO, clozapine; OLZ, olanzapine; QUE, quetiapine; PANSS, Positive and Negative Syndrome Scale.

schizophrenia and 4 with schizoaffective disorder. In a chart review of 11 patients in a state-operated psychiatric hospital (4 with schizophrenia and 4 with schizo-affective disorder), adjunctive gabapentin was associated with a reduction in agitation (71). Negative reports exist, including a case report of a patient with schizophrenia who experienced increased hallucinations and delusions when gabapentin was added to his regimen of clozapine, procyclidine, divalproex, and fluoxetine (72). There is some interest regarding the use of gabapentin for movement disorders associated with schizophrenia treatments, including akathisia (73) and tardive dyskinesia (74).

Oxcarbazepine

Oxcarbazepine was launched in the United States in 2000 for the management of seizures. It does not have FDA approval for any psychiatric disorder per se. No controlled studies are available regarding adjunctive oxcarbazepine for the treatment of schizophrenia. Because it is an analogue of carbamazepine, it was anticipated that it would have a similar efficacy profile and yet not be as problematic in terms of liver enzyme induction as carbamazepine. A retrospective medical record review of the use of oxcarbazepine in 56 hospitalized psychiatric patients (14 with schizophrenia or "other idiopathic psychotic disorders" and 6 with schizoaffective disorder) found the agent to be well tolerated and simpler to use than carbamazepine (75). There is an open-label case series of six male inpatients where oxcarbazepine was added to antipsychotic treatment, starting with 300 mg/day and ending with a final dose of 900 to 2100 mg/day (76). After 42 days of combination treatment, BPRS scores decreased substantially. A negative case report is also available where worsening of dysphoria and irritability was observed with adjunctive oxcarbazepine in a patient with schizophrenia and obsessive-compulsive traits (77). The patient's clinical deterioration was attributed to pharmacokinetic interactions (77).

ANTIEPILEPTIC DRUGS FOR AGGRESSION?

A common rationale for using adjunctive AEDs in patients with schizophrenia is to manage persistent aggressive behavior (78,79). In a prior iteration of a set of guidelines for the treatment of schizophrenia, adjunctive valproate was ranked first for the problem of aggression/violence and for agitation/excitement (with a history of substance abuse) (80). The above discussions of carbamazepine and valproate have described some of the evidence supporting this use of AEDs, but there remains little in the way of controlled clinical trials that specifically study patients with hostile behavior. These studies are logistically difficult to conduct given the imprecise definitions of aggression, the difficulty of measuring outcome because of the relative rarity of aggressive events, and the challenges of selecting appropriate patients for study, which includes determining allowable comorbidities and concomitant medications (81). Since the usual outcome measure is the aggressive event rate, a large sample size and lengthy baseline and trial periods are required when this rate is low (81). Furthermore, formidable practical and ethical obstacles interfere with the many sound techniques (e.g., randomization) used in typical designs of psychopharmacological clinical trials (81). Thus, most of the evidence supporting the notion that adjunctive AEDs are helpful in managing aggressive behavior in patients with schizophrenia comes from uncontrolled observations or is generalized from studies of other disorders (82).

The use of combinations of AEDs in patients with schizophrenia and aggression has also been reported in the literature. A retrospective study was carried out in a sample of 45 patients with schizophrenia, schizoaffective and bipolar disorder, and hospitalized in a forensic psychiatric facility in Canada (83). Patients were placed on adjunctive AEDs only if they failed to respond adequately to antipsychotic agents alone. Patients treated with topiramate, valproate, or the combination of topiramate and valproate showed a decrease in Overt Aggression Scale scores and a decrease in the number of episodes of agitation. However, valproate therapy, but not topiramate therapy, decreased the intensity of agitation episodes as measured by the Agitation-Calmness Evaluation Scale.

CLINICAL RECOMMENDATIONS

Unlike for the treatment of bipolar mania (84), combinations of antipsychotics and AEDs are not FDA approved for the treatment of schizophrenia. Such "off-label" use makes it imperative for the clinician to be able to articulate a solid rationale for choosing the combination therapy and to document that reason in the medical record. Diagnostic reassessment is also worthwhile to "rule in" a mood disorder (as per DSM-IV-TR, a diagnosis of schizophrenia cannot be made if there is evidence of the presence of schizoaffective disorder or a mood disorder with psychotic features). Another diagnostic possibility is the presence of a comorbid psychiatric or somatic disorder that is complicating treatment response. A common example is that of comorbid alcohol abuse. Before prescribing combination treatment, adherence to the current therapy must be assessed. If lack of response to treatment is due to noncompliance, adding another medication is unlikely to help.

Not all AEDs have the same evidence base for the treatment of schizophrenia. Data supporting the use of augmentation strategies is not robust to begin with, but a lack of controlled trials in patients with schizophrenia for the use of adjunctive gabapentin or for oxcarbazepine, and weak support for topiramate, make the choice of these agents less compelling than for carbamazepine, valproate, or lamotrigine. The data for carbamazepine and valproate make those agents a possible choice for patients with aggressive or impulsive behavior, and that for lamotrigine as a possible adjunctive medication for use with clozapine in patients with treatment-refractory schizophrenia. Special considerations include the need for plasma level monitoring of carbamazepine and possible dose adjustment of the antipsychotic prescribed with it. Worsening with adjunctive lamotrigine has been reported and may necessitate discontinuation of that agent even before an adequate dose of lamotrigine has been achieved.

The use of adjunctive AEDs in patients with schizophrenia can be considered as a mini-clinical trial with that patient. Specific target symptoms need to be identified and measured before starting the combination treatment and then periodically reassessed. If both the clinician and the patient cannot conclude that a substantial benefit is accruing, then that combination needs to be expeditiously discontinued. The ongoing additional risk of multiple medication treatment cannot be justified unless there is tangible and documentable therapeutic benefit.

SUMMARY

The coprescribing of AEDs with antipsychotics among patients with schizophrenia is common practice. Clinicians resort to combination therapies when monotherapies are inadequate in controlling symptoms or maintaining response.

The evidence base supporting the use of augmentation strategies with AEDs in the treatment of schizophrenia is limited. Although case reports and open uncontrolled studies have been published for carbamazepine, valproate, gabapentin, lamotrigine, topiramate, and oxcarbazepine, these have not always led to the conduct of double-blind and/or randomized clinical trials. Carbamazepine has been assessed in several small controlled studies, but the overall number of patients who have participated in published augmentation studies over the past 25 years is only approximately 300. It is possible that the best use of carbamazepine with antipsychotics is for patients with schizophrenia and aggression, but no adequately powered studies have been conducted to specifically test this. Adjunctive valproate has been widely used as a treatment strategy for patients with residual symptoms, but the largest reported trials have focused on patients with acute exacerbations of schizophrenia rather than on the more refractory patient. For both valproate and lamotrigine, the industry-conducted clinical trials have essentially failed to support the use of combination treatment.

There remains a need for the clinician to be nimble enough to consider novel combinations of medications in an effort to reduce persistent symptoms of schizophrenia. "Absence of evidence" is not the same as "evidence of absence" for the possibility that an individual patient may benefit from adjunctive AEDs. However, this means the clinician must make an attempt to quantify improvement, help the patient assess the value of the treatment while balancing benefits and adverse effects, and be prepared to abandon the combination if substantial advantages for the use of the combination are not forthcoming.

REFERENCES

1. Citrome L, Levine J, Allingham B. Utilization of valproate: extent of inpatient use in the New York State Office of Mental Health. Psychiatr Q 1998; 69(4):283–300.
2. Citrome L, Levine J, Allingham B. Changes in use of valproate and other mood stabilizers for patients with schizophrenia from 1994 to 1998. Psychiatr Serv 2000; 51(5): 634–638.
3. Citrome L, Jaffe A, Levine J. Datapoints - mood stabilizers: utilization trends in patients diagnosed with schizophrenia 1994–2001. Psychiatr Serv 2002; 53(10):1212.
4. Citrome L. Antipsychotic polypharmacy versus augmentation with anticonvulsants: the US Perspective. Paper presented at: XXIV CINP Congress, Paris, France, 2004, June 20–24. Int J Neuropsychopharmacol 2004, 7(suppl 1):S69 (abstr).
5. Wessels T, Grunler D, Bunk C, et al. Changes in the treatment of acute psychosis in a German public hospital from 1998 to 2004. Psychiatr Q 2007; 78(2):91–99.
6. Davids E, Bunk C, Specka M, et al. Psychotropic drug prescription in a psychiatric university hospital in Germany. Prog Neuropsychopharmacol Biol Psychiatry 2006; 30(6): 1109–1116.
7. Grohmann R, Engel RR, Geissler KH, et al. Psychotropic drug use in psychiatric inpatients: recent trends and changes over time-data from the AMSP study. Pharmacopsychiatry 2004; 37(suppl 1):S27–S38.
8. Mallinger JB, Lamberti JS. Racial differences in the use of adjunctive psychotropic medications for patients with schizophrenia. J Ment Health Policy Econ 2007; 10(1):15–22.
9. Xiang YT, Weng YZ, Leung CM, et al. Clinical and social determinants of psychotropic drug prescription for schizophrenia outpatients in China. Prog Neuropsychopharmacol Biol Psychiatry 2007; 31(3):756–760.
10. Kreyenbuhl JA, Valenstein M, McCarthy JF, et al. Long-term antipsychotic polypharmacy in the VA health system: patient characteristics and treatment patterns. Psychiatr Serv 2007; 58(4):489–495.

11. Hakola HP, Laulumaa VA. Carbamazepine in treatment of violent schizophrenics. Lancet 1982; 1(8285):1358.
12. Luchins DL. Carbamazepine in violent non-epileptic schizophrenics. Psychopharmacol Bull 1984; 20(3):569–571.
13. Neppe VM. Carbamazepine as adjunctive treatment in nonepileptic chronic inpatients with EEG temporal lobe abnormalities. J Clin Psychiatry 1983; 44(9):326–331.
14. Dose M, Apelt S, Emrich HM. Carbamazepine as an adjunct of antipsychotic therapy. Psychiatry Res 1987; 22(4):303–310.
15. Okuma T, Yamashita I, Takahashi R, et al. A double-blind study of adjunctive carbamazepine versus placebo on excited states of schizophrenic and schizoaffective disorders. Acta Psychiatr Scand 1989; 80(3):250–259.
16. Nachshoni T, Levin Y, Levy A, et al. A double-blind trial of carbamazepine in negative symptom schizophrenia. Biol Psychiatry 1994; 35(1):22–26.
17. Simhandl C, Meszaros K, Denk E, et al. Adjunctive carbamazepine or lithium carbonate in therapy-resistant chronic schizophrenia. Can J Psychiatry 1996; 41(5):317.
18. Hesslinger B, Normann C, Langosch JM, et al. Effects of carbamazepine and valproate on haloperidol plasma levels and on psychopathologic outcome in schizophrenic patients. J Clin Psychopharmacol 1999; 19(4):310–315.
19. Ohlmeier MD, Jahn K, Wilhelm-Gossling C, et al. Perazine and carbamazepine in comparison to olanzapine in schizophrenia. Neuropsychobiology 2007; 55(2):81–88.
20. Leucht S, Kissling W, McGrath J, et al. Carbamazepine for schizophrenia. Cochrane Database Syst Rev 2007; 3:CD001258.
21. Fenn HH, Robinson D, Luby V, et al. Trends in pharmacotherapy of schizoaffective and bipolar affective disorders: a 5-year naturalistic study. Am J Psychiatry 1996; 153(5):711–713.
22. Weisler RH, Hirschfeld R, Cutler AJ, et al. Extended-release carbamazepine capsules as monotherapy in bipolar disorder: pooled results from two randomised, double-blind, placebo-controlled trials. CNS Drugs 2006; 20(3):219–231.
23. Citrome L, Macher JP, Salazar DE, et al. Pharmacokinetics of aripiprazole and concomitant carbamazepine. J Clin Psychopharmacol 2007; 27(3):279–283.
24. Linnoila M, Viukari M, Kietala O. Effect of sodium valproate on tardive dyskinesia. Br J Psychiatry 1976; 129):114–119.
25. Nagao T, Ohshimo T, Mitsunobu K, et al. Cerebrospinal fluid monoamine metabolites and cyclic nucleotides in chronic schizophrenic patients with tardive dyskinesia or drug-induced tremor. Biol Psychiatry 1979; 14(3):509–523.
26. Wassef AA, Hafiz NG, Hampton D, et al. Divalproex sodium augmentation of haloperidol in hospitalized patients with schizophrenia: clinical and economic implications. J Clin Psychopharmacol 2001; 21(1):21–26.
27. Chong SA, Tan CH, Lee EL, et al. Augmentation of risperidone with valproic acid. J Clin Psychiatry 1998; 59(8):430.
28. Ko GN, Korpi ER, Freed WJ, et al. Effect of valproic acid on behavior and plasma amino acid concentrations in chronic schizophrenia patients. Biol Psychiatry 1985; 20(2):209–215.
29. Fisk GG, York SM. The effect of sodium valproate on tardive dyskinesia revisited. Br J Psychiatry 1987; 150:542–546.
30. Dose M, Hellweg R, Yassouridis A, et al. Combined treatment of schizophrenic psychoses with haloperidol and valproate. Pharmacopsychiatry 1998; 31(4):122–125.
31. Wassef AA, Dott SG, Harris A, et al. Randomized, placebo-controlled pilot study of divalproex sodium in the treatment of acute exacerbations of chronic schizophrenia. J Clin Psychopharmacol 2000; 20(3):357–361.
32. Casey DE, Daniel DG, Wassef AA, et al. Effect of divalproex combined with olanzapine or risperidone in patients with an acute exacerbation of schizophrenia. Neuropsychopharmacology 2003; 28(1):182–192.
33. Abbott Laboratories. ABT-711 M02-547 Clinical Study Report. Available at: http://www.clinicalstudyresults.org/documents/company-study_782_0.pdf. Accessed November 20, 2006.
34. Citrome L, Shope CB, Nolan KA, et al. Risperidone alone versus risperidone plus valproate in the treatment of patients with schizophrenia and hostility. Int Clin Psychopharmacol 2007; 22(6):356–362.

35. Citrome L, Casey DE, Daniel DG, et al. Effects of adjunctive valproate on hostility in patients with schizophrenia receiving olanzapine or risperidone: a double-blind multicenter study. Psychiatr Serv 2004; 55(3):290–294.

36. Sajatovic M, Coconcea N, Ignacio RV, et al. Adjunct extended-release valproate semisodium in late life schizophrenia. Int J Geriatr Psychiatry 2008; 23(2):142–147.

37. Kelly DL, Conley RR, Feldman S, et al. Adjunct divalproex or lithium to clozapine in treatment-resistant schizophrenia. Psychiatr Q 2006; 77(1):81–95.

38. Yoshimura R, Shinkai K, Ueda N, et al. Valproic acid improves psychotic agitation without influencing plasma risperidone levels in schizophrenic patients. Pharmacopsychiatry 2007; 40(1):9–13.

39. Cramer JA, Sernyak M. Results of a naturalistic study of treatment options: switching atypical antipsychotic drugs or augmenting with valproate. Clin Ther 2004; 26(6): 905–914.

40. Wassef AA, Winkler DE, Roache AL, et al. Lower effectiveness of divalproex versus valproic acid in a prospective, quasi-experimental clinical trial involving 9,260 psychiatric admissions. Am J Psychiatry 2005; 162(2):330–339.

41. Abbott Laboratories. Depakote ER Divalproex Sodium Extended-Release Tablets, Formulary Information. Abbott Park, IL: Abbott Laboratories, 2000.

42. Dutta S, Zhang Y, Selness DS, et al. Comparison of the bioavailability of unequal doses of divalproex sodium extended-release formulation relative to the delayed-release formulation in healthy volunteers. Epilepsy Res 2002; 49(1):1–10.

43. Citrome L, Tremeau F, Wynn PS, et al. A study of the safety, efficacy, and tolerability of switching from the standard delayed release preparation of divalproex sodium to the extended release formulation in patients with schizophrenia. J Clin Psychopharmacol 2004; 24(3):255–259.

44. Basan A, Leucht S. Valproate for schizophrenia. Cochrane Database Syst Rev 2003; 3: CD004028.

45. Dursun SM, McIntosh D, Milliken H. Clozapine plus lamotrigine in treatment-resistant schizophrenia. Arch Gen Psychiatry 1999; 56(10):950.

46. Dursun SM, Deakin JF. Augmenting antipsychotic treatment with lamotrigine or topiramate in patients with treatment-resistant schizophrenia: a naturalistic case-series outcome study. J Psychopharmacol 2001; 15(4):297–301.

47. Thomas R, Howe V, Foister K, et al. Adjunctive lamotrigine in treatment-resistant schizophrenia. Int J Neuropsychopharmacol 2006; 9(1):125–127.

48. Heck AH, de Groot IW, van Harten PN. Addition of lamotrigine to clozapine in inpatients with chronic psychosis. J Clin Psychiatry 2005; 66(10):1333.

49. Chan YC, Miller KM, Shaheen N, et al. Worsening of psychotic symptoms in schizophrenia with addition of lamotrigine: a case report. Schizophr Res 2005; 78(2–3):343–345.

50. Stuve W, Wessels A, Timmerman L. Remission of positive symptomatology of a schizophrenic psychosis after withdrawing lamotrigine: a case report. Eur Psychiatry 2004; 19(1):59–61.

51. Kalyoncu A, Mirsal H, Pektas O, et al. Use of lamotrigine to augment clozapine in patients with resistant schizophrenia and comorbid alcohol dependence: a potent anticraving effect? J Psychopharmacol 2005; 19(3):301–305.

52. Tiihonen J, Hallikainen T, Ryynanen OP, et al. Lamotrigine in treatment-resistant schizophrenia: a randomized placebo-controlled crossover trial. Biol Psychiatry 2003; 54 (11):1241–1248.

53. Kremer I, Vass A, Gorelik I, et al. Placebo-controlled trial of lamotrigine added to conventional and atypical antipsychotics in schizophrenia. Biol Psychiatry 2004; 56(6): 441–446.

54. Akhondzadeh S, Mackinejad K, Ahmadi-Abhari SA, et al. Does the addition of lamotrigine to risperidone improve psychotic symptoms and cognitive impairments in chronic schizophrenia? Therapy 2005; 2(3):399–406.

55. Zoccali R, Muscatello MR, Bruno A, et al. The effect of lamotrigine augmentation of clozapine in a sample of treatment-resistant schizophrenic patients: a double-blind, placebo-controlled study. Schizophr Res 2007; 93(1–3):109–116.

56. Glaxo-Smith-Kline. A multicenter, double-blind, placebo-controlled, randomized, parallel group evaluation of the efficacy of a flexible dose of lamotrigine versus placebo as

add-on therapy in schizophrenia. Study No. SCA30926. Available at: http://ctr.gsk.co. uk/Summary/lamotrigine/III_SCA30926.pdf. Accessed November 5, 2005.

57. Glaxo-Smith-Kline. A multicenter, randomized, double-blind, parallel group study to evaluate the efficacy and safety of a flexible dose of lamotrigine compared to placebo as an adjunctive therapy to an atypical antipsychotic agent(s) in subjects with schizophrenia. Study No. SCA101464. Available at: http://ctr.gsk.co.uk/Summary/lamotrigine/III_ SCA101464.pdf. Accessed May 27, 2006.

58. Goff DC, Keefe R, Citrome L, et al. Lamotrigine as add-on therapy in schizophrenia: results of two placebo-controlled trials. J Clin Psychopharmacol 2007; 27(6):582–589.

59. Premkumar TS, Pick J. Lamotrigine for schizophrenia. Cochrane Database Syst Rev 2006; 4:CD005962.

60. Dursun SM, Devarajan S. Clozapine weight gain, plus topiramate weight loss. Can J Psychiatry 2000; 45(2):198.

61. Lévy E, Agbokou C, Ferreri F, et al. Topiramate-induced weight loss in schizophrenia: a retrospective case series study. Can J Clin Pharmacol 2007; 14(2):E234–E239.

62. Kim JH, Yim SJ, Nam JH. A 12-week, randomized, open-label, parallel-group trial of topiramate in limiting weight gain during olanzapine treatment in patients with schizophrenia. Schizophr Res 2006; 82(1):115–117.

63. Ko YH, Joe SH, Jung IK, et al. Topiramate as an adjuvant treatment with atypical anti-psychotics in schizophrenic patients experiencing weight gain. Clin Neuropharmacol 2005; 28(4):169–175.

64. Drapalski AL, Rosse RB, Peebles RR, et al. Topiramate improves deficit symptoms in a patient with schizophrenia when added to a stable regimen of antipsychotic medication. Clin Neuropharmacol 2001; 24(5):290–294.

65. Millson RC, Owen JA, Lorberg GW, et al. Topiramate for refractory schizophrenia. Am J Psychiatry 2002; 159(4):675.

66. Hofer A, Fleischhacker WW, Hummer M. Worsening of psychosis after replacement of adjunctive valproate with topiramate in a schizophrenia patient. J Clin Psychiatry 2003; 64(10):1267–1268.

67. Duggal HS. Psychotic symptoms associated with topiramate: cognitive side effects or worsening of psychosis? J Clin Psychiatry 2004; 65(8):1145.

68. Huguelet P, Morand-Collomb S. Effect of topiramate augmentation on two patients suffering from schizophrenia or bipolar disorder with comorbid alcohol abuse. Pharmacol Res 2005; 52(5):392–394.

69. Tiihonen J, Halonen P, Wahlbeck K. Topiramate add-on in treatment-resistant schizo-phrenia: a randomized, double-blind, placebo-controlled, crossover trial. J Clin Psychiatry 2005; 66(8):1012–1015.

70. Chouinard G, Beauclair L, Belanger MC. Gabapentin: long-term antianxiety and hyp-notic effects in psychiatric patients with comorbid anxiety-related disorders. Can J Psychiatry 1998; 43(3):305.

71. Megna JL, Devitt PJ, Sauro MD, et al. Gabapentin's effect on agitation in severely and persistently mentally ill patients. Ann Pharmacother 2002; 36(1):12–16.

72. Jablonowski K, Margolese HC, Chouinard G. Gabapentin-induced paradoxical exacer-bation of psychosis in a patient with schizophrenia. Can J Psychiatry 2002; 47(10):975–976.

73. Pfeffer G, Chouinard G, Margolese HC. Gabapentin in the treatment of antipsychotic-induced akathisia in schizophrenia. Int Clin Psychopharmacol 2005; 20(3):179–181.

74. Hardoy MC, Carta MG, Carpiniello B, et al. Gabapentin in antipsychotic-induced tardive dyskinesia: results of 1-year follow-up. J Affect Disord 2003; 75(2):125–130.

75. Centorrino F, Albert MJ, Berry JM, et al. Oxcarbazepine: clinical experience with hospitalized psychiatric patients. Bipolar Disord 2003; 5(5):370–374.

76. Leweke FM, Gerth CW, Koethe D, et al. Oxcarbazepine as an adjunct for schizophrenia. Am J Psychiatry 2004; 161(6):1130–1131.

77. Baird P. The interactive metabolism effect of oxcarbazepine coadministered with tricyclic antidepressant therapy for OCD symptoms. J Clin Psychopharmacol 2003; 23(4): 419.

78. Citrome L. Use of lithium, carbamazepine, and valproic acid in a state-operated psychiatric hospital. J Pharm Technol 1995; 11(2):55–59.

79. Citrome L, Volavka J. Clinical management of persistent aggressive behavior in schizophrenia. Part II: Long-term pharmacotherapeutic strategies. Essent Psychopharmacol 2002; 5(1):17–30.
80. McEvoy JP, Scheifler PL, Frances A. The expert consensus guideline series, treatment of schizophrenia. J Clin Psychiatry 1999; 60(suppl 11):43.
81. Volavka J, Citrome L. Atypical antipsychotics in the treatment of the persistently aggressive psychotic patient: methodological concerns. Schizoph Res 1999, 35(suppl): S23–S33.
82. Citrome L. Schizophrenia and valproate. Psychopharmacol Bull 2003; 37(suppl 2):74–88.
83. Gobbi G, Gaudreau PO, Leblanc N. Efficacy of topiramate, valproate, and their combination on aggression/agitation behavior in patients with psychosis. J Clin Psychopharmacol 2006; 26(5):467–473.
84. Citrome L, Goldberg JF, Stahl SM. Toward convergence in the medication treatment of bipolar disorder and schizophrenia. Harv Rev Psychiatry 2005; 13(1):28–42.
85. Krawiecka M, Goldberg D, Vaughan M. A standardized psychiatric assessment scale for rating chronic psychotic patients. Acta Psychiatr Scand 1977; 55(4):299–308.

7 Antiepileptic Drugs in the Treatment of Anxiety Disorders: Role in Therapy

Michael Van Ameringen and Catherine Mancini
Department of Psychiatry and Behavioural Neurosciences, McMaster University and Anxiety Disorders Clinic, McMaster University Medical Centre—HHS, Hamilton, Ontario, Canada

Beth Patterson and Christine Truong
Anxiety Disorders Clinic, McMaster University Medical Centre—HHS, Hamilton, Ontario, Canada

INTRODUCTION

Pharmacological treatments for anxiety disorders have been evolving rapidly. A variety of drug groups have been shown to be effective. Benzodiazepines have long been used to treat anxiety; however, the development of tolerance to these drugs has made them less favorable treatments (1,2). Serotonin selective reuptake inhibitors (SSRIs) and serotonin-norepinephrine reuptake inhibitors (SNRIs) have emerged to become the current gold standard. Despite such widespread use, these agents are only effective in approximately 50% to 60% of patients and can be associated with significant side effects (3). There is a clinical need for alternative medication treatments for anxiety disorders, in the form of either monotherapy or as augmentation agents.

Antiepileptic drugs (AEDs) have been widely used in the treatment of mood disorders and have become first-line treatments for bipolar disorder (4,5). The successful use of AEDs in mood disorders has led clinicians and researchers to investigate their potential efficacy in other psychiatric disorders, in particular, in anxiety disorders.

This chapter attempts to review the small but emerging literature on the use of AEDs in anxiety disorders. Information for this review was obtained from a MEDLINE search and a review of abstracts from major psychiatric congresses (including the Annual Meeting of the American Psychiatric Association, the National Conference of the Anxiety Disorders Association of America, the Annual Meeting of the American College of Neuropsychopharmacology, and the International Forum on Mood and Anxiety Disorders). Each anxiety disorder will be reviewed, focusing on available data that have been presented or published for each AED that has been studied in that disorder.

The notion of using AEDs in anxiety disorders can find a basis in emerging constructs, describing fear circuits in the brain. Numerous brain regions are likely involved in the expression of fear; however, the amygdala is thought to play a key role because of its ability to link sensory stimuli with affective outcomes and initiate emotionally appropriate behaviors (6). Various pathologies, such as anxiety disorders and addiction, could be a manifestation of an "overexpression" of these amygdala-based, conditioned emotional associations (7). This overexpression may result from a failure of proper inhibitory control in the amygdala.

Gamma-aminobutyric acid (GABA) is the primary inhibitory neurotransmitter in the central nervous system (CNS). The inhibitory action of GABA counterbalances the excitatory activity of the neurotransmitter glutamate. The homeostasis between GABA and glutamate controls CNS arousal and neuronal excitability. Maintaining this balance prevents overexcitability, which is known to occur in seizure disorders but is also thought to play a role in pathological anxiety (8), potentially through the overexpression of conditioned fear associations, as previously mentioned.

Abnormalities in both the GABAergic and glutamatergic systems have been associated with various anxiety disorders. For example, decreased occipital GABA levels in panic disorder patients, by as much as 22% compared with healthy controls, have been found (9). A dysfunction in GABA-A receptor binding is also thought to play a role in anxiety disorders, stemming from the observation of diminished response to exogenous benzodiazepines in individuals with anxiety (10). A potential glutamatergic dysfunction has recently been associated with obsessive-compulsive disorder (OCD) on the basis of a neuroimaging study describing an increased level of caudate glutamatergic concentrations in treatment-naïve pediatric OCD patients (11). It has also been hypothesized that a glutamatergic abnormality in social anxiety may be a key component in the dysfunctional neurocircuitry. Increased levels of glucocorticoids in response to stress are thought to stimulate the release of hippocampal glutamate, which may inhibit neurogenesis. A decrease in neurogenesis may be associated with social phobia, as found in animal models of social dominance with subordinate status being linked with a marked decrease in new cells in the dentate gyrus (12).

Various AEDs are thought to modulate GABA and glutamate function, and treating anxious patients with such agents may therefore restore the homeostasis between these two neurotransmitters and decrease neuronal overexcitability, particularly in the amygdala. The following is a summary of the AEDs that have been examined in the treatment of anxiety disorders.

Carbamazepine is indicated for epilepsy and is useful in treating partial and complex seizures. It is also indicated for treatment of acute mania and prophylaxis in bipolar disorder. Its primary mechanism of action is through blockade of voltage-gated sodium channels in neuronal cell membranes, thus preventing the release of excitatory neurotransmitters from nerve terminals (13–16).

Gabapentin is an AED that increases the release of nonsynaptic GABA from glial cells, thereby decreasing neuronal overexcitability (8). Although it was initially synthesized as a GABA analogue, its exact mechanism of action is unclear (17). A gabapentin-binding site has been demonstrated in neocortical and hippocampal areas with unclear functional significance (17).

Lamotrigine is used as either an adjunct or monotherapy agent for epilepsy. It is thought to produce antiseizure effects by its action on voltage-sensitive sodium channels, and subsequent inhibition of the release of glutamate and aspartate. It has been studied in mood disorders and has been found to be effective for the treatment of bipolar depression (18).

Levetiracetam reduces currents through high-voltage-activated calcium channels, and acts via unique binding sites on CNS membranes. Although the exact mechanism of action is unknown, levetiracetam does not have a direct effect on GABA concentrations or GABA receptors, but promotes chloride influx at $GABA_A$ receptors by inhibiting zinc and β-carbolines in the same manner as valproate and clonazepam (19).

Oxcarbazepine is structurally related to carbamazepine; however, it is not metabolized to the 10,11-epoxide, which is thought to be responsible for a decrease in the side effects typically seen with carbamazepine. Its primary mechanism of action is thought to involve blockade of voltage dependent sodium channels (20–22).

Phenytoin is used to control generalized tonic-clonic and psychomotor seizures. It appears to inhibit seizure activity through its action on the motor cortex. Its anticonvulsive effects likely come from its promotion of sodium efflux thus stabilizing firing thresholds against hyperexcitability (23,24).

Pregabalin is a structural analogue to GABA, although it is not active at GABA receptors, nor does it acutely alter GABA uptake or degradation (25). It may have a novel mechanism of action by binding to a subunit of voltage-dependent calcium channels in CNS tissues (26) and acts as a presynaptic modulator of several excitatory neurotransmitters (25).

Tiagabine is the only selective GABA reuptake inhibitor (SGRI). It increases synaptic GABA availability by selective inhibition of the GABA transporter-1, the most abundant GABA transporter (26,27). It has been indicated for add-on treatment of partial seizures.

Topiramate appears to have several mechanisms of action. It has been shown to enhance the activity of GABA at non-benzodiazepine sites, to inhibit glutamate via α-amino-3 hydroxy-5-methyl-4-isoxazole propionic acid (AMPA)/kainate subreceptors, and to block voltage-gated sodium channels. It is also a weak inhibitor of carbonic anhydrase isoenzymes CAII and CAIV (28).

Valproate is primarily used as sole or adjunctive therapy for the treatment of simple or complex absence seizures and generalized seizures with tonic-clonic manifestations. It is used adjunctively for patients with multiple seizure types. Valproate is also indicated for the treatment of mania in bipolar disorder. Although its exact mechanism of action is unknown, it has been suggested that valproate increases brain concentrations of GABA by promoting chloride influx at $GABA_A$ receptors, in turn, by inhibiting the $GABA_A$ receptor modulators zinc and β-carbolines (19).

Vigabatrin, a specific GABA transaminase inhibitor, is used as an anticonvulsant and also to treat hyperekplexia (startle disease) in neonates (29,30).

SOCIAL PHOBIA

Social phobia (social anxiety disorder) is characterized by a marked and persistent fear of social or performance situations due to an excessive fear of embarrassment or humiliation (31). Individuals with social phobia typically fear and avoid public speaking, participating in small groups, dating, speaking to authority figures, attending parties, and speaking with and meeting strangers.

Numerous drug classes have been found to be efficacious in social phobia, including SSRIs (32,33), SNRIs (34), monoamine oxidase inhibitors (MAOIs) (35–37), reversible inhibitors of monoamine oxidase-A (RIMAs) (38,39), and benzodiazepines, as well as AEDs.

Topiramate

Van Ameringen et al. (40) evaluated the effectiveness of topiramate in treating social phobia in a 16-week open-label trial of 23 patients with generalized social phobia. The mean dose of topiramate at end point was 222.8 ± 141.8 mg/day, with a dose range of 25 to 400 mg/day. In the intent-to-treat (ITT) sample, 12(45.1%) patients were responders [defined as a Clinical Global Impression of Improvement (CGI-I) scale score of ≤2] and significant improvement was found from baseline to end point on the Liebowitz Social Anxiety Scale (LSAS). Significant changes in self-report measures of social anxiety were also demonstrated. However, no changes were found on measures of depression or generalized anxiety. Six of the twenty-three participants (26.1%) achieved remission status, defined as an end point LSAS score less than or equal to 30. The most common adverse events included weight loss, paresthesia, and headache, with only five patients dropping out of the study as a result of them. Although this was an open-label design, these results suggest that topiramate may have a specific effect on symptoms of social phobia. This finding is particularly intriguing given the purported mechanism of action of topiramate involving both glutamate and GABA neurotransmitter systems. The remission rate in this study was similar to that found in a recent placebo-controlled trial of venlafaxine in the treatment of social phobia (41). However, a major drawback with topiramate may be individuals' ability to tolerate its bothersome side effects, particularly cognitive impairment.

Gabapentin
The effectiveness of gabapentin in treating social phobia was examined in a placebo-controlled study by Pande et al. (42). Sixty-nine patients were randomly assigned to a 14-week double-blind treatment of either gabapentin, with a varying dose of 900 to 3600 mg/day or a placebo. The treatment group demonstrated significantly more symptom reduction then the control group, as measured by the LSAS ($p = 0.008$), the Brief Social Phobia Scale (BSPS; $p = 0.007$), and the Social Phobia Inventory (SPIN; $p = 0.008$). In the ITT analysis, twice as many patients taking gabapentin were considered responders (32% for gabapentin vs. 14% for placebo), defined as a decrease of at least 50% on the LSAS; however, this difference in response rate did not reach significance ($p = 0.08$). The Clinical Global Impression of Change (CGI-C) scale response rate (defined as "much" or "very much improved") was 38.2% for the gabapentin group as compared with 17.1% for the placebo group. Adverse events that occurred significantly more in the gabapentin group included dizziness, somnolence, nausea, flatulence, and decreased libido. Of the 44% of individuals who withdrew from this study before completion, 21% of those taking gabapentin withdrew because of adverse events, compared with 11% of the placebo group. Although gabapentin did not separate for placebo on the primary outcome measure (≥50% decrease in LSAS baseline scores), there was a suggestion from secondary outcome measures that there may be a treatment effect of gabapentin on social phobic symptoms, though moderate.

The effects of gabapentin on anxiety induced by simulated public speaking were investigated in 32 normal male volunteers, aged 17 to 30 years, who were randomly assigned to gabapentin 400 mg/day ($N = 11$), 800 mg/day ($N = 10$), or placebo ($N = 11$) (43). The self-rated Visual Analogue Mood Scale (VAMS) and Profile of Mood States (POMS) were used as primary outcome measures along with physiological measures of heart rate and blood pressure and were obtained at five time points throughout the procedure. Two hours after receiving study treatment, subjects were given two minutes to prepare a four-minute improvised speech that would be recorded on video camera. Subjects were given their choice of several sensitive topics to speak about. Treatment with gabapentin at 800 mg/day attenuated the anxiety of subjects that had a decrease on the VAMS item calm-excited ($p < 0.05$) as compared with gabapentin 400 mg/day and to placebo ($p = 0.036$). In addition, volunteers receiving both doses of gabapentin showed a decrease in the hostility score on the POMS. No significant drug effect was found in differences between physiological measures. These results are in agreement with other studies, suggesting an anxiolytic potential of gabapentin.

Pregabalin

The effectiveness of pregabalin in treating social phobia was demonstrated by a double-blind, placebo-controlled study conducted by Pande et al. (44). In this study, 135 patients with social phobia were randomly assigned to 10 weeks of high-dose pregabalin (600 mg/day; $N = 47$), low-dose pregabalin (150 mg/day; $N = 42$), or a placebo ($N = 46$). Using the ITT sample, pregabalin 600 mg/day was found to be significantly better than placebo on the primary outcome measure of change from baseline to end point in the LSAS total score ($p = 0.024$), as well as on the secondary measures the LSAS subscales of total fear, total avoidance, social fear, and social avoidance, and the BSPS fear subscale. The rate of response (defined as a CGI-I rating of much or very much improved) was 43% (20 of 47) for the high-dose group, compared with 22% (10 of 46) for the placebo group. The low-dose group showed greater improvement over the placebo group, but the difference did not reach statistical significance. Pregabalin was also found to be relatively well tolerated, with mild-to-moderate somnolence and dizziness being the most common side effects associated with the high-dose group. Of the 30.4% of patients who withdrew from the study, 23.4% of those in the high-dose pregabalin group withdrew because of adverse events, compared with 9.5% in the low-dose group and 8.7% in the placebo group. The results of this study suggest that pregabalin may be a promising new agent in the treatment of social phobia.

Valproate

Valproate has shown mixed results in the treatment of social phobia, as described in two reports. Nardi et al. treated 16 generalized social phobics in an open trial of valproate with doses of 500 to 1500 mg/day (mean dose = 1071 ± 75 mg/day) for one to nine months. All patients were considered to be nonresponders (45). In another study, Kinrys et al. treated 17 social phobics in a 12-week open trial of valproate with doses of 500 to 2500 mg/day (mean dose = 1985 ± 454 mg/day). In the ITT analysis, 41.1% were considered responders by the CGI-I, with a mean drop in the LSAS of 19.1 points. Adverse events included nausea, somnolence, dizziness, and fatigue. Only 1 of 17 participants dropped out because of adverse events (46). Conclusions that can be drawn from this study are limited because of the small sample size and open-label design. The contradicting results of these two studies suggest the need for further investigations of valproate in social phobia.

Tiagabine

Tiagabine monotherapy (mean dose = 10 mg/day) for social phobia was investigated by Dunlop et al. (47) in a 12-week open-trial of 63 social phobia patients followed by a double-blind relapse-prevention phase. The mean dose of tiagabine was 12.2 ± 4.0 mg/day. Twenty-seven patients completed the open-label phase but 54 were included in the ITT analyses. Of the 36 patients who withdrew from the study, 12 discontinued because of adverse events and 4 because of lack of efficacy. In the ITT analysis, significant reductions in social phobia symptoms were found as measured by the LSAS and SPIN. Significant improvements in quality of life were also found as measured by the Sheehan Disability Scale (SDS). In the ITT analysis, 40.7% (22/54) were considered to be responders (defined as a CGI ≤ 2 at end point) compared with 63.0% (17/27) of the completers. The most common adverse events were somnolence (32%) and dizziness (25%). Seventeen responders were randomized to the relapse prevention phase, where they were randomly assigned to continue on tiagabine ($N = 6$), or switch to placebo ($N = 11$). Seven patients completed this phase and the results were not reported because of the low statistical power of the small sample. (47)

Kinrys et al. (48) conducted a retrospective analysis of 14 patients treated with adjunctive tiagabine after nonresponse to an SSRI. Tiagabine was taken for a mean duration of 30.6 weeks at a mean dose of 16.4 ± 6.9 mg/day, ranging from 8 to 83 mg/day, with the SSRI and sometimes with other medications, including quetiapine, clonazepam, and bupropion. In this cohort, nine (64.2%) patients met the response criteria (defined as a CGI ≤ 2 at end point), and five (35.7%) met remission criteria (defined as a LSAS ≤ 30). Symptom response and remission were maintained in these patients at 28 weeks (48).

These two open-label reports suggest that tiagabine may be useful as a monotherapy or an augmentation therapy for treatment-resistant social phobia. However, the small sample-size, open-label design, and, in the augmentation study, the use of a variety of concomitant medications limit the generalizability of these results.

Levetiracetam

Recently, Simon et al. (49) gave levetiracetam to 20 patients with generalized social phobia for eight weeks, with doses initiated at 250 mg/day and flexibly titrated to 3000 mg/day (mean dose = 2013mg/day). Thirteen of the twenty patients completed the trial, and of those patients, three discontinued because of adverse events (drowsiness and nervousness). In the ITT analysis, there was a significant decrease in mean LSAS score from baseline to end point (20.5 points). Significant decreases in Hamilton Anxiety Scale (HAM-A) and the CGI-Severity (CGI-S) Scale scores were also found (49).

In a seven-week study of Diagnostic and Statistical Manual of Mental Disorders (DSM)-IV social anxiety disorder, 18 patients were randomly assigned (in a 2:1 ratio) to double-blind treatment with either levetiracetam (500–3000 mg/day) or placebo (50). Study medication was started at 500 mg at bedtime for four days, and increased as tolerated at the rate of 500 mg every three to four days, to 2000 mg/day by day 14, and to a maximum daily dose of 3000 mg (1500 mg b.i.d.). The mean dose of levetiracetam at the final visit was 2279 mg/day ($N = 9$), compared with 2786 mg/day for placebo ($N = 7$). The primary outcomes were the change in the BSPS from baseline and the rate of response (defined as a final CGI-I score of 1 or 2). Analyses were performed on the ITT sample using the last observation carried forward (LOCF). No statistically significant differences were observed on any measures of social anxiety, including the BSPS, LSAS, and SPIN. Response rates by CGI-I were 22% for levetiracetam and 14% for placebo ($p = $ NS). Although the differences between drug and placebo were not statistically significant, the actual magnitude of reduction was twofold greater for levetiracetam than for placebo on all three social phobia scales. The effect sizes of levetiracetam compared with placebo were 0.33 for the BSPS and 0.50 for the LSAS, representing mild-to-moderate effects. The authors noted that the low placebo response rate suggested they had a somewhat treatment-refractory group that might present a harder test for a putative treatment to demonstrate efficacy. Other limitations included the small sample size and short treatment duration. Adverse events were experienced in two of nine subjects ($N = 1$ severe headache and drowsiness, $N = 1$ disinhibition and inebriation) in the levetiracetam group, suggesting that a lower initial dose and slower titration may be preferable.

The current levetiracetam studies do not support its routine use in social phobia, but given their small sample sizes, further trials in larger samples may be warranted.

POSTTRAUMATIC STRESS DISORDER

Posttraumatic stress disorder (PTSD) is a pathological response resulting from exposure to a traumatic stressor. Three clusters of symptoms occur in PTSD: (1) persistent re-experiencing of the traumatic event (i.e., dreams and distressing recollections), (2) avoidance of stimuli associated with the trauma as well as numbing or detachment, and (3) persistent symptoms of increased arousal (31).

Evidence from placebo-controlled trials has demonstrated the efficacy of SSRIs and SNRIs in treating PTSD, making these agents first-line treatments for PTSD (51). Fluoxetine (52,53), sertraline (54–57), paroxetine, (58–60) and venlafaxine extended release (61) have all demonstrated efficacy in placebo-controlled trials. Other medications with demonstrated efficacy in PTSD include the MAOI, phenelzine (62,63), and the tricyclic antidepressants amitriptyline (64,65) and imipramine (62,63,65). Recent evidence, as described below, suggests that AEDs may be a tolerable and efficacious alternative treatment for PTSD.

Lamotrigine

A placebo-controlled trial was conducted by Hertzberg et al. (66) to evaluate the effectiveness of lamotrigine in treating PTSD. Ten patients received lamotrigine and four patients received placebo for up to 10 weeks (mean dose at end point = 380 mg/day). Improvements in avoidance or numbing and re-experiencing (i.e., flashbacks, nightmares) symptoms, as measured by the Duke Global Rating for PTSD (DGRP), were found with lamotrigine while no improvements were measured in the control group. Five (50%) patients treated with lamotrigine were classified as responders compared with one (25%) in the placebo group. Two of the ten lamotrigine patients developed a rash leading to discontinuation, while two of four placebo patients also discontinued the study due to a rash. Other side effects were judged to be mild and included sweating, drowsiness, poor concentration, thirst, restlessness, and sexual dysfunction (66). Although this study used a placebo-controlled design, the results must be interpreted with caution. The small sample size did not allow for statistical analysis of the quantifiable measures, and only one placebo patient completed the study. More studies with larger samples would allow further assessment of the potential benefits of lamotrigine in PTSD.

Topiramate

Two open-label trials of topiramate in PTSD has been reported. In the first study by Berlant et al. (67), 35 PTSD patients were given topiramate as monotherapy or as adjunctive therapy for a mean duration of treatment of 33 weeks. It was found that topiramate reduced nightmares in 79% of patients and reduced intrusions or flashbacks in 86% of patients based on self-report at end point. Fourteen of the seventeen patients who had completed the PTSD Checklist-Civilian Version (PCL-C) after four weeks of treatment had a score of 50 of less (which is below the standard cutoff score for active PTSD). Symptom improvements were reported with both topiramate monotherapy and adjunctive therapy, with a mean mono-therapy dose for full response of 43 mg/day (range 25–75 mg/day), compared with 97 mg/day (range 25–500 mg/day) for a full response with adjunctive therapy. Nine patients discontinued treatment because of side effects. These included urticaria, eating cessation, acute narrow-angle glaucoma, severe head-ache, overstimulation/panic, memory concerns, and one occurrence of emergent suicidal ideation. The topiramate doses used in this study were quite low as compared with what have been used in other psychiatric illnesses (68). Various methodological limitations make the results of this study difficult to interpret. Only half the sample completed a standardized self-report measure of PTSD, and this measure was included in the results after four weeks of treatment, which is not likely an adequate duration in order to assess response. The study also included a heterogeneous population, including different subtypes of PTSD (i.e., hallucinatory versus nonhalucinatory PTSD) and significant comorbidity (i.e., comorbid bipolar disorder), and used topiramate as both adjunctive and monotherapy.

In an effort to address some of these methodological limitation, this study was replicated in a sample of 33 consecutive civilians with PTSD, where halluci-nations were excluded, treatment lasted up to 12 weeks, and the PCL-C was used to assess all patients (69). Topiramate was administered as either monotherapy ($N = 5$) or adjunctive treatment ($N = 28$) in flexible doses and response was measured after four weeks. Results revealed a mean reduction in the PCL-C score of 49% ($p < 0.001$) and a response rate of 77% at week 4. The median time to respond was nine days, and the mean dose for those reporting a full response was 60 mg/day $\pm$ 47. By week 4, 94% of patients with nightmares and 79% of patients with intrusions at baseline reported complete cessation of their symptoms. These results are quite promising but should be interpreted with caution given the open-label design and that the monotherapy and augmentation group data are presented together (69).

Topiramate monotherapy has been evaluated in two controlled studies of PTSD. In the first, Tucker et al. (70) randomized 38 patients with noncombat-related PTSD to flexible doses of topiramate (median dose 150 mg/day, range 25–400 mg/day) or placebo for 12 weeks. No significant difference was found on the primary efficacy measure of change from baseline in the total Clinician-Administered PTSD Scale (CAPS) score (71). However, significant effects on sec-ondary outcome measures were found in favor of topiramate on the Treatment Outcome PTSD scale (TOP-8) (decrease in overall severity 68% vs. 41.6%, $p = 0.025$) and end point CGI-I scores (1.9 ± 1.2 vs. 2.6 ± 1.1, $p = 0.055$). In the second study (72), 40 veterans with PTSD were randomized to 12 weeks of topiramate or placebo. Topiramate was found to be superior on the CGI-I at weeks 6 and 8 ($p = 0.021$) as well as on the CAPS-D (hyperarousal) subscale change from baseline ($p = 0.019$).

No significant differences were found in CAPS total score, TOP 8, or other symptom severity measures.

In short, there is some evidence to indicate the helpfulness of topiramate in treating PTSD symptoms. However, available results do not show overall efficacy based on primary PTSD outcome measures. Further placebo-controlled trials that either specifically utilize monotherapy or adjunctive therapy with more homogeneous samples would allow for a better evaluation of the usefulness of topiramate in PTSD.

Gabapentin

Case reports have described the successful treatment of PTSD with gabapentin (73,74). Brannon et al. reported a reduction in nightmares and anxiety in patients suffering from PTSD and comorbid depression treated with gabapentin 1200 mg/day (73). Hamner et al. (74) conducted a retrospective chart review of 30 patients with PTSD who were treated with adjunctive gabapentin. Sixty-seven percent of patients had comorbid major depressive disorder. In nearly every case gabapentin was added to target sleep disturbance symptoms associated with PTSD. It was found that 77% of patients demonstrated "moderate" or "marked" improvements in sleep duration, as well as a decrease in the frequency of nightmares. The most common adverse events were sedation and mild dizziness (74). The results of this study should be interpreted with caution, given its retrospective nature as well as the inclusion of patients receiving multiple concomitant sedating medications. Controlled research is needed to evaluate the efficacy of gabapentin in treating the core symptoms of PTSD, as well as its usefulness as an adjunctive agent to treat nightmares and insomnia.

Valproate

Open-label data thus suggest valproate may be helpful in PTSD, but there are conflicting reports regarding its effectiveness in treating all of the core-symptom clusters of PTSD.

Symanski and Olympia (75) recorded two cases demonstrating improvements in PTSD with valproate treatment of 1000 mg/day and 1500 mg/day respectively, showing prominent reductions in irritability. In an open-trial, Fesler (76) treated 16 Vietnam veterans with valproate (mean dose = 109.3 mg/day) for one year. The majority of patients experienced significant improvements in hyperarousal and avoidant symptoms; however, little improvement was found in re-experiencing or intrusive symptoms. Gastrointestinal complaints were the most common adverse events and included abdominal cramps, indigestion, nausea, and constipation. In another study, 16 veteran outpatients with PTSD were prescribed valproate alone or adjunctively (mean dose of 1,365 mg/day) for eight weeks. Three patients dropped out because of adverse events. Of the 13 patients who completed the trial, 11 were considered responders, defined by a CGI-I less than or equal to 2. Significant improvement was also found on the CAPS total score, on the CAPS subscale scores of intrusion and hyperarousal, and on the HAM-A and Hamilton Depression Scale (HAM-D) scale scores (77). Another open-label trial of 21 patients with combat-induced PTSD treated with valproate (mean dose = 1840 mg/day) found similar results (78). Reduction was measured in all three symptom clusters using the CAPS. Six patients discontinued valproate because of intolerable side effects including rash, diarrhea, and nausea.

In a retrospective chart analysis, a sample of 325 veterans was identified through a computerized search as having both a PTSD diagnosis and having had treatment with any form of valproate (79). Fifty patients met eligibility criteria; three were treated with valproate monotherapy and 47 were treated adjunctively with a variety of psychotropic agents. The primary outcome measures were CGI-I and change in baseline CGI-S as scored by raters who were blinded to the order of visits, medication names and doses, and serum valproic acid levels. The mean valproate dose was 1070 ± 455 mg/day. Twenty-five patients (50%) were rated as very much or much improved on the CGI-I. The improved end point CGI-I differed significantly from "no change" ($p < 0.000001$). The change in CGI-S ratings differed significantly from 0, but the average change was not considered large. Patients treated in primary care had a greater improvement compared with those in the mental health setting ($p < 0.005$). Valproate dosage and serum valproic acid levels ($N = 37$) were well correlated ($r = 0.57$, $p < 0.0005$). The authors concluded that valproate treatment improves the global clinical function of veterans with PTSD.

In a more recent open-trial (80), however, valproate was not found to be effective in noncombat related PTSD. In a trial of 10 patients with PTSD related to accidents, witnessing the death of a loved one, and sexual or physical abuse, valproate monotherapy was initiated at 250 mg/day and increased up to 2000 mg/day (mean dose = 1400 ± 380 mg/day). No improvements were found in PTSD or depressive symptoms using the Posttraumatic Diagnostic Scale (PDS), the Impact of Event Scale-Revised (IES-R), and the Beck Depression Inventory (BDI), after four and eight weeks of treatment.

In a recently reported randomized controlled trial of valproate monotherapy, 86 Vietnam veterans (98% male; 95% had combat-related trauma) with a mean duration of illness of 28 years were randomized to valproate or placebo (81). No significant differences were found in the CAPS total score or in scores on the CAPS-B (re-experiencing), CAPS-D (hyperarousal), TOP-8, CGI-I, or HAM-A scales. Significant improvement was found in the reduction of CAPS-C (avoidance) and Montgomery Åsberg Depression Rating Scale (MADRS) scores as well as on symptoms of avoidance. The authors concluded that valproate was ineffective in treating PTSD in an older, male veteran population (81).

Tiagabine

Open-label studies have suggested adjunctive tiagabine may be helpful in some PTSD symptoms. An open-label case series conducted by Lara (82) examined the use of tiagabine to augment antidepressant therapy in PTSD. Six patients were included in the case series; two with comorbid bipolar depression and four with comorbid major depression. Patients started tiagabine at 2 to 4 mg/day, increasing to a maximum of 16 mg/day. Significant reduction in anxiety was found after one week of therapy, and the effect was maintained at six weeks, as measured by the change in the baseline score of the Davidson Trauma Scale (DTS) (82). Aggression levels were also significantly reduced. Similar success in treating one patient with PTSD and comorbid major depression with adjunctive tiagabine was reported by Berigan (83). In this case report, a reduction of re-experiencing symptoms was accredited to the addition of tiagabine. In addition, an open-label trial found positive results using tiagabine (mean dose = 7.3 mg/day) in six (86%) of the seven patients evaluated using the PCL-C ($p < 0.05$) (84). Of the six patients whose symptoms improved, five had an end point CGI-I score of less than or equal to 2.

Two controlled studies, however, do not support the efficacy of tiagabine monotherapy in PTSD. Davidson and et al. (85) examined the efficacy of tiagabine in PTSD utilizing a 12-week open-label phase followed by a double-blind randomization of patients who completed the open-label phase to either tiagabine continuation or switching to placebo after tapering off tiagabine for an additional 12-weeks. In the ITT sample of the open phase ($N = 26$) of tiagabine (mean dose 12.8 ± 4.3 mg/day), significant improvements were observed in all measures of PTSD, depression, general anxiety, social anxiety, resilience, and disability. After the double-blind, placebo-controlled discontinuation phase ($N = 18$), there were no significant differences between the two groups, with gains being maintained on all outcomes (85).

Davidson et al. (86) recently reported a 12-week, randomized, multicenter, double-blind study of 232 patients with PTSD who were randomly assigned to treatment with tiagabine ($N = 116$) or placebo ($N = 116$). Tiagabine was initiated at 4 mg/day (2 mg b.i.d.) and individually titrated by 4 mg/day per week to a maximum dose of 16 mg/day. The mean dose of tiagabine at end point was 11.2 mg/day (range 2.0–16.0 mg/day); for placebo equivalent the mean dose was 11.8 mg/day (range 2.0–16.0 mg/day). Efficacy was assessed using the change from baseline in the total scores on the CAPS, DTS, and TOP-8. Additional assessments included the CGI-C, Connor-Davidson Resilience Scale, SDS, and a patient-rated evaluation of sleep (sleep questionnaire). There were no significant differences between treatment groups in change from baseline in the CAPS total score or on the other efficacy outcome measures. The authors concluded that tiagabine was not significantly different from placebo in the treatment of symptoms of PTSD.

Carbamazepine

Several open-label studies have suggested that carbamazepine may be a useful treatment for PTSD. Lipper et al. (87) reported that 7 of 10 patients who met DSM-III criteria for PTSD and a comorbid personality disorder were rated as "moderately" or "very much" improved on the CGI-I scale after treatment with carbamazepine (mean dose = 780 mg/day). Patients also demonstrated a reduction in the frequency and intensity of flashbacks, nightmares, and intrusive thoughts, as measured by interview-rated and self-report scales (87). Wolf et al. (88) described improvements in the clinical condition of 10 patients with PTSD treated with carbamazepine, as assessed by staff observations and self-report, with particular improvements in violent behavior. No standardized measures, were, however, used to assess symptom improvement. The use of carbamazepine (300–1200 mg/day) in a group of 28 sexually abused children, aged 8 to 17 years with PTSD including with comorbidity [e.g., attention deficit hyperactivity disorder (ADHD), depression, oppositional defiant disorder, and polysubstance abuse), has also been reported. Of the 28 patients, 22 became free of PTSD symptoms, while 6 patients reported infrequent abuse-related nightmares (89). No standardized measures were used. These studies support the potential use of carbamazepine in PTSD, but double-blind, placebo-controlled studies are needed.

Phenytoin

In a small open-label study examining the effects of phenytoin on memory, cognition, and brain structure in PTSD, nine adult male and female patients were treated with phenytoin for a three-month period (90). Treatment was started at

300 mg/day in three divided doses and increased to 400 mg/day if plasma levels were subtherapeutic. Plasma levels of phenytoin were measured at weeks 1, 2, 3, 4, 8, and 12, and dose was adjusted to be within the therapeutic range used in the treatment of epilepsy (10–20 mg/mL). Subjects underwent magnetic resonance imaging (MRI) for measurement of whole-brain and hippocampal volume, as well as neuropsychological testing of memory and cognition, before and after treatment. Subjects showed a significant improvement in PTSD symptoms with pheytoin treatment as measured by the CAPS, showing reductions in each of the symptom clusters of intrusions, avoidance, and hyperarousal ($p < 0.05$). No significant effects were found on HAM-D or HAM-A scores.

In a subsequent publication, neuropsychological testing revealed no significant changes in memory or cognition in this sample with phenytoin treatment (91). By contrast, phenytoin administration resulted in a significant 6% increase in right whole-brain volume as measured with volumetric MRI ($p < 0.05$), as well as a 5% nonsignificant increase in right hippocampal volume. Moreover, there were significant correlations between increases in hippocampal volume and reduction of PTSD symptoms as measured with the CAPS for the intrusion cluster for both the left ($r = -0.70$, df $= 8$, $p = 0.037$) and right ($r = -0.73$, df $= 8$, $p = 0.026$) hippocampus, and for the hyperarousal cluster for right ($r = -0.70$, df $= 8$, $p = 0.048$) hippocampal volume. Correlations with total CAPS score were not significant. There was no correlation between changes in whole-brain volumes and improvements on the CAPS.

This study suggests that phenytoin may be an effective treatment for PTSD and may also be associated with changes in brain structure, particularly in right whole-brain volume. This study further indicates that medications used in the treatment of neurological and psychiatric disorders may have effects on the brain that were previously unanticipated. Of note, the mechanism by which phenytoin may affect brain structure in PTSD is not fully understood and requires further investigation.

Vigabatrin

A series of five PTSD cases augmented with vigabatrin has been reported. Vigabatrin, 250 mg to 500 mg at bedtime, was introduced to treat hypervigilance and startle which had not improved with other treatments. All five patients tolerated vigabatrin well and had a rapid amelioration of their exaggerated startle responses. No changes were found in other PTSD symptoms (92).

Oxcarbazepine

Two case reports have described improvements in PTSD symptoms with oxcarbazepine augmentation. One report describes the case of a 46-year-old man with chronic PTSD who had been unresponsive or intolerant to numerous pharmacological treatments including carbamazepine and valproate. The patient was augmented with 300 mg/day of oxcarbazepine, titrated up to 900 mg/day, along with 150 mg/day of sertraline and 0.5 mg/day of clonazepam. The patient reported experiencing less frequent and severe nightmares, as well as improvements in all areas of functioning. Gains were maintained at four-month follow-up (93). In another case report, a 38-year-old woman with PTSD and bipolar disorder who had partially responded to carbamazepine was treated with oxcarbazepine. Within a month of initiation of oxcarbazepine, she reported progressive improvement in her

PTSD symptoms. As oxcarbazepine monotherapy 750 mg b.i.d. continued, she reported significant reduction of her PTSD symptoms and stabilization of her mood without adverse effects (94).

Levetiracetam

Kinrys et al. (95) recently reported a retrospective analysis of 23 patients with DSM-IV diagnoses of PTSD who, after being deemed inadequate responders to antidepressant therapy, received adjunctive levetiracetam in a naturalistic fashion. Existing medication regimes were supplemented with a starting dose of 250 mg of levetiracetam at bedtime with a weekly dose escalation of 250 to 500 mg. The target dosage range was 1000 to 3000 mg/day given in a b.i.d. or nightly regimen, on the basis of each patient's individual response and tolerability to the drug. The primary outcome measure was the PCL-C and secondary efficacy measures included the HAM-D, CGI-S, and CGI-I. Significant improvement was found on all measures ($p < 0.001$). Thirteen (56%) patients met responder criteria at end point, as defined by PCL-C mean change $= 23.5$ and CGI-I score less than 2. Six (26%) patients met remission criteria (final CGI-S score <2). Adverse events were generally mild, and no patient stopped levetiracetam therapy because of side effects. This study indicates levetiracetam may be an effective treatment in combination with antidepressant therapy for patients with PTSD who remain symptomatic after initial intervention, but needs to be confirmed by double-blind, placebo-controlled trials.

PANIC DISORDER

Panic disorder is characterized by recurrent, unexpected panic attacks, defined as discrete periods of intense anxiety and feelings of fearfulness, terror, and often impending doom. There is persistent concern regarding future panic attacks and their consequences and the panic attacks may lead to agoraphobic avoidance. Typically avoided situations include being outside the home alone, being in a crowd, being on a bridge, or traveling in a bus, train, or automobile (31).

Tricyclic antidepressants and MAOIs were among the first pharmacological agents shown to be efficacious in the treatment of panic disorder (96–98). Currently, benzodiazepines (99–110), SSRIs (111–115), and SNRIs (116–119), either alone or in combination, are used as standard treatments for panic disorder. Among the SSRIs, fluoxetine (114,120–122), fluvoxamine (123–131) paroxetine, sertraline (132–135), citalopram (136), and escitalopram (136) have all been demonstrated efficacious in randomized clinical trials.

Gabapentin

Successful treatment of panic disorder with gabapentin has been described in case reports (17). In the only double-blind, placebo-controlled study published to date (137), Pande et al. randomly assigned 103 patients with panic disorder to gabapentin (600–3600 mg/day) or placebo for eight weeks. Although the difference in symptom severity, as measured by the Panic and Agoraphobia Scale (PAS), was insignificant between the drug and placebo groups for the entire patient sample, a significant improvement was found in an analysis of a severely ill subsample (those with a PAS baseline ≥ 20; $p = 0.04$) (137). However, no significant difference in rate of responders was found between drug and placebo in those with a baseline PAS of 20 or more (37% gabapentin versus 26.9% placebo $p = 0.437$), or between those with a baseline PAS less than 20 (45% gabapentin versus 66.7% placebo $p = 0.223$). Twelve percent of the gabapentin group discontinued the study due to adverse events compared with 4% of the placebo group (137). Common adverse events included somnolence, headache, and dizziness. Given this negative result, gabapentin should probably be reserved for use as an adjunctive therapy or for treatment nonresponders to standard therapies.

Valproate

The antipanic effects of valproate have been described in several case reports, which have included documenting the successful treatment of panic disorder with comorbid alcoholism (138), substance abuse (139), benzodiazepine withdrawal (140), and multiple sclerosis (141). A case series by Ontiveros and Fountaine (142) described the improvement of four patients with treatment-resistant panic disorder using a combination of valproate and clonazepam.

Further support for the effectiveness of valproate in treating panic disorder has come from open-label studies. Primeau et al. (143) conducted an open trial in 10 patients with panic disorder or agoraphobia with panic attacks. Patients were treated with valproate for seven weeks with an initial dose of 500 mg/day that was increased to a maximum of 2,250 mg/day. Significant improvements were noted for both panic and anxiety symptoms. Similar results were found in a six-week open-label study of valproate in 12 patients with panic disorder conducted by Woodman and Noyles (144). All 12 patients demonstrated moderate or marked improvement after the six-week trial, and the improvements gained were sustained at six-month and 18-month follow-up. Other open-trials have demonstrated the ability of valproate to block lactate-induced panic attacks (145) and to treat patients with panic disorder and mood instability resistant to conventional therapy (146).

In the only controlled study of valproate in panic disorder, Lum et al. (147) treated 12 patients in a double-blind, placebo-controlled, 2×2 crossover design with doses achieving a plasma valproic acid level between 60 and 120 mg/mL. Significant improvements in the valproate group as compared with the placebo group were noted on the CGI-S and CGI-I scales, with marked reductions in the length and intensity of panic attacks, as well as a decrease in psychic and somatic symptoms of anxiety as measured by the HAM-A scale. Five patients reported adverse events while taking valproate, which included gastrointestinal discomfort, dizziness, and somnolence (147). These preliminary results suggest that VPA may be an effective treatment for panic disorder that demonstrates a long-term effect. Larger placebo-controlled trials with long-term follow-up, however, are needed to confirm these findings.

Tiagabine

In an open-trial of five patients with panic disorder, including with comorbidity, Gruener (148) reported improvement with tiagabine (20 mg/day). Anxiety was significantly reduced in all patients at two weeks, and improvement was maintained for the entire eight-week treatment period. Similar success was found in a case series of four patients treated with tiagabine, where reductions in anxiety, agoraphobia, and panic attacks were noted (149).

Tiagabine has also been reported to reduce cholecystokinin-tetrapeptide (CCK-4)-induced panic in healthy subjects. Zwanzger et al. (150) administered

15 mg/day of tiagabine to 15 healthy volunteers for seven days. A CCK-4 challenge was given before and after the one-week treatment. A significant reduction in panic was found after the second CCK-4 challenged. A significant decrease in heart rate was also found after tiagabine treatment; however, adrenocorticotropic hormone (ACTH) and cortisol concentrations did not change.

These small studies suggest a potential antipanic effect of tiagabine. The efficacy and tolerability of this agent in panic disorder, however, must be determined with large scale double-blind, placebo-controlled trials.

Carbamazepine

The use of carbamazepine in patients with panic disorder and benzodiazepine withdrawal has suggested that carbamazepine may have antipanic effects (151). In an open trial by Tondo et al. (152), 34 patients with panic disorder with or without agoraphobia were treated with carbamazepine at a mean dose of 419 mg/day for 2 to 12 months. Patients' response was rated as "absent/scarce" or "good" on the basis of a global rating of frequency of panic attacks, degree of avoidance behavior, and adaptive functioning. Using these criteria, 20(58%) patients were rated as having a good response to medication (152).

However, in a controlled study of 14 patients with panic disorder conducted by Uhde et al. (152,153), carbamazepine was not effective. Carbamazepine treatment did not result in a significant change on any outcome measure. Forty percent of patients had a decrease in the frequency of panic attacks, 50% had an increase in panic attack frequency, and 10% demonstrated no change. Neither EEG abnormalities nor prominent psychosensory symptoms in this study predicted response to carbamazepine.

Phenytoin

McNamara and Fogel (154) described three patients who experienced a complete cessation of panic attacks with phenytoin treatment. These patients also had abnormal temporal lobe EEG patterns, comparable to interictal temporal lobe epilepsy. It is unclear whether these observations can be applied to individuals with panic disorder, as it is highly unusual for panic disorder patients to have EEG abnormalities.

Levetiracetam

A recent open-label, fixed-flexible dose study was conducted in two outpatient clinics where 18 patients with panic disorder with or without agoraphobia were treated with levetiracetam for 12 weeks (155). The mean daily dose of levetiracetam during the last two weeks of the study was 1138 mg ($\pm$627 mg; range 306 mg–2386 mg). Participants showed significant improvement on the primary efficacy measure of the CGI-S with mean scores decreasing from 4.8 ($\pm$0 0.4) to 2.7 ($\pm$1.1) ($t = 6.5$; df = 16; $p < 0.00$). Panic attack frequency decreased from 2.9 ($\pm$0.8) to 1.2 ($\pm$1.2) ($t = 5.9$; df = 12; $p < 0.00$) on the Agoraphobia, Avoidance Behavior Scale (item B of the PAS), and the mean HAM-A score decreased from 23.4 ($\pm$5.6) to 7.6 ($\pm$5.9) ($t = 8.9$; df = 12; $p < 0.00$). This small open-label study suggests levetiracetam may have anxiolytic effects in panic disorder, but needs to be confirmed in large double-blind, placebo-controlled studies.

Vigabatrin

Zwanzger et al. (156) reported successful vigabatrin treatment in three patients meeting DSM-IV criteria for panic disorder. After a medication-free period of at least two weeks, patients received vigabatrin at a daily dose of 2 g for six months. All patients showed a marked reduction in anxiety on the HAM-A and clear improvement in agoraphobia on the PAS after two weeks. Maximal effects of vigabatrin on anxiety as assessed by the HAM-A and PAS were observed within 4 weeks of treatment. In addition, the anxiolytic effect of vigabatrin was maintained during subsequent therapy throughout the next six months, with the occurrence of very few panic attacks.

Similar results were shown in 10 healthy volunteers who received vigabatrin 2 g per day for seven days after placebo-controlled administration of 50 μg of CCK-4 to induce panic symptoms (157). Panic symptom severity was evaluated with the Acute Panic Inventory (API) and a DSM-IV derived panic-symptom scale (PSS). Additionally, a 100-mm visual analogue scale (VAS) was used for evaluation of subjective anxiety. All subjects reported a marked reduction of CCK-4–induced panic and anxiety symptoms after one week of vigabatrin treatment. Compared with the first CCK-4 challenge, the number of reported PSS symptoms decreased by 50% from 9.4 ± 0.9 (range 5–13) to 4.7 ± 1.0 (range 0–6) after vigabatrin treatment ($F(1,9) = 45.08$, $p < 0.001$). PSS sumscores decreased by 54% from 19.7 ± 2.8 (range 3–31) to 9 ± 2.2 (range 0–25) ($F(1,9) = 9.2$, $p < 0.014$). The mean API sumscore decreased significantly by 45% from 24.0 ± 3.3 (range 10–38) to 13.2 ± 3.5 (range 0–42) ($F(1,9) = 18.96$, $p < 0.002$). Moreover, subjects reported a significant reduction of VAS-scores for anxiety from 52.0 ± 6.6 (range 30–90) to 26.5 ± 5.7 (range 0–60) ($F(1,9) = 9.56$, $p < 0.013$).

GENERALIZED ANXIETY DISORDER

Generalized anxiety disorder (GAD) is characterized by excessive and uncontrollable anxiety and worry that has been present for at least six months. The anxiety and worry is centered on a number of day to day life events, including family life, work, health and finances, and is associated with feelings of restlessness, feeling on edge, being easily tired, poor concentration, irritability, muscle tension, and sleep problems (31).

A wide spectrum of drug classes has been shown to be efficacious in the treatment of GAD. Benzodiazepines (158–167) have demonstrated safety and efficacy in more placebo-controlled trials then any other medication, but rebound and withdrawal symptoms as well as lack of efficacy in common comorbid conditions have limited their use (168). Other efficacious medications include the tricyclic imipramine (169–172), buspirone (158,164,173–176), the SSRIs, paroxetine (170,177–179), escitalopram (85,180–182), and sertraline (179,183,184), the SNRI venlafaxine (158,170,174,185–188), and the antihistamine hydroxyzine (162,176).

Gabapentin

Two case reports have described improvements in patients with GAD following the addition of gabapentin (189). Improvements in both anxiety and arousal were noted.

Pregabalin

To date, at least seven double-blind, placebo-controlled studies have demonstrated the efficacy of pregabalin in GAD. Pande et al. (190) compared the effectiveness and tolerability of pregabalin in treating GAD to that of lorazepam and a placebo. Two hundred and seventy-six patients were randomly assigned to one of four treatment groups: pregabalin 150 mg/day ($N = 69$), pregabalin 600 mg/day ($N = 70$), lorazepam 6 mg/day ($N = 68$), and placebo ($N = 69$). Significant improvements from baseline to end point were found on the HAM-A for all active treatment groups, with the high-dose pregabalin and lorazepam groups demonstrating similar anxiolytic effects. There were also significantly more responders ($\geq 50\%$ decrease in HAM-A) in patients receiving pregabalin 600 mg/day (46%) and lorazepam 6 mg/day (61%) than in those given placebo (27%). Although the side effects of pregabalin and lorazepam were similar, those in the pregabalin treatment group found the side effects more tolerable. The most common side effects for both treatments were dizziness (38.6% for 600 mg/day pregabalin and 13.2.3% for 6 mg/day lorazepam) and somnolence (35.7% for 600 mg/day pregabalin and 54.4% for 6 mg/day lorazepam). Only the lorazepam group demonstrated significantly more withdrawal effects then placebo (191).

In a double-blind, fixed-dose, placebo- and active-controlled study, Feltner et al. (163) randomized 271 patients to receive pregabalin 50 mg t.i.d. ($N = 70$), pregabalin 200 mg t.i.d. ($N = 66$), placebo ($N = 67$), or lorazepam 2 mg t.i.d. ($N = 68$) for four weeks. Adjusted mean change scores on the HAM-A (primary outcome measure) were significantly improved for pregabalin 200 mg t.i.d. [difference of 3.90 between drug and placebo; $p \leq 0.0013$ analysis of covariance (ANCOVA), df $= 252$] and for lorazepam [difference of 2.35; $p \leq 0.0483$ (ANCOVA), df $= 252$], with the significant difference between the pregabalin 200 mg t.i.d. and placebo groups seen at week 1 of treatment [$p \leq 0.0001$ (ANCOVA), df $= 238$].

Similar results were found in another double-blind, placebo-controlled, active comparator trial, where patients were randomized to four weeks of treatment with pregabalin 300 mg/day ($N = 91$), 450 mg/day ($N = 90$), or 600 mg/day ($N = 89$); alprazolam 1.5 mg/day ($N = 93$); or placebo ($N = 91$) (161). The end point response criterion was a 50% or greater reduction in the baseline HAM-A total score. Study drug was administered in divided doses using a t.i.d. schedule. Pregabalin and alprazolam produced a significantly greater reduction in mean $\pm$ SE HAM-A total score at LOCF end point compared with placebo: pregabalin 300 mg/day (-12.2 ± 0.8, $p < 0.001$), 450 mg/day (-11.0 ± 0.8, $p = 0.02$), and 600 mg/day (-11.8 ± 0.8, $p = 0.002$); alprazolam (-10.9 ± 0.8, $p = 0.02$); and placebo (-8.4 ± 0.8). By week 1 and at LOCF end point, the three pregabalin groups and the alprazolam group had significantly ($p < 0.01$) improved HAM-A psychic anxiety symptoms compared with the placebo group. HAM-A somatic anxiety symptoms were also significantly ($p < 0.02$) improved in the 300 and 600 mg/day pregabalin groups, but not in the 450 mg/day pregabalin (week 1, $p = 0.06$; week 4, $p = 0.32$) and the alprazolam groups (week 1, $p = 0.21$; week 4, $p = 0.15$), as compared with placebo. Of the five treatment groups, the 300 mg/day pregabalin group was the only medication group that differed statistically in global improvement at treatment end point, not only from the placebo group, but also from the alprazolam group.

Pohl et al. (191) evaluated the anxiolytic efficacy of b.i.d. versus t.i.d. dosing of pregabalin in patients with GAD. Outpatients with GAD were randomized to six weeks of double-blind treatment with pregabalin 200 mg/day (b.i.d.; $N = 78$), 400 mg/day (b.i.d.; $N = 89$), 450 mg/day (t.i.d.; $N = 88$), or placebo ($N = 86$). Mean improvement in end point HAM-A total score was significantly greater for pregabalin 200 mg/day ($p = 0.006$), 400 mg/day ($p = 0.001$), and 450 mg/day ($p = 0.005$) compared with placebo (LOCF). Pairwise comparisons of b.i.d. with t.i.d. dosing found no difference in HAM-A change score at end point. Improvement on both psychic and somatic factors of the HAM-A was rapid: significance versus placebo was achieved as early as the first assessment at week 1, with 30% or more reduction in HAM-A severity and equal or greater improvement for every subsequent visit in 38% or more patients in all three pregabalin dosage groups ($p \leq 0.001$). This study showed similar efficacy and comparable tolerability of pregabalin in GAD with b.i.d. and t.i.d. dosing.

Montgomery et al. (192) showed that pregabalin was safe, well tolerated, and rapidly efficacious across both the physical-somatic and emotional symptoms of GAD in a six-week, multicenter, randomized, double-blind, placebo-controlled comparison of pregabalin and venlafaxine. Outpatients ($N = 421$) were randomly assigned to pregabalin 400 or 600 mg/day, venlafaxine 75 mg/day, or placebo. Pregabalin at both dosages (400 mg/day, $p = 0.008$; 600 mg/day, $p = 0.03$) and venlafaxine ($p = 0.03$) produced significantly greater improvement in HAM-A total scores at LOCF end point than did placebo. Only the pregabalin 400-mg/day treatment group experienced significant improvement in all a priori primary and secondary efficacy measures. Pregabalin in both dosage treatment groups (400 mg/day, $p < 0.01$; 600 mg/day, $p < 0.001$) significantly improved HAM-A total scores at week 1, with significant improvement through LOCF end point. Statistically significant improvement began at week 2 for venlafaxine.

Khan et al. (193) evaluated the efficacy of pregabalin 150 to 600 mg/day in the elderly ($N = 277$) in an eight-week, multicenter, randomized, placebo-controlled, double-blind, parallel-group study. Patients were 65 years and older. On the primary outcome measure (change from baseline in HAM-A least squares mean total score), pregabalin-treated patients achieved a significantly greater reduction at LOCF end point than did patients who received placebo (–12.84 vs. –10.65; $p = 0.0437$). A significant reduction from baseline in mean HAM-A total score was found in favor of pregabalin at weeks 2 ($p = 0.0052$), 4 ($p = 0.0043$), 6 ($p = 0.0011$), and 8 ($p = 0.0070$). Significantly, more pregabalin-treated patients were responders at week 4 (defined as a $\geq 50\%$ reduction in HAM-A total score) (49.3% vs. 32.9%, $p < 0.05$) and over half of pregabalin-treated patients were responders at week 8, with results approaching significance (52.6% vs. 41.1%, $p \leq 0.07$). The most common side effects among pregabalin-treated patients were dizziness (20%), somnolence (13%), headache (10%), and nausea (9%). The authors concluded that pregabalin was a safe and effective treatment of GAD in an elderly population.

Finally, the long-term efficacy of pregabalin in GAD was investigated by Smith, et al. in a treatment-discontinuation study (194). Six hundred twenty-four adult patients with DSM-IV GAD and a mean HAM-A score of 25.2 received open-label pregabalin 150 mg t.i.d. for eight weeks. Responders who had a HAM-A score of 11 or less for the weeks 7 and 8, visits were then randomized to double-blind treatment with either pregabalin ($N = 168$) or placebo ($N = 170$) for an additional 26 weeks. The primary efficacy parameter was time to relapse, defined as either: (1) a HAM-A of 20 or more and a diagnosis of GAD at two successive visits one week apart; (2) a CGI-I rated "much worse" or "very much worse" and a diagnosis of GAD at two successive visits one week apart; or (3) symptomatic worsening of anxiety which required clinical intervention. There was a significant difference between pregabalin and placebo in time to relapse ($p = 0.0001$). Significantly, more pregabalin-treated patients maintained efficacy through the double-blind period (defined as an end point CGI-I ≤ 5) as compared with placebo-treated patients (pregabalin 57.1%, placebo 36.5%; $p = 0.001$). Statistical significance in favor of pregabalin was also demonstrated on the HAM-A and the SDS (both total and individual subscale scores). Pregabalin was well tolerated, with no unexpected adverse events occurring during the eight months of the study. The results of this study clearly demonstrate the efficacy of pregabalin for the prevention of relapse of GAD during long-term treatment.

These positive, large-scale, placebo-controlled trials of pregabalin in GAD make pregabalin a new treatment alternative for GAD. Further study of its ability to treat commonly comorbid conditions, such as depressive symptoms, would allow for a better understand of its role in treating GAD, whether as a first-line agent or a strategy reserved for treatment-resistant cases, patients who cannot tolerate antidepressants, or patients for whom benzodiazepines are not indicated.

Tiagabine

There are two published case series examining tiagabine augmentation in the treatment of GAD (148,195). Five patients with GAD and comorbid major depression and/or neuropathic pain received tiagabine 6 mg/day. (148). After two weeks of tiagabine, a significant reduction in HAM-A score was found that was maintained for the eight-week treatment trial. Tiagabine was generally well tolerated. In a case series of five treatment-refractory patients (4 with GAD and 1 with major depressive and severe anxiety due to antidepressant withdrawal), tiagabine in 1-mg incremental doses was initiated either as a monotherapy or adjunctive treatment (195). Tiagabine improved anxiety and was well tolerated by all patients, including the patient with anxiety secondary to acute antidepressant withdrawal.

Similar findings were reported by Papp and Ray (196) using a mean dose of 9 mg/day of tiagabine in an eight-week treatment trial of 25 patients with GAD. Seven (37%) patients rated as much or very much improved by the CGI-I. Six (24%) patients withdrew because of adverse events, which included abnormal thinking, nausea, amnesia, anemia, asthenia, colitis, diarrhea, hallucinations, headache, migraine, and somnolence.

Rosenthal and Dolnak (197) conducted a 10-week, open-label, blind rater study of 40 patients randomized to tiagabine or paroxetine. Tiagabine and paroxetine significantly reduced measures of anxiety and depression, along with improving sleep and overall functioning. Forty percent of the tiagabine group was considered responders (defined as a ≥50% decrease in baseline HAM-A scores) compared with 60% of the paroxetine group. In both groups, 20% of patients achieved remission (defined as an end point HAM-A score ≤7). Both treatments where well tolerated, with one patient withdrawing due to adverse events while taking tiagabine and two withdrawing while taking paroxetine (197).

A recently completed double-blind, placebo-controlled trial examined tiagabine monotherapy in the treatment of GAD (198). Two hundred seventy-two patients were randomized to tiagabine ($N = 134$) (mean dose 10.5 mg/day) or placebo ($N = 132$) for eight weeks. In those who completed the trial ($N = 198$), there was a significant reduction in the primary outcome measure (HAM-A) favoring tiagabine; however, in the ITT analysis the difference did not reach statistical significance. Fifty-seven percent of patients in the tiagabine group were considered responders (much or very much improved on the CGI-I), compared with 44% of the placebo group ($p = 0.08$). Tiagabine reduced GAD symptoms according to the observed case and mixed models repeated-measures (MMRM) analyses but not the primary LOCF analysis. In a post hoc MMRM analysis, a significant difference in the mean reduction in HAM-A total score over the efficacy evaluation period was found, favoring tiagabine over placebo ($p < 0.01$). Tiagabine had an early onset of effect, as shown by significant reduction from baseline in mean HAM-A total score compared with placebo at week 1 (observed cases, $p < 0.05$). Tiagabine was generally well tolerated with dizziness, headache, and nausea as the most common adverse events. Although tiagabine did not separate from placebo in the ITT analysis, the improvements seen in the observed case and MMRM analyses suggest that tiagabine may reduce symptoms in GAD. Further placebo-controlled studies have been completed but results are not yet available. Once these results become available, we will be better able to ascertain the role of tiagabine in the treatment of GAD.

Levetiracetam

One case report has described the adjunctive use of levetiracetam in GAD. Levetiracetam 250 mg/day was added to citalopram in a 42-year-old female with GAD. Levetiracetam was associated with reduced anxiety after four days with sustained improvement at six months (199).

OBSESSIVE-COMPULSIVE DISORDER

OCD is characterized by persistent, intrusive thoughts and/or images (obsessions), and repetitive, ritualistic behaviors that the individual feels he or she must complete (compulsions) (31).

SSRIs are considered the gold standard treatment for OCD. Paroxetine (200–202), fluoxetine (203–208), citalopram (209,210), fluvoxamine (205,207,208, 211–213), sertraline (204,205,207,208,214–216) and escitalopram (217) have all demonstrated efficacy in placebo-controlled trials. Other agents shown to demonstrate efficacy are clomipramine (205,207,208,217–220) and the MAOI phenelzine (221). In treatment-resistant cases, placebo-controlled trials support the augmenting of an SSRI with haloperidol (222), pindolol (223), risperidone (224), quetiapine, (225), and olanzapine. (226) As OCD is a chronic and disabling condition, a continued search for treatment possibilities for partial responders and refractory patients is necessary.

Gabapentin

Cora-Locatelli et al. (227) described the use of gabapentin in the treatment of five patients with OCD who were partial responders to fluoxetine. Gabapentin (mean dose = 2520 mg/day) and fluoxetine (mean dose = 68 mg/day) were taken simultaneously for six weeks and the combination was relatively well tolerated. All patients demonstrated improvements in anxiety, obsessive-compulsive symptoms, sleep, and mood on the basis of clinical evaluations. However, patients experienced a rebound of psychiatric symptoms once gabapentin was discontinued (228).

Valproate

The use of valproate in treating OCD has been documented only in patients who have ceased treatment of conventional antiobsessional medication because of side effects such as anxiety, irritability, confusion, psychosis, and other cognitive impairments (229,230). Deltito (229) described the use of valproate in 10 patients with OCD who discontinued the use of medications including clomipramine, fluoxetine, sertraline, and paroxetine. Valproate was used as pretreatment, with an initial dose of 250 mg/day that was increased to a final dose of approximately 2500 mg/day. Treatment was then completed with the addition of typical anti-obsessional pharmacotherapy without the previously mentioned side effects. Successful outcomes, determined by clinical evaluation, were noted in 8 of the 10 patients. A case-report by Cora-Locatelli et al. (230) described the use of valproate 750 mg/day in combination with 1 mg/day fluoxetine. Both treatments were started at the same time and marked changes in Yale-Brown Obsessive-Compulsive Scale (Y-BOCS), HAM-A, and HAM-D scores were found. The authors discontinued the fluoxetine as they suspected valproate to be responsible for the improvement. The patients' symptoms continued to improve with valproate monotherapy.

Carbamazepine
Three reports have described the use of carbamazepine in OCD. In a case report, a 27-year-old woman with OCD receiving inpatient treatment with a combination of carbamazepine (500 mg/day) and clomipramine (200 mg/day) displayed significant improvements in anxiety, distress, and habitual checking that allowed her to be discharged from the hospital (231). Previous psychopharmacological treatments were not effective. In an open-label trial of four patients with OCD and temporal EEG abnormalities, improvement was demonstrated in only one patient (232). In a series of nine patients treated with carbamazepine (400 to 1600 mg/day), only one of the eight who completed the trial demonstrated any improvement (233). These preliminary finding suggest that carbamazepine is likely not an effective monotherapy for OCD; however, controlled investigations are need to adequately evaluate its efficacy.

Topiramate
To date, topiramate has been evaluated in one case report and 2 open-label trials in treatment-resistant OCD. The case report described a nine-week topiramate augmentation of paroxetine, where a significant change from baseline was found on the Y-BOCS and the CGI-I (234). In one of the open-label trials, Van Ameringen et al. (235) augmented 16 patients with topiramate (mean dose = 253.1 mg/day) for between 14 and 26 weeks. At end point, 11 (68.8%) patients were considered responders, defined as a CGI-I rating of much or very much improved. Significant improvement on the CGI-S scale was also found ($p < 0.001$). Most patients experienced one or more adverse event, which included weight loss, sedation/fatigue, paresthesia, and memory/word finding problems (235). In the other open-label trial, topiramate (mean dose of 237.5 ± 29.1 mg/day) was added to the serotonin reuptake inhibitor (SRI) of subjects with treatment-resistant OCD for 16 weeks (236). Significant changes from baseline were found in both of the primary outcome measures, the Y-BOCS ($p = 0.002$) and GAF scores ($p = 0.002$). Response, defined as an end point Y-BOCS score of less than 30% of the baseline score, was achieved by 86% of the sample. Weight loss, sedation, memory/word-finding difficulties, and paresthesias were the most common adverse events. These preliminary data may suggest a potential role for topiramate as an augmenting agent for treatment-resistant OCD, but they must be verified in double-blind, placebo-controlled trials.

Lamotrigine

There is one report of lamotrigine treatment for SRI-resistant OCD. Eight patients with an inadequate response to at least 200 mg/day of sertraline or 225 mg/day of clomipramine for a mean period of 14 weeks had lamotrigine added for at least four weeks up to a maximum dose of 100 mg/day. The SRI dose remained unchanged throughout the study period. No significant changes where found on the CGI-S or CGI-I scales. The mean baseline and end point Y-BOCS scores were 24.0 and 18.9, respectively (237). This small trial suggests that lamotrigine augmentation may not be a useful strategy for SRI-refractory OCD. However, given the potential effectiveness of topiramate, another agent with anti-glutamatergic properties, further evaluation of lamotrigine is warranted using the higher doses that are found to be effective in treating bipolar depression (238).

MIXED ANXIETY CONDITIONS

In this section, "mixed anxiety conditions" refers to studies that included patients with varying anxiety disorders.

Tiagabine

In a case series of 10 patients with an anxiety disorder or a comorbid anxiety condition considered refractory to previous antianxiety treatments, tiagabine was given as monotherapy ($N = 5$) or in combination with other medications ($N = 5$), including risperidone, citralopram, paroxetine, and clomipramine. Patients in the series had a primary diagnosis of GAD ($N = 5$), PTSD ($N = 1$), major depressive disorder ($N = 2$), bipolar disorder ($N = 1$), or schizophrenia ($N = 1$). All patients were rated as much improved or very much improved on the CGI-C scale after four weeks of tiagabine treatment, with most patients reporting marked improvement in anxiety after one week of treatment (239).

Schwartz et al. (240) conducted an eight-week open-trial of tiagabine augmentation in a sample of mixed anxiety disorders, including GAD, panic disorder, PTSD, and social phobia. Concomitant medications included SSRIs, venlafaxine, nefazodone, and alprazolam. Significant improvements from baseline in anxiety were found as measured by the HAM-A and the Beck Anxiety Inventory (BAI). At end point, 76% of patients were considered responders ($\geq$50% reduction in HAM-A), and 59% achieved remission (HAM-A total score $\leq$7).

These open trials of tiagabine in mixed anxiety disorders suggest tiagabine may have general anxiolytic effects. Conversely, the inclusion of multiple anxiety diagnoses and multiple concomitant medications significantly limits the conclusions that can be drawn from them. Moreover, placebo-controlled trials examining the efficacy of tiagabine as monotherapy and as combination therapy in individual anxiety disorders have not been robust and indicate that tiagabine may have moderate anxiolytic effects at best.

SUMMARY

A summary of the studies described in this chapter can be found in Table 1. In Table 2, we have included the level of evidence associated with each AED for each anxiety disorder. As detailed in the Canadian Clinical Practice Guidelines (241), levels of evidence are ranked from 1 to 4, which are as follows: (1) meta-analysis or

(text continues on page 126)

TABLE 1 Summary of Open and Controlled Trials of Anticonvulsants in Anxiety Disorders

Author(s) and yr (Ref.)	Drug	Disorder	Sample size	Design	Concomitant psychotropic medications	Outcomes	Adverse events
Van Ameringen et al., 2004 (40)	Topiramate (monotherapy)	Social phobia	23	Open trial		45.1% considered responders (CGI-I ≤ 2); 26.1% achieved remission (LSAS ≤ 30); significant decrease in LSAS	Somnolence
Pande et al., 1999 (42)	Gabapentin (monotherapy)	Social phobia	69	Double-blind, placebo-controlled trial		No significant difference in response (≥50% decrease on LSAS)	Nausea Somnolence Dizziness Fatigue
De-Paris et al., 2003 (43)	Gabapentin (monotherapy)	Social phobia	32	Open-label trial		Gabapentin at 800 mg > Gabapentin 400 mg (visual analogue mood scale item calm-excite)	Somnolence Dizziness Nausea Headaches
Pande et al., 2004 (44)	Pregabalin (monotherapy)	Social phobia	135	Double-blind, placebo-controlled trial		Significant decrease in LSAS in high-dose group (600 mg/day) Significantly more responders in high-dose group than placebo	Dizziness Somnolence Nausea Flatulence Decreased libido
Nardi et al., 1997 (44,45)	Valproic acid (monotherapy)	Social phobia	16	Open-label trial		All nonresponders	Rash, GI symptoms
Kinrys et al., 2003 (46)	Valproic acid (monotherapy)	Social phobia	17	Open-label trial		41.1% response by CGI-I	Sedation Headache Tremor GI discomfort Weight gain
Dunlop et al., 2007 (47)	Tiagabine (monotherapy)	Social phobia	54	Open-label trial		Significant reduction in LSAS and SPIN; 40.7% were responders (CGI-I ≤ 2) in the ITT sample	Somnolence Dizziness Insomnia Nausea

(Continued)

TABLE 1 Summary of Open and Controlled Trials of Anticonvulsants in Anxiety Disorders (*Continued*)

Author(s) and yr (Ref.)	Drug	Disorder	Sample size	Design	Concomitant psychotropic medications	Outcomes	Adverse events
Kinrys et al., 2004 (48)	Tiagabine (augmentation)	Treatment refractory social phobia	14	Retrospective analysis, open-label trial	SSRIs, quetiapine, clonazepam, bupropion	64.2% (9/14) met response criteria (CGI-I ≤ 2); 35.7% (5/14) met remission criteria (LSAS ≤ 30)	Sedation Tiredness Headaches
	Levetiracetam (monotherapy)	Social phobia	20	Open-label trial		Significant reduction in LSAS, CGI-S, HAM-A and HAM-D	Drowsiness Nervousness
Simon et al., 2004 (49)	Levetiracetam (monotherapy)	Social phobia	18	Double-blind, placebo-controlled pilot study		Levetiracetam = PBO Effect sizes of LEV (0.33) BSPS and 0.50 for the LSAS compared with PBO	Headaches Drowsiness Disinhibition Inebreation
Zhang et al., 2005 (50)	Lamotrigine (monotherapy)	PTSD	14	Double-blind, placebo-controlled trial		50% (5/10) of the lamotrigine group vs. 25% (1/4) of placebo group rated as "much" or "very much improved" on the DGRP	Dizziness Dry mouth Nausea Headache
Hertzberg et al., 1997 (66)	Topiramate (monotherapy and augmentation)	PTSD	33	Open-label trial	SSRIs, benzodiazepine, stimulants, atypical neuroleptics, gabapentin, lamotrigine, mirtazapine, venlafaxine, verapamil	Mean reduction in PCL-C of 49% ($p < 0.001$) and a response rate of 77% at wk 4.	Panic Nervousness Overstimulation Shakiness Clumsiness Cognitive impairment Severe headache
Berlant, 2004 (69)	Topiramate (monotherapy)	Noncombat related PTSD	38	Double-blind, placebo-controlled trial		Topiramate = PBO (CAPS—primary efficacy measure) Topiramate > PBO (TOP-8, = 0.025) Topiramate > PBO (end point CGI-I scores $p = 0.055$).	Headache Sinusitis Taste perversion Language problems Insomnia Dyspepsia Nervousness Fatigue Hypertension Difficulty with concentration/attention

Study	Drug	Condition	N	Design	Results	Side effects
Tucker et al., 2007 (70)	Topiramate (monotherapy)	Combat-related PTSD	40	Double-blind, placebo-controlled trial	Topiramate = PBO (CAPS total, CAPS-B, CAPS-C, TOP 8, HAM-D, or HAM-A). Topiramate > PBO (wk 6 and 8 CGI-I, $p = 0.021$) Topiramate > PBO (CAPS-D, $p = 0.019$)	
Davis et al. (unpublished) (72)	Topiramate (augmentation)	PTSD	35	Open trial	76% had reduced nightmares; 86% had reduced flashbacks. After 4 wk 82% did not meet criteria for active PTSD	Antidepressants neuroleptics anticonvulsants benzodiazepines lithium
Berlant et al., 2002 (67)	Gabapentin (augmentation)	PTSD	30	Retrospective chart review	77% of patients reported moderate or marked improvements in sleep duration	Antidepressants antipsychotics β-blockers antiepileptics benzodiazepine
Hamner et al., 2001 (74)	Valproic acid (augmentation)	PTSD	16	Open-label trial	Decreased hyperarousal	Antidepressants benzodiazepines neuroleptics
Fesler et al., 1991 (76)	Valproic acid (monotherapy and augmentation)	Combat-related PTSD	16	Open-label clinical trial	Significant improvement on CAPS total score ($p < 0.01$), on CAPS subscale scores of intrusion ($p < 0.05$) and hyperarousal ($p < .01$) and on the HAM-A and HAM-D ($p < 0.01$).	Fluoxetine bupropion buspirone lorazepam temazepam nefazadone	Drowziness Dizziness Irritability Headaches Vomiting Dry mouth Flushing
Clark et al., 1999 (77)	Valproic acid (augmentation)	Combat-related PTSD	21	Open-label trial	Symptom reduction in all three clusters	Benzodiazepines	
Petty et al., 2002 (78)	Valproic acid (monotherapy)	Noncombat-related PTSD	10	Open-label trial	No improvements in PTSD or depressive symptoms		Sedation Mild dizziness

(Continued)

TABLE 1 Summary of Open and Controlled Trials of Anticonvulsants in Anxiety Disorders (*Continued*)

Author(s) and yr (Ref.)	Drug	Disorder	Sample size	Design	Concomitant psychotropic medications	Outcomes	Adverse events
Otte et al., 2004 (79)	Valproic acid (augmentation and monotherapy)	PTSD	325	Retrospective chart review	Benzodiazepines Trazodone other antidepressants neuroleptics lithium buspirone other anticonvulsants methylphenidate	50% (25/50) patients were rated as "very much" or "much" improved on the CGI-I. The improved end point CGI-I differed significantly from "no change" ($p < 0.000001$)	Sedation Gastrointestinal distress
Davis et al., 2005 (80)	Divalproate (monotherapy)	PTSD	86	Randomized, placebo-controlled trial		Divalproate = PBO (CAPS total score, CAPS-B, CAPS-D, TOP-8, CGI-I or HAM-A) Divalproate > PBO (CAPS-C and MADRS)	
Davis et al. (submitted) (81)	Tiagabine (augmentation)	PTSD	6	Open-label trial	Antidepressants	Significant reduction in DTS	Urticaria Eating cessation Acute narrow-angle glaucoma Headache Memory difficulties
Lara, 2002 (82)	Tiagabine (augmentation)	PTSD with comorbidity	7	Open-label trial	Antidepressants valproic acid benzodiazepines buspirone	6/7 patients rated "markedly improved" in CGI-C	Drowsiness
Taylor, 2003 (84)	Tiagabine (monotherapy)	PTSD	26	Open-label followed by randomization to tiagabine or placebo trial		Significant reductions in open-label phase on all measures of PTSD, depression, general anxiety, social anxiety, resilience, and disability Gain, where maintained, in both tiagabine and placebo group	

Study	Drug	Disorder	N	Study design	Other drugs	Results	Side effects
Davidson et al., 2004 (85)	Tiagabine (monotherapy)	PTSD	232	Randomized, multicenter, double-blind trial		Tiagabine = PBO	Dizziness Headache Somnolence Nausea
Davidson et al., 2007 (86)	Carbamazepine (monotherapy)	PTSD	10	Open-label trial		Decrease in intensity of nightmares, flashbacks and intrusive thoughts. 7/10 responded "moderately" to "very much" on CGI-I	
Lipper et al., 1986 (87)	Carbamazepine	PTSD	10	Open-label trial		Decrease in staff observation of violent behavior and self report measures	Headache Tremor
Wolf et al., 1988 (88)	Carbamazepine (augmentation)	Childhood PTSD	28	Open-label trial	Methylphenidate clonidine sertraline fluoxetine imipramine	22/28 free of PTSD symptoms	Gastrointestinal symptoms
Looff et al., 1995 (89)	Phenytoin (monotherapy)	PTSD	9	Open-label trial		Significant improvement in PTSD (CAPS) No significant effects were found on depression (HAM-D) or anxiety (HAM-A) scores	
Bremner et al., 2004 (90)	Phenytoin (monotherapy)	PTSD	9	Open-label trial		Significant correlation between increased hippocampal volume and reduction of PTSD symptoms. PTSD patients treated with phenytoin resulted in significant (6%) increase in right whole-brain volume ($p < 0.05$)	
	Levetiracetam (augmentation)	PTSD	23	Retrospective analysis		Significant improvement was found on all measures	Sedation Tiredness Light-headedness Dry mouth Dyspepsia
Bremner et al., 2005 (91)	Gabapentin (monotherapy)	Panic disorder	103	Double-blind, placebo-controlled trial		No significant difference in response, significant improvement in PAS for severely-ill	Headache Nausea Somnolence

(Continued)

TABLE 1 Summary of Open and Controlled Trials of Anticonvulsants in Anxiety Disorders (*Continued*)

Author(s) and yr (Ref.)	Drug	Disorder	Sample size	Design	Concomitant psychotropic medications	Outcomes	Adverse events
Kinrys et al., 2006 (95)	Valproic acid (monotherapy)	Panic disorder with/without agoraphobia	10	Open-label trial		Significant reduction in CGI-S, HAM-A, Covi Anxiety Scale, and SCL-90-Panic factor	Nausea Dizziness Drowsiness Tremor Diarrhea
Pande et al., 2000 (137)	Valproic acid (monotherapy)	Panic disorder	12	Open-label trial		Significant improvement based on CGI-S and CGI-I, HAM-A, BSI	Sedation Nausea Dry mouth
Primeau et al., 1990 (143)	Valproic acid (Monotherapy)	Panic disorder	16	Open-label trial		Significant reduction in HAM-A, 71% decrease in frequency of attacks, 43% remitted	
Woodman and Noyles, 1994 (144)	Valproic acid (monotherapy)	Panic disorder	12	Double-blind, placebo-controlled trial		Significant improvements on CGI-S, and CGI-I scales	Gastrointestinal dysfunction Dizziness Somnolence
	Valproic acid (augmentation)	Panic disorder with comorbid mood instability	13	Open-label trial	Antidepressants benzodiazepines haloperidol	Decrease in panic frequency, HAM-A, and on BAI, BDI	Nausea Increased appetite
Keck et al., 1993 (145)	Tiagabine (monotherapy)	Panic disorder	15	Open-label trial		A significant reduction in panic was found after the second CCK-4 challenge	Visual field constriction (long-term use)
Lum et al., 1990 (147)	Carbamazepine (monotherapy)	Panic disorder with/without agoraphobia	34	Open-label trial		58.8% rated as having a "good response" by at least 5 independent investigators	
Baetz and Bowen, 1998 (146)	Carbamazepine (monotherapy)	Panic disorder	14	Controlled trial		40% had a completed cessation of panic attacks, 50% had an increase, 10% had no change	Restlessness Dizziness Blurred vision Rash

Study	Drug	Disorder	N	Study design	Results	Side effects
Zwanzger et al., 2003 (150)	Levetiracetam (monotherapy)	Panic disorder	18	Open-label, fixed-flexible dose study trial	Significant improvement on the CGI-S (primary efficacy measure) Panic attack frequency also significantly decreased	Insomnia, Irritability, Headaches
Tondo et al., 1989 (152)	Viagabatrin (monotherapy)	Panic disorder	3	Open-label trial	Marked reduction in agoraphobia and anxiety (HAM-A) as early as 2 wk, and maintained during subsequent therapy throughout the next 6 mo	Dizziness, Fatigue, Visual field-constrictions (long-term use)
Uhde et al., 1988 (153)	Viagabatrin (monotherapy)	Panic disorder	10	Placebo-controlled (CCK-4), followed by open-label	A significant reduction in panic was found after the second CCK-4 challenge.	Visual field constrictions (long-term use)
Papp, 2006 (155)	Pregabalin (monotherapy)	GAD	276	Double-blind, placebo and active—controlled trial	Pregabalin 600 mg > PBO, Lorazepam > PBO, Pregabalin 600 mg = Lorazepam	Somnolence, Dizziness
Zwanzger et al., 2001 (156)	Pregabalin (monotherapy)	GAD	271	Double-blind, fixed-dose, parallel-group, placebo and active-controlled trial	Pregabalin 600 mg > PBO, Lorazepam > PBO	Somnolence, Dizziness, Weight gain
Zwanzger et al., 2001 (157)	Pregabalin (monotherapy)	GAD	454	Double-blind, placebo-controlled, active comparator trial	Pregabalin 300 mg, 450 mg and 600 mg > PBO, Alprazolam > PBO	Dizziness, Weight gain
Pande et al., 2003 (190)	Pregabalin (monotherapy)	GAD	341	Double-blind, placebo-controlled trial	All 3 pregabalin dosage groups > PBO	Dizziness, Somnolence, Dry mouth, Euphoria, Blurred vision, Incoordination, Flatulence, Infection, Abnormal thinking
Feltner et al., 2003 (163)	Pregabalin (monotherapy)	GAD	421	Multicenter, randomized, double blind, placebo-controlled trial	Pregabalin 400 mg/day, 600 mg/day > PBO (HAM-A total score), Venlafaxine > PBO, Pregabalin 400 mg/day > PBO (all primary and secondary measures)	Dizziness, Somnolence, Nausea

(Continued)

TABLE 1 Summary of Open and Controlled Trials of Anticonvulsants in Anxiety Disorders (*Continued*)

Author(s) and yr (Ref.)	Drug	Disorder	Sample size	Design	Concomitant psychotropic medications	Outcomes	Adverse events
Rickels et al., 2005 (161)	Pregabalin (monotherapy)	GAD	277	Multicenter, randomized, placebo-controlled, double-blind, parallel-group study		Pregabalin > PBO	Dizziness Somnolence Headaches Nausea
Pohl et al., 2005 (191)	Pregabalin (monotherapy)	GAD	624	Open-label, double-blind trial		Pregabalin > PBO (time to relapse) Pregabalin > PBO (efficacy maintained through the double blind period as compared with double blind baseline) Pregabalin > PBO (HAM-A and the Sheehan Disability Scale)	
Montgomery et al., 2006 (192)	Tiagabine (monotherapy)	GAD	25	Open-label trial		Significant reduction in HAM-A, HADS, and LSAS; 37% responded (CGI-I ≤ 2)	Somnolence Asthenia Abnormal thinking
Khan et al., 2006 (193)	Tiagabine (monotherapy)	GAD	40	Open-label, blind rater, positive-controlled trial		Tiagabine and paroxetine significantly improved HAM-A scores and improved sleep quality	Headache Nausea Anorexia Dizziness
Smith et al., 2002 (194)	Tiagabine (monotherapy)	GAD	272	Double-blind, placebo-controlled trial		ITT: Tiagabine = PBO Completers: Tiagabine > PBO	Dizziness Headache Nausea
Papp and Ray, 2003 (196)	Gabapentin (augmentation)	OCD	5	Open-label trial	Fluoxetine	Significant improvement in OCD, anxiety and mood symptoms as well as sleep	
Rosenthal, 2003 (197)	Carbamazepine (monotherapy)	OCD with temporal EEG abnormalities	4	Open-label trial		1/4 demonstrated improvement	
Van Ameringen et al., 2004 (198)	Carbamazepine (monotherapy)	OCD	9	Open-label trial		1/8 who completed demonstrated improvement	Sedation

Study	Drug	Condition	N	Design	Comparators	Results	Side effects
Cora-Locatelli et al.,1998 (227)	Topiramate (augmentation)	OCD	16	Retrospective, open-label case series	SSRIs fluvoxamine fluoxetine citalopram paroxetine	68.8% (11/16) of patients were rated "very much" or "much" improved on the CGI-I at end point. A significant improvement on the CGI-S score was also found ($p < 0.001$).	Weight loss Sedation/fatigue Paresthesia Memory/word-finding problems
Jenike and Brotman, 1984 (232)	Topiramate (augmentation)	OCD	12	Open-label trial	Antidepressants fluoxetine fluvoxamine citalopram paroxetine sertraline venlafaxine	Significant changes from baseline in both Y-BOCS ($p = .002$) and the GAF scores ($p = .002$).	Weight loss Sedation/fatigue Paresthesia Memory/word-finding problems
	Lamotrigine (augmentation)	OCD	8		Sertraline clomipramine	No significant changes as rated by CGI-I scale	
Joffe and Swinson, 1987 (233)	Tiagabine (monotherapy and augmentation)	Mixed conditions: GAD, PTSD, MDD, bipolar disorder, schizophrenia	10	Open-label trial	Risperidone citalopram paroxetine clomipramine	All patients rated as "much" or "very much improved" on the CGI-C after 4 wk	
Van Ameringen et al., 2006 (235)	Tiagabine (augmentation)	Mixed conditions: GAD, PTSD, panic disorder, social phobia	18	Open-label trial	SSRIs SNRI nefazodone alprazolam	Significant improvements on HAM-A and BAI; 76% of patients where responders ($\geq 50\%$ decrease on HAM-A); 59% achieved remission HAM-A ≤ 7.	Cognitive slowness Somnolence Headache

Abbreviations: CGI-I, Clinical Global Impression-Improvement Score; CGI-S, Clinical Global Impression-Severity Score; HAM-A, Hamilton Anxiety Rating Scale; HAM-D, Hamilton Depression Rating Scale; PBO, placebo; BSPS, Brief Social Phobia Scale; PTSD, posttraumatic stress disorder; DGRP, Duke Global Rating Scale for PTSD; PCL-C, TPSD Checklist—Civilian Version; CAPS, Clinician-Administered PTSD Scale; TOP-8, Treatment Outcome PTSD; DTS, Davidson Trauma Scale; CGI-C, Clinical Global Impression-Change score; PAS, Panic and Agoraphobia Scale; SCL-90, Symptom Checklist-90; BSI, Brief Symptom Inventory; BAI, Beck Anxiety Inventory; BDI, Beck Depression Inventory; CCK-4, cholecystokinin-tetrapeptide; GAD, generalized anxiety disorder; OCD, obsessive-compulsive disorder; EEG, electroencephalogram; Y-BOCS, Yale-Brown Obsessive-Compulsive Scale; GAF, Global Assessment of Functioning; HADS, Hospital Anxiety and Depression Scale.

TABLE 2 Levels of Evidence for Epileptic Use in Anxiety Disorders

Drug	Panic disorder	OCD	PTSD	Social phobia	GAD
Lamotrigine		Level 4	Level 2		
Topiramate		Level 3	Level 1(–ve)[a]	Level 3	
Gabapentin	Level 2 (–ve)[a]	Level 4	Level 3	Level 2	Level 4
Pregabalin				Level 2	Level 1
Valproic acid	Level 2	Level 4	Level 2 (–ve)[a]	Level 3	
Tiagabine	Level 3		Level 3	Level 3	Level 2
Carbamazepine	Level 3	Level 4	Level 3		
Levetiracetam	Level 3		Level 4	Level 2	Level 4
Phenytoin	Level 4		Level 4		
Vigabatrin	Level 3		Level 4		
Oxcarbazepine			Level 4		

Note: Level of evidence criteria (241) are as follows:
Level 1: Meta-analysis or replicated randomized controlled trial (RCT) that includes a placebo condition.
Level 2: At least 1 RCT with placebo or active comparison condition.
Level 3: Uncontrolled trial with 10 or more subjects.
Level 4: Anecdotal case reports.
[a]Negative results of RCT.

replicated, randomized controlled trial that includes a placebo condition (the highest level of evidence); (2) at least one randomized controlled trial with placebo or active comparison condition; (3) uncontrolled trial with at least 10 or more subjects; and (4) anecdotal reports or expert opinions.

The psychotropic use of AEDs is an active area of research, with a number of case reports, case series, and open trials suggesting the potential efficacy of these treatments in a variety of anxiety disorders (Table 1). The strongest evidence, level 1, can be found for pregabalin in GAD (Table 2). Level 2 evidence suggests efficacy of lamotrigine in PTSD, gabapentin in social phobia, pregabalin in social phobia and generalized anxiety with comorbidity, and valproate in panic disorder (Table 2). Of note, despite level 1 evidence criteria being met for lamotrigine in PTSD and valproate in panic disorder, these results need to be viewed with caution, given the very small sample sizes used in the supporting studies.

The remainder of the evidence for AEDs in the treatment of anxiety disorders remains at level 3 or 4. Although there have been numerous studies and reports describing the use of AEDS in anxiety disorders, they have suffered from a number of methodological problems. These include inadequate sample size, lack of placebo controls, heterogeneous patients samples, use of inadequate doses of medication, lack of controlling for patient variables such as comorbidity, disorder subtype and use of concomitant medications, as well as the reliance on impressionistic outcome measures such as the CGI-scale.

Although AEDS seem to be promising treatments for anxiety disorders, it is not yet clear where their place will be in the spectrum of treatments available for these conditions. Given the very preliminary data on the efficacy of AEDs in anxiety disorders, their current clinical use should be reserved for treatment-refractory individuals, as augmentation strategies for partial responders, and as alternative treatments for those individuals who cannot tolerate first-line treatments, such as SSRIs, or those who are not appropriate candidates for benzodiazepines. There is currently no evidence to support the use of AEDs as first-line treatments with the exception of pregabalin in GAD. In addition, for AEDs that have thus far shown some evidence of benefit in the treatment of anxiety disorders, their potential use in combination with mood stabilizers in bipolar disorder patients who suffer from a comorbid anxiety disorder should be considered.

Future research examining the potential use of AEDs in anxiety disorders will require large-scale controlled trials in a number of these disorders, including head-to-head comparisons with first-line treatments and examinations of clinical subgroups that may preferentially respond to AEDs. In addition, it may be warranted to evaluate the potential use of AEDs in youth with anxiety disorders given the current concerns about the safety and efficacy of SSRIs in this age group.

REFERENCES

1. van Steveninck AL, Wallnofer AE, Schoemaker RC, et al. A study of the effects of long-term use on individual sensitivity to temazepam and lorazepam in a clinical population. Br J Clin Pharmacol 1997; 44:267–275.
2. Cowley DS, Roy-Byrne PP, Radant A, et al. Benzodiazepine sensitivity in panic disorder: Effects of chronic alprazolam treatment. Neuropsychopharmacology 1995; 12: 147–157.
3. Rapport DJ, Calabrese JR. Tolerance to fluoxetine. J Clin Psychopharmacol 1993; 13: 361–361.
4. Pope HG, Mcelroy SL, Keck PE, et al. Valproate in the treatment of acute mania: a placebo-controlled study. Arch Gen Psychiatry 1991; 48:62–68.
5. Lerer B, Moore N, Meyendorff E, et al. Carbamazepine versus lithium in mania: a double-blind study. J Clin Psychiatry 1987; 48:89–93.
6. Quirk GJ, Gehlert DR. Inhibition of the amygdala: key to pathological states? Ann N Y Acad Sci 2003; 985:263–272.
7. LeDoux JE. The Emotional Brain. New York, NY: Simon & Schuster, 1996.
8. Lydiard RB. The role of GABA in anxiety disorders. J Clin Psychiatry 2003; 64(suppl 3): 21–27.
9. Goddard AW, Mason GF, Almai A, et al. Reductions in occipital cortex GABA levels in panic disorder detected with 1h-magnetic resonance spectroscopy. Arch Gen Psychiatry 2001; 58:556–561.
10. Smith TA. Type A gamma-aminobutryric acid (GABAA) receptors subunits and benzodiazepines binding site sensitivity. Nature 1978; 274:383–385.
11. Rosenberg DR, MacMaster FP, Keshavan MS, et al. Decrease in caudate glutamatergic concentrations in pediatric obsessive-compulsive disorder patients taking paroxetine. J Am Acad Child Adolesc Psychiatry 2000; 39:1096–1103.
12. Mathew SJ, Coplan JD, Gorman JM. Neurobiological mechanisms of social anxiety disorder. Am J Psychiatry 2001; 158:1558–1567.
13. Satoh M, Foong FW. A mechanism of carbamazepine-analgesia as shown by bradykinin-induced trigeminal pain. Brain Res Bull 1983; 10:407–409.
14. Burchiel KJ. Carbamazepine inhibits spontaneous activity in experimental neuromas. Exp Neurol 1988; 102:249–253.
15. Chapman V, Suzuki R, Chamarette HL, et al. Effects of systemic carbamazepine and gabapentin on spinal neuronal responses in spinal nerve ligated rats. Pain 1998; 75: 261–272.
16. Tanelian DL, Cousins MJ. Combined neurogenic and nociceptive pain in a patient with pancoast tumor managed by epidural hydromorphone and oral carbamazepine. Pain 1989; 36:85–88.
17. Pollack MH, Matthews J, Scott EL. Gabapentin as a potential treatment for anxiety disorders. Am J Psychiatry 1998; 155:992–993.
18. Calabrese JR, Bowden CL, Sachs GS, et al. A double-blind placebo-controlled study of lamotrigine monotherapy in outpatients with bipolar I depression. lamictal 602 study group. J Clin Psychiatry 1999; 60:79–88.
19. Rigo JM, Hans G, Nguyen L, et al. The anti-epileptic drug levetiracetam reverses the inhibition by negative allosteric modulators of neuronal GABA- and glycine-gated currents. Br J Pharmacol 2002; 136:659–672.

20. Grant SM, Faulds D. Oxcarbazepine. A review of its pharmacology and therapeutic potential in epilepsy, trigeminal neuralgia and affective disorders. Drugs 1992; 43: 873–888.

21. McAuley JW, Biederman TS, Smith JC, et al. Newer therapies in the drug treatment of epilepsy. Ann Pharmacother 2002; 36:119–129.

22. Tecoma ES. Oxcarbazepine. Epilepsia 1999; 40:S37–S46.

23. Wamil AW, McLean MJ. Phenytoin blocks N-methyl-D-aspartate responses of mouse central neurons. J Pharmacol Exp Ther 1993; 267:218–227.

24. Kawano H, Sashihara S, Mita T, et al. Phenytoin, an antiepileptic drug, competitively blocked non-NMDA receptors produced by xenopus oocytes. Neurosci Lett 1994; 166: 183–186.

25. Frampton JE, Foster RH. Pregabalin: in the treatment of generalised anxiety disorder. CNS Drugs 2006; 20:685–693 (discussion 694–695).

26. Fink-Jensen A, Suzdak PD, Swedberg MD, et al. The gamma-aminobutyric acid (GABA) uptake inhibitor, tiagabine, increases extracellular brain levels of GABA in awake rats. Eur J Pharmacol 1992; 220:197–201.

27. Borden LA, Murali Dhar TG, Smith KE, et al. Tiagabine, SK&F 89976-A, CI-966, and NNC-711 are selective for the cloned GABA transporter GAT-1. Eur J Pharmacol 1994; 269:219–224.

28. Biton V, Edwards KR, Montouris GD, et al. Topiramate titration and tolerability. Ann Pharmacother 2001; 35:173–179.

29. Harden CL. New antiepileptic drugs. Neurology 1994; 44:787–795.

30. Ben-Menachem E. Pharmacokinetic effects of vigabatrin on cerebrospinal fluid amino acids in humans. Epilepsia 1989; 30(suppl 3):S12–S14.

31. American Psychiatric Association. Diagnostic and Statistical Manual of Mental Disorders. 4th ed. Washington, DC: American Psychiatric Association, 1994.

32. Stein MB, Fyer AJ, Davidson JRT, et al. Fluvoxamine treatment of social phobia (social anxiety disorder): a double-blind, placebo-controlled study. Am J Psychiatry 1999; 156: 756–760.

33. Van Ameringen MA, Lane RM, Walker JR, et al. Sertraline treatment of generalized social phobia: a 20-week, double-blind, placebo-controlled study. Am J Psychiatry 2001; 158: 275–281.

34. Liebowitz MR, Mangano R. Comparison of venlafaxine extended-release (ER) and paroxetine in the short-term treatment of SAD. Arch Gen Psychiatry 2005; 62: 190–198.

35. Gelernter CS, Uhde TW, Cimbolic P, et al. Cognitive-behavioral and pharmacological treatments of social phobia: a controlled-study. Arch Gen Psychiatry 1991; 48:938–945.

36. Liebowitz MR, Schneier F, Campeas R, et al. Phenelzine vs atenolol in social phobia. A placebo-controlled comparison. Arch Gen Psychiatry 1992; 49:290–300.

37. Heimberg RG, Liebowitz MR, Hope DA, et al. Cognitive behavioral group therapy vs phenelzine therapy for social phobia: 12-week outcome. Arch Gen Psychiatry 1998; 55: 1133–1141.

38. Fahlen T, Nilsson HL, Borg K, et al. Social phobia: the clinical efficacy and tolerability of the monoamine oxidase -A and serotonin uptake inhibitor brofaromine. A double-blind placebo-controlled study. Acta Psychiatr Scand 1995; 92:351–358.

39. Schneier FR, Goetz D, Campeas R, et al. Placebo-controlled trial of moclobemide in social phobia. Br J Psychiatry 1998; 172:70–77.

40. Van Ameringen M, Mancini C, Pipe B, et al. An open trial of topiramate in the treatment of generalized social phobia. J Clin Psychiatry 2004; 65:1674–1678.

41. Stein MB, Pollack MH, Mangano R. Long-term treatment of generalized SAD with venlafaxine extended release. Poster presented at: The 23rd Annual Conference of the Anxiety Disorders Association of America; March 27–30, 2003; Toronto, Canada.

42. Pande AC, Davidson JR, Jefferson JW, et al. Treatment of social phobia with gabapentin: a placebo-controlled study. J Clin Psychopharmacol 1999; 19:341–348.

43. de-Paris F, Sant'Anna MK, Vianna MR, et al. Effects of gabapentin on anxiety induced by simulated public speaking. J Psychopharmacol 2003; 17:184–188.

44. Pande AC, Feltner DE, Jefferson JW, et al. Efficacy of the novel anxiolytic pregabalin in social anxiety disorder: a placebo-controlled, multicenter study. J Clin Psychopharmacol 2004; 24:141–149.

45. Nardi AE, Mendolwicz M, Versiani FM. Valproic acid in social phobia: an open trial. Biol Psychiatry 1997; 42:S118.

46. Kinrys G, Pollack MH, Simon NM, et al. Valproic acid for the treatment of social anxiety disorder. Int Clin Psychopharmacol 2003; 18:169–172.

47. Dunlap BW, Papp L, Garlow SJ, et al. Tiagabine for social anxiety disorder. Human Psychopharmacol 2007; 22:241–244.

48. Kinrys G, Soldani F, Hsu D, et al. Adjunctive tiagabine for treatment refractory social anxiety disorder. Poster presented at: The 157th Annual Meeting of the American Psychiatric Association; May 1–6, 2004; New York, NY.

49. Simon NM, Worthington JJ, Doyle AC, et al. An open-label study of levetiracetam for the treatment of social anxiety disorder. J Clin Psychiatry 2004; 65:1219–1222.

50. Zhang W, Connor KM. Levetiracetam in social phobia: a placebo controlled pilot study. J Psychopharmacol 2005; 19:551–553.

51. Ballenger JA, Davidson JRT, Lecrubier Y, et al. Consensus statement on posttraumatic stress disorder from the international consensus group on depression and anxiety. J Clin Psychiatry 2000; 61:60–66.

52. Connor KM, Sutherland SM, Tupler LA, et al. Fluoxetine in post-traumatic stress disorder. Randomised, double-blind study. Br J Psychiatry 1999; 175:17–22.

53. van der Kolk BA, Dreyfuss D, Michaels M, et al. Fluoxetine in posttraumatic stress disorder. J Clin Psychiatry 1994; 55:517–522.

54. Davidson JR, Rothbaum BO, van der Kolk BA, et al. Multicenter, double-blind comparison of sertraline and placebo in the treatment of posttraumatic stress disorder. Arch Gen Psychiatry 2001; 58:485–492.

55. Brady K, Pearlstein T, Asnis GM, et al. Efficacy and safety of sertraline treatment of posttraumatic stress disorder: a randomized controlled trial. JAMA 2000; 283:1837–1844.

56. Zohar J, Amital D, Miodownik C, et al. Double-blind placebo-controlled pilot study of sertraline in military veterans with posttraumatic stress disorder. J Clin Psychopharmacol 2002; 22:190–195.

57. Tucker P, Potter-Kimball R, Wyatt DB, et al. Can physiologic assessment and side effects tease out differences in PTSD trials? A double-blind comparison of citalopram, sertraline, and placebo. Psychopharmacol Bull 2003; 37:135–149.

58. Tucker P, Zaninelli R, Yehuda R, et al. Paroxetine in the treatment of chronic posttraumatic stress disorder: results of a placebo-controlled, flexible-dosage trial. J Clin Psychiatry 2001; 62:860–868.

59. Marshall RD, Beebe KL, Oldham M, et al. Efficacy and safety of paroxetine treatment for chronic PTSD: a fixed-dose, placebo-controlled study. Am J Psychiatry 2001; 158: 1982–1988.

60. Stein DJ, Davidson J, Seedat S, et al. Paroxetine in the treatment of post-traumatic stress disorder: pooled analysis of placebo-controlled studies. Expert Opin Pharmacother 2003; 4:1829–1838.

61. Davidson J, Lipschitz A, Musgnung J. Venlafaxinw XR and sertraline in PTSD: a placebo-controlled study. Eur Neuropsychopharmacol 2003; 13:S380.

62. Kosten TR, Frank JB, Dan E, et al. Pharmacotherapy for posttraumatic stress disorder using phenelzine or imipramine. J Nerv Ment Dis 1991; 179:366–370.

63. Frank JB, Kosten TR, Giller EL Jr., et al. A randomized clinical trial of phenelzine and imipramine for posttraumatic stress disorder. Am J Psychiatry 1988; 145:1289–1291.

64. Davidson J, Kudler H, Smith R, et al. Treatment of posttraumatic-stress-disorder with amitriptyline and placebo. Arch Gen Psychiatry 1990; 47:259–266.

65. Davidson JR, Kudler HS, Saunders WB, et al. Predicting response to amitriptyline in posttraumatic stress disorder. Am J Psychiatry 1993; 150:1024–1029.

66. Hertzberg MA, Butterfield MI, Feldman ME, et al. A preliminary study of lamotrigine for the treatment of posttraumatic stress disorder. Biol Psychiatry 1999; 45:1226–1229.

67. Berlant J, van Kammen DP. Open-label topiramate as primary or adjunctive therapy in chronic civilian posttraumatic stress disorder: a preliminary report. J Clin Psychiatry 2002; 63:15–20.
68. Chengappa KN, Rathore D, Levine J, et al. Topiramate as add-on treatment for patients with bipolar mania. Bipolar Disord 1999; 1:42–53.
69. Berlant JL. Prospective open-label study of add-on and monotherapy topiramate in civilians with chronic nonhallucinatory posttraumatic stress disorder. BMC Psychiatry 2004; 4:24.
70. Tucker P, Trautman RP, Wyatt DB, et al. Efficacy and safety of topiramate monotherapy in civilian posttraumatic stress disorder: a randomized, double-blind, placebo-controlled study. J Clin Psychiatry 2007; 68:201–206.
71. Blake DD, Weathers FW, Nagy LM, et al. The development of a clinician-administered PTSD scale. J Trauma Stress 1995; 8:75–90.
72. Davis EA. Topiramate for PTSD. Presented at: The 160th Annual Meeting of the American Psychiatric Association; May 19–24, 2007; San Diego, California.
73. Brannon N, Labbate L, Huber M. Gabapentin treatment for posttraumatic stress disorder. Can J Psychiatry 2000; 45:84.
74. Hamner MB, Brodrick PS, Labbate LA. Gabapentin in PTSD: A retrospective, clinical series of adjunctive therapy. Ann Clin Psychiatry 2001; 13:141–146.
75. Szymanski HV, Olympia J. Divalproex in posttraumatic stress disorder. Am J Psychiatry 1991; 148:1086–1087.
76. Fesler FA. Valproate in combat-related posttraumatic stress disorder. J Clin Psychiatry 1991; 52:361–364.
77. Clark RD, Canive JM, Calais LA, et al. Divalproex in posttraumatic stress disorder: an open-label clinical trial. J Trauma Stress 1999; 12:395–401.
78. Petty F, Davis LL, Nugent AL, et al. Valproate therapy for chronic, combat-induced posttraumatic stress disorder. J Clin Psychopharmacol 2002; 22:100–101.
79. Davis LL, Ambrose SM, Newell JM, et al. Divalproex for the treatment of posttraumatic stress disorder: a retrospective chart review. Int J Psychiatry Clin Pract 2005; 9:278–283.
80. Otte C, Wiedemann K, Yassouridis A, et al. Valproate monotherapy in the treatment of civilian patients with non-combat-related posttraumatic stress disorder: An open-label study. J Clin Psychopharmacol 2004; 24:106–108.
81. Davis EA. Divalporex for PTSD. Presented at: The 160th Annual Meeting of the American Psychiatric Association; May 19–24, 2007; San Diego, California.
82. Lara ME. Tiagabine for augmentation of antidepressant treatment of post-traumatic stress disorder. Presented at: The 22nd National Conference of the Anxiety Disorders Association of America; March 21–24, 2002; Austin, TX.
83. Berigan T. Treatment of posttraumatic stress disorder with tiagabine. Can J Psychiatry 2002; 47:788.
84. Taylor FB. Tiagabine for posttraumatic stress disorder: a case series of 7 women. J Clin Psychiatry 2003; 64:1421–1425.
85. Connor KM, Davidson JR, WEisler RH, et al. Tiagabine for posttraumatic stress disorder: effects of open-label and double-blind discontinuation treatment. Psychopharmacology (Berl) 2006; 184:21–26.
86. Davidson JR, Brady K, Mellman TA, et al. The efficacy and tolerability of tiagabine in adult patients with post-traumatic stress disorder. J Clin Psychopharmacol 2007; 27:85–88.
87. Lipper S, Davidson JR, Grady TA, et al. Preliminary study of carbamazepine in post-traumatic stress disorder. Psychosomatics 1986; 27:849–854.
88. Wolf ME, Alavi A, Mosnaim AD. Posttraumatic stress disorder in vietnam veterans clinical and EEG findings; possible therapeutic effects of carbamazepine. Biol Psychiatry 1988; 23:642–644.
89. Looff D, Grimley P, Kuller F, et al. Carbamazepine for PTSD. J Am Acad Child Adolesc Psychiatry 1995; 34:703–704.
90. Bremner JD, Mletzko T, Welter S, et al. Treatment of posttraumatic stress disorder with phenytoin: an open-label pilot study. J Clin Psychiatry 2004; 65:1559–1564.

91. Bremner JD, Mletzko T, Welter S, et al. Effects of phenytoin on memory, cognition and brain structure in post-traumatic stress disorder: a pilot study. J Psychopharmacol 2005; 19:159–165.
92. Macleod AD. Vigabatrin and posttraumatic stress disorder. J Clin Psychopharmacol 1996; 16:190–191.
93. Berigan T. Oxcarbazepine treatment of posttraumatic stress disorder. Can J Psychiatry 2002; 47:973–974.
94. Malek-Ahmadi P, Hanretta AT. Possible reduction in posttraumatic stress disorder symptoms with oxcarbazepine in a patient with bipolar disorder. Ann Pharmacother 2004; 38:1852–1854.
95. Kinrys G, Wygat LE, Pardo TB, et al. Levetiracetam for treatment-refactory PTSD. J Clin Psychiatry 2006; 67:211–214.
96. Andersch S, Rosenberg NK, Kullingsjo H, et al. Efficacy and safety of alprazolam, imipramine and placebo in treating panic disorder. A Scandinavian multicenter study. Acta Psychiatr Scand Suppl 1991; 365:18–27.
97. Modigh K, Westberg P, Eriksson E. Superiority of clomipramine over imipramine in the treatment of panic disorder: a placebo-controlled trial. J Clin Psychopharmacol 1992; 12: 251–261.
98. Sheehan DV, Ballenger J, Jacobsen G. Treatment of endogenous anxiety with phobic, hysterical, and hypochondriacal symptoms. Arch Gen Psychiatry 1980; 37:51–59.
99. Tesar GE, Rosenbaum JF, Pollack MH, et al. Double-blind, placebo-controlled comparison of clonazepam and alprazolam for panic disorder. J Clin Psychiatry 1991; 52:69–76.
100. Boyer W. Serotonin uptake inhibitors are superior to imipramine and alprazolam in alleviating panic attacks: a meta-analysis. Int Clin Psychopharmacol 1995; 10:45–49.
101. Schweizer E, Pohl R, Balon R, et al. Lorazepam vs. alprazolam in the treatment of panic disorder. Pharmacopsychiatry 1990; 23:90–93.
102. Beauclair L, Fontaine R, Annable L, et al. Clonazepam in the treatment of panic disorder: a double-blind, placebo-controlled trial investigating the correlation between clonazepam concentrations in plasma and clinical response. J Clin Psychopharmacol 1994; 14:111–118.
103. Moroz G, Rosenbaum JF. Efficacy, safety, and gradual discontinuation of clonazepam in panic disorder: a placebo-controlled, multicenter study using optimized dosages. J Clin Psychiatry 1999; 60:604–612.
104. Rosenbaum JF, Moroz G, Bowden CL. Clonazepam in the treatment of panic disorder with or without agoraphobia: a dose-response study of efficacy, safety, and discontinuance. Clonazepam panic disorder dose-response study group. J Clin Psychopharmacol 1997; 17:390–400.
105. Valenca AM, Nardi AE, Nascimento I, et al. Double-blind clonazepam vs placebo in panic disorder treatment. Arq Neuropsiquiatr 2000; 58:1025–1029.
106. Charney DS, Woods SW. Benzodiazepine treatment of panic disorder: a comparison of alprazolam and lorazepam. J Clin Psychiatry 1989; 50:418–423.
107. de Jonghe F, Swinkels J, Tuynman-Qua H, et al. A comparative study of suriclone, lorazepam and placebo in anxiety disorder. Pharmacopsychiatry 1989; 22:266–271.
108. Dunner DL, Ishiki D, Avery DH, et al. Effect of alprazolam and diazepam on anxiety and panic attacks in panic disorder: a controlled study. J Clin Psychiatry 1986; 47:458–460.
109. Noyes R Jr., Anderson DJ, Clancy J, et al. Diazepam and propranolol in panic disorder and agoraphobia. Arch Gen Psychiatry 1984; 41:287–292.
110. Noyes R Jr., Burrows GD, Reich JH, et al. Diazepam versus alprazolam for the treatment of panic disorder. J Clin Psychiatry 1996; 57:349–355.
111. Ballenger JC, Wheadon DE, Steiner M, et al. Double-blind, fixed-dose, placebo-controlled study of paroxetine in the treatment of panic disorder. Am J Psychiatry 1998; 155:36–42.
112. Londborg PD, Wolkow R, Smith WT, et al. Sertraline in the treatment of panic disorder. A multi-site, double-blind, placebo-controlled, fixed-dose investigation. Br J Psychiatry 1998; 173:54–60.
113. Asnis GM, Hameedi FA, Goddard AW, et al. Fluvoxamine in the treatment of panic disorder: a multi-center, double-blind, placebo-controlled study in outpatients. Psychiatry Res 2001; 103:1–14.

114. Michelson D, Allgulander C, Dantendorfer K, et al. Efficacy of usual antidepressant dosing regimens of fluoxetine in panic disorder: randomised, placebo-controlled trial. Br J Psychiatry 2001; 179:514–518.

115. Pollack M, Mangano R, Entsuah R, et al. A randomized controlled trial of venlafaxine ER and paroxetine in the treatment of outpatients with panic disorder. Psychopharmacology (Berl) 2007; 194(2):233–242.

116. Liebowitz M, Asnis G, Tzanis E, et al. Venlafaxine extended release versus placebo in the short-term treatment of panic disorders [abstract NR194] In: American Psychiatric Association. New Research Abstracts, Annual Meeting of the American Psychiatric Association; May 1–6; Washington (DC): American Psychiatric Association; 2004.

117. Pollack MH, Worthington JJ III, Otto MW, et al. Venlafaxine for panic disorder: results from a double-blind, placebo-controlled study. Psychopharmacol Bull 1996; 32:667–670.

118. Bradwejn J, Ahokas A, Stein DJ, et al. Venlafaxine extended-release capsules in panic disorder: flexible-dose, double-blind, placebo-controlled study. Br J Psychiatry 2005; 187: 352–359.

119. Michelson D, Lydiard RB, Pollack MH, et al. Outcome assessment and clinical improvement in panic disorder: evidence from a randomized controlled trial of fluoxetine and placebo. The fluoxetine panic disorder study group. Am J Psychiatry 1998; 155:1570–1577.

120. Ribeiro L, Busnello JV, Kauer-Sant'Anna M, et al. Mirtazapine versus fluoxetine in the treatment of panic disorder. Braz J Med Biol Res 2001; 34:1303–1307.

121. Tiller JWG, Bouwer C, Behnke K. Moclobemide and fluoxetine for panic disorder. International Panic Disorder Study Group. Eur Arch Psychiatry Clin Neurosci 1999; 249: S7–S10.

122. Sharp DM, Power KG, Simpson RJ, et al. Global measures of outcome in a controlled comparison of pharmacological and psychological treatment of panic disorder and agoraphobia in primary care. Br J Gen Pract 1997; 47:150–155.

123. Black DW, Wesner R, Bowers W, et al. A comparison of fluvoxamine, cognitive therapy, and placebo in the treatment of panic disorder. Arch Gen Psychiatry 1993; 50:44–50.

124. Bakish D, Hooper CL, Filteau MJ, et al. A double-blind placebo-controlled trial comparing fluvoxamine and imipramine in the treatment of panic disorder with or without agoraphobia. Psychopharmacol Bull 1996; 32:135–141.

125. Den Boer JA, Westenberg HG. Serotonin function in panic disorder: a double blind placebo controlled study with fluvoxamine and ritanserin. Psychopharmacology (Berl) 1990; 102:85–94.

126. Hoehn-Saric R, McLeod DR, Hipsley PA. Effect of fluvoxamine on panic disorder. J Clin Psychopharmacol 1993; 13:321–326.

127. Bakker A, van Balkom AJ, Spinhoven P. SSRIs vs. TCAs in the treatment of panic disorder: a meta-analysis. Acta Psychiatr Scand 2002; 106:163–167.

128. Oehrberg S, Christiansen PE, Behnke K, et al. Paroxetine in the treatment of panic disorder. A randomised, double-blind, placebo-controlled study. Br J Psychiatry 1995; 167:374–379.

129. Bakker A, van Dyck R, Spinhoven P, et al. Paroxetine, clomipramine, and cognitive therapy in the treatment of panic disorder. J Clin Psychiatry 1999; 60:831–838.

130. Lecrubier Y, Bakker A, Dunbar G, et al. A comparison of paroxetine, clomipramine and placebo in the treatment of panic disorder. Collaborative paroxetine panic study investigators. Acta Psychiatr Scand 1997; 95:145–152.

131. Sheehan DV, Burnham DB, Iyengar MK, et al. Efficacy and tolerability of controlled-release paroxetine in the treatment of panic disorder. Panic Disorder Study Group. J Clin Psychiatry 2005; 66:34–40.

132. Pohl RB, Wolkow RM, Clary CM. Sertraline in the treatment of panic disorder: a double-blind multicenter trial. Am J Psychiatry 1998; 155:1189–1195.

133. Pollack MH, Otto MW, Worthington JJ, et al. Sertraline in the treatment of panic disorder: a flexible-dose multicenter trial. Arch Gen Psychiatry 1998; 55:1010–1016.

134. Pollack MH, Rapaport MH, Clary CM, et al. Sertraline treatment of panic disorder: response in patients at risk for poor outcome. J Clin Psychiatry 2000; 61:922–927.

135. Lepola U, Arato M, Zhu Y, et al. Sertraline versus imipramine treatment of comorbid panic disorder and major depressive disorder. J Clin Psychiatry 2003; 64:654–662.

136. Stahl SM, Gergel I, Li D. Escitalopram in the treatment of panic disorder: a randomized, double-blind, placebo-controlled trial. J Clin Psychiatry 2003; 64:1322–1327.

137. Pande AC, Pollack MH, Crockatt J, et al. Placebo-controlled study of gabapentin treatment of panic disorder. J Clin Psychopharmacol 2000; 20:467–471.

138. Brady KT, Sonne S, Lydiard RB. Valproate treatment of comorbid panic disorder and affective disorders in two alcoholic patients. J Clin Psychopharmacol 1994; 14:81–82.

139. Roberts JM, Malcolm R, Santos AB. Treatment of panic disorder and comorbid substance abuse with divalproex sodium. Am J Psychiatry 1994; 151:1521.

140. McElroy SL, Keck PE Jr., Lawrence JM. Treatment of panic disorder and benzodiazepine withdrawal with valproate. J Neuropsychiatry Clin Neurosci 1991; 3:232–233.

141. Marazziti D, Cassano GB. Valproic acid for panic disorder associated with multiple sclerosis. Am J Psychiatry 1996; 153:842–843.

142. Ontiveros A, Fontaine R. Sodium valproate and clonazepam for treatment-resistant panic disorder. J Psychiatry Neurosci 1992; 17:78–80.

143. Primeau F, Fontaine R, Beauclair L. Valproic acid and panic disorder. Can J Psychiatry 1990; 35:248–250.

144. Woodman CL, Noyes R Jr. Panic disorder: treatment with valproate. J Clin Psychiatry 1994; 55:134–136.

145. Keck PE Jr., Taylor VE, Tugrul KC, et al. Valproate treatment of panic disorder and lactate-induced panic attacks. Biol Psychiatry 1993; 33:542–546.

146. Baetz M, Bowen RC. Efficacy of divalproex sodium in patients with panic disorder and mood instability who have not responded to conventional therapy. Can J Psychiatry 1998; 43:73–77.

147. Lum M, Fontaine R, Elie R, et al. Divalproex sodium's antipanic effect in panic disorder: a placebo-controlled study. Biol Psychiatry 1990; 27:164A.

148. Gruener D. Tiagabine as an augmenting agent for the treatment of anxiety. Presented at: The 22nd National Conference of the Anxiety Disorders Association of America; 2002; Austin, TX.

149. Zwanzger P, Baghai TC, Schule C, et al. Tiagabine improves panic and agoraphobia in panic disorder patients. J Clin Psychiatry 2001; 62:656–657.

150. Zwanzger P, Eser D, Padberg F, et al. Effects of tiagabine on cholecystokinin-tetrapeptide (CCK-4)-induced anxiety in healthy volunteers. Depress Anxiety 2003; 18:140–143.

151. Lawlor BA. Carbamazepine, alprazolam withdrawal, and panic disorder. Am J Psychiatry 1987; 144:265–266.

152. Tondo L, Burrai C, Scamonatti L, et al. Carbamazepine in panic disorder. Am J Psychiatry 1989; 146:558–559.

153. Uhde TW, Stein MB, Post RM. Lack of efficacy of carbamazepine in the treatment of panic disorder. Am J Psychiatry 1988; 145:1104–1109.

154. McNamara ME, Fogel BS. Anticonvulsant-responsive panic attacks with temporal lobe EEG abnormalities. J Neuropsychiatry Clin Neurosci 1990; 2:193–196.

155. Papp LA. Safety and efficacy of levetiracetam for patients with panic disorder: results of an open-label, fixed-flexible dose study. J Clin Psychiatry 2006; 67:1573–1576.

156. Zwanzger P, Baghai T, Boerner RJ, et al. Anxiolytic effects of vigabatrin in panic disorder. J Clin Psychopharmacol 2001; 21:539–540.

157. Zwanzger P, Baghai TC, Schuele C, et al. Vigabatrin decreases cholecystokinin-tetrapeptide (CCK-4) induced panic in healthy volunteers. Neuropsychopharmacology 2001; 25:699–703.

158. Mitte K, Noack P, Steil R, et al. A meta-analytic review of the efficacy of drug treatment in generalized anxiety disorder. J Clin Psychopharmacol 2005; 25:141–150.

159. Lydiard RB, Ballenger JC, Rickels K. A double-blind evaluation of the safety and efficacy of abecarnil, alprazolam, and placebo in outpatients with generalized anxiety disorder. Abecarnil Work Group. J Clin Psychiatry 1997; 58(suppl 11):11–18.

160. Moller HJ, Volz HP, Reimann IW, et al. Opipramol for the treatment of generalized anxiety disorder: a placebo-controlled trial including an alprazolam-treated group. J Clin Psychopharmacol 2001; 21:59–65.

161. Rickels K, Pollack MH, Feltner DE, et al. Pregabalin for treatment of generalized anxiety disorder: a 4-week, multicenter, double-blind, placebo-controlled trial of pregabalin and alprazolam. Arch Gen Psychiatry 2005; 62:1022–1030.
162. Llorca PM, Spadone C, Sol O, et al. Efficacy and safety of hydroxyzine in the treatment of generalized anxiety disorder: a 3-month double-blind study. J Clin Psychiatry 2002; 63: 1020–1027.
163. Feltner DE, Crockatt JG, Dubovsky SJ, et al. A randomized, double-blind, placebo-controlled, fixed-dose, multicenter study of pregabalin in patients with generalized anxiety disorder. J Clin Psychopharmacol 2003; 23:240–249.
164. Laakmann G, Schule C, Lorkowski G, et al. Buspirone and lorazepam in the treatment of generalized anxiety disorder in outpatients. Psychopharmacology (Berl) 1998; 136: 357–366.
165. Fresquet A, Sust M, Lloret A, et al. Efficacy and safety of lesopitron in outpatients with generalized anxiety disorder. Ann Pharmacother 2000; 34:147–153.
166. Rickels K, Schweizer E, DeMartinis N, et al. Gepirone and diazepam in generalized anxiety disorder: a placebo-controlled trial. J Clin Psychopharmacol 1997; 17:272–277.
167. Rickels K, DeMartinis N, Aufdembrinke B. A double-blind, placebo-controlled trial of abecarnil and diazepam in the treatment of patients with generalized anxiety disorder. J Clin Psychopharmacol 2000; 20:12–18.
168. Rickels K, Rynn M. Pharmacotherapy of generalized anxiety disorder. J Clin Psychiatry 2002; 63:9–16.
169. Rickels K, Downing R, Schweizer E, et al. Antidepressants for the treatment of generalized anxiety disorder. A placebo-controlled comparison of imipramine, trazodone, and diazepam. Arch Gen Psychiatry 1993; 50:884–895.
170. Kanczinski F, Lima MS, Souza JS, et al. Antidepressants for generalized anxiety disorder. Cochrane Database Syst Rev 2003; 2:CD003592.
171. Hoehn-Saric R, McLeod DR, Zimmerli WD. Differential effects of alprazolam and imipramine in generalized anxiety disorder: somatic versus psychic symptoms. J Clin Psychiatry 1988; 49:293–301.
172. Rocca P, Fonzo V, Scotta M, et al. Paroxetine efficacy in the treatment of generalized anxiety disorder. Acta Psychiatr Scand 1997; 95:444–450.
173. Strand M, Hetta J, Rosen A, et al. A double-blind, controlled trial in primary care patients with generalized anxiety: a comparison between buspirone and oxazepam. J Clin Psychiatry 1990; 51(suppl):40–45.
174. Davidson JR, DuPont RL, Hedges D, et al. Efficacy, safety, and tolerability of venlafaxine extended release and buspirone in outpatients with generalized anxiety disorder. J Clin Psychiatry 1999; 60:528–535.
175. Pollack MH, Worthington JJ, Manfro GG, et al. Abecarnil for the treatment of generalized anxiety disorder: a placebo-controlled comparison of two dosage ranges of abecarnil and buspirone. J Clin Psychiatry 1997; 58(suppl 11):19–23.
176. Lader M, Scotto JC. A multicentre double-blind comparison of hydroxyzine, buspirone and placebo in patients with generalized anxiety disorder. Psychopharmacology (Berl) 1998; 139:402–406.
177. Pollack MH, Zaninelli R, Goddard A, et al. Paroxetine in the treatment of generalized anxiety disorder: results of a placebo-controlled, flexible-dosage trial. J Clin Psychiatry 2001; 62:350–357.
178. Rickels K, Zaninelli R, McCafferty J, et al. Paroxetine treatment of generalized anxiety disorder: a double-blind, placebo-controlled study. Am J Psychiatry 2003; 160: 749–756.
179. Ball SG, Kuhn A, Wall D, et al. Selective serotonin reuptake inhibitor treatment for generalized anxiety disorder: a double-blind, prospective comparison between paroxetine and sertraline. J Clin Psychiatry 2005; 66:94–99.
180. Goodman WK, Bose A, Wang Q. Treatment of generalized anxiety disorder with escitalopram: pooled results from double-blind, placebo-controlled trials. J Affect Disord 2005; 87:161–167.

181. Baldwin DS, Huusom AK, Maehlum E. Escitalopram and paroxetine in the treatment of generalised anxiety disorder: randomised, placebo-controlled, double-blind study. Br J Psychiatry 2006; 189:264–272.
182. Goodman WK, Bose A, Wang Q. Treatment of generalized anxiety disorder with Escitalopram: pooled results from double-blind, placebo-controlled trials. J Affect Disord 2005; 87:161–167.
183. Rynn MA, Siqueland L, Rickels K. Placebo-controlled trial of sertraline in the treatment of children with generalized anxiety disorder. Am J Psychiatry 2001; 158:2008–2014.
184. Allgulander C, Dahl AA, Austin C, et al. Efficacy of sertraline in a 12-week trial for generalized anxiety disorder. Am J Psychiatry 2004; 161:1642–1649.
185. Sheehan DV. Venlafaxine extended release (XR) in the treatment of generalized anxiety disorder. J Clin Psychiatry 1999; 60(suppl 22):23–28.
186. Rickels K, Pollack MH, Sheehan DV, et al. Efficacy of extended-release venlafaxine in nondepressed outpatients with generalized anxiety disorder. Am J Psychiatry 2000; 157: 968–974.
187. Nimatoudis I, Zissis NP, Kogeorgos J, et al. Remission rates with venlafaxine extended release in Greek outpatients with generalized anxiety disorder: a double-blind, randomized, placebo controlled study. Int Clin Psychopharmacol 2004; 19:331–336.
188. Katz IR, Reynolds CF III, Alexopoulos GS, et al. Venlafaxine ER as a treatment for generalized anxiety disorder in older adults: pooled analysis of five randomized placebo-controlled clinical trials. J Am Geriatr Soc 2002; 50:18–25.
189. Pollack MH, Matthews J, Scott EL. Gabapentin as a potential treatment for anxiety disorders. Am J Psychiatry 1998; 155:992–993.
190. Pande AC, Crockatt JG, Feltner DE, et al. Pregabalin in generalized anxiety disorder: a placebo-controlled trial. Am J Psychiatry 2003; 160:533–540.
191. Pohl RB, Feltner DE, Fieve RR, et al. Efficacy of pregabalin in the treatment of generalized anxiety disorder: double-blind, placebo-controlled comparison of BID versus TID dosing. J Clin Psychopharmacol 2005; 25:151–158.
192. Montgomery SA, Tobias K, Zornberg GL, et al. Efficacy and safety of pregabalin in the treatment of generalized anxiety disorder: a 6-week, multicenter, randomized, double-blind, placebo-controlled comparison of pregabalin and venlafaxine. J Clin Psychiatry 2006; 67:771–782.
193. Khan A, Farfel GM, Brock JD, et al. Efficacy and safety of pregabalin in the treatment of generalized anxiety disorder in elderly patients. 2006.
194. Smith W, Feltner D, Kavoussi R. Pregabalin in generalized anxiety disorder: long term efficacy and relapse prevention. Eur Neuropsychopharmacol 2002; 12:S350–S350.
195. Schaller JL, Thomas J, Rawlings D. Low-dose tiagabine effectiveness in anxiety disorders. MedGenMed 2004; 6:8.
196. Papp LA, Ray S. Tiagabine treatment of generalized anxiety disorder. Presented at: The 156th Annual Meeting of the American Psychiatric Association; 2003; San Francisco, CA.
197. Rosenthal M. Tiagabine for the treatment of generalized anxiety disorder: a randomized, open-label, clinical trial with paroxetine as a positive control. J Clin Psychiatry 2003; 64:1245–1249.
198. Van Ameringen M, Pollack MH, Roy-Byrne. A randomized, double-blind, placebo-controlled study of tiagabine in patients with generalized anxiety disorder. 2004.
199. Pollack M. Levetiractam (keppra) for anxiety. Curbside Consultant 2002; 1(4):468–474.
200. Zohar J, Judge R. Paroxetine versus clomipramine in the treatment of obsessive-compulsive disorder. OCD paroxetine study investigators. Br J Psychiatry 1996; 169: 468–474.
201. Denys D, van der Wee N, van Megen HJ, et al. A double blind comparison of venlafaxine and paroxetine in obsessive-compulsive disorder. J Clin Psychopharmacol 2003; 23:568–575.
202. Hollander E, Allen A, Steiner M, et al. Acute and long-term treatment and prevention of relapse of obsessive-compulsive disorder with paroxetine. J Clin Psychiatry 2003; 64: 1113–1121.

203. Tollefson GD, Rampey AH Jr., Potvin JH, et al. A multicenter investigation of fixed-dose fluoxetine in the treatment of obsessive-compulsive disorder. Arch Gen Psychiatry 1994; 51:559–567.
204. Bergeron R, Ravindran AV, Chaput Y, et al. Sertraline and fluoxetine treatment of obsessive-compulsive disorder: results of a double-blind, 6-month treatment study. J Clin Psychopharmacol 2002; 22:148–154.
205. Piccinelli M, Pini S, Bellantuono C, et al. Efficacy of drug treatment in obsessive-compulsive disorder. A meta-analytic review. Br J Psychiatry 1995; 166:424–443.
206. Zitterl W, Meszaros K, Hornik K, et al. Efficacy of fluoxetine in Austrian patients with obsessive-compulsive disorder. Wien Klin Wochenschr 1999; 111:439–442.
207. Greist JH, Jefferson JW, Kobak KA, et al. Efficacy and tolerability of serotonin transport inhibitors in obsessive-compulsive disorder: a meta-analysis. Arch Gen Psychiatry 1995; 52:53–60.
208. Ackerman DL, Greenland S. Multivariate meta-analysis of controlled drug studies for obsessive-compulsive disorder. J Clin Psychopharmacol 2002; 22:309–317.
209. Montgomery SA, Kasper S, Stein DJ, et al. Citalopram 20 mg, 40 mg and 60 mg are all effective and well tolerated compared with placebo in obsessive-compulsive disorder. Int Clin Psychopharmacol 2001; 16:75–86.
210. Pallanti S, Quercioli L, Bruscoli M. Response acceleration with mirtazapine augmentation of citalopram in obsessive-compulsive disorder patients without comorbid depression: a pilot study. J Clin Psychiatry 2004; 65:1394–1399.
211. Goodman WK, Kozak MJ, Liebowitz M, et al. Treatment of obsessive-compulsive disorder with fluvoxamine: a multicentre, double-blind, placebo-controlled trial. Int Clin Psychopharmacol 1996; 11:21–29.
212. Mundo E, Maina G, Uslenghi C. Multicentre, double-blind, comparison of fluvoxamine and clomipramine in the treatment of obsessive-compulsive disorder. Int Clin Psychopharmacol 2000; 15:69–76.
213. Mundo E, Rouillon F, Figuera ML, et al. Fluvoxamine in obsessive-compulsive disorder: similar efficacy but superior tolerability in comparison with clomipramine. Hum Psychopharmacol 2001; 16:461–468.
214. Kronig MH, Apter J, Asnis G, et al. Placebo-controlled, multicenter study of sertraline treatment for obsessive-compulsive disorder. J Clin Psychopharmacol 1999; 19:172–176.
215. Hoehn-Saric R, Ninan P, Black DW, et al. Multicenter double-blind comparison of sertraline and desipramine for concurrent obsessive-compulsive and major depressive disorders. Arch Gen Psychiatry 2000; 57:76–82.
216. Bisserbe J, Lane R, Flament M. A double-blind comparison of sertraline and clomipramine in outpatients with obsessive compulsive disorder. Eur Psychiatry 1997; 12:82–93.
217. Fineberg NA, Pampaloni I, Pallanti S, et al. Escitalopram in obsessive-compulsive disorder: a randomized, placebo-controlled, paroxetine-referenced, fixed-dose, 24-week study. Curr Med Res Opin. 2007; Apr; 23(4):701–711.
218. Kobak KA, Greist JH, Jefferson JW, et al. Behavioral versus pharmacological treatments of obsessive compulsive disorder: a meta-analysis. Psychopharmacology (Berl) 1998; 136: 205–216.
219. The Clomipramine Collaborative Study Group. Clomipramine in the treatment of patients with obsessive-compulsive disorder. Arch Gen Psychiatry 1991; 48:730–738.
220. Vallejo J, Olivares J, Marcos T, et al. Clomipramine versus phenelzine in obsessive-compulsive disorder. A controlled clinical trial. Br J Psychiatry 1992; 161:665–670.
221. Jenike MA, Baer L, Minichiello WE, et al. Placebo-controlled trial of fluoxetine and phenelzine for obsessive-compulsive disorder. Am J Psychiatry 1997; 154:1261–1264.
222. McDougle CJ, Goodman WK, Leckman JF, et al. Haloperidol addition in fluvoxamine-refractory obsessive-compulsive disorder: a double-blind, placebo-controlled study in patients with and without tics. Arch Gen Psychiatry 1994; 51:302–308.
223. Dannon PN, Sasson Y, Hirschmann S, et al. Pindolol augmentation in treatment-resistant obsessive compulsive disorder: a double-blind placebo controlled trial. Eur Neuropsychopharmacol 2000; 10:165–169.

224. McDougle CJ, Epperson CN, Pelton GH, et al. A double-blind, placebo-controlled study of risperidone addition in serotonin reuptake inhibitor-refractory obsessive-compulsive disorder. Arch Gen Psychiatry 2000; 57:794–801.
225. Denys D, de Geus F, van Megen HJ, et al. A double-blind, randomized, placebo-controlled trial of quetiapine addition in patients with obsessive-compulsive disorder refractory to serotonin reuptake inhibitors. J Clin Psychiatry 2004; 65:1040–1048.
226. Bystritsky A, Ackerman DL, Rosen RM, et al. Augmentation of serotonin reuptake inhibitors in refractory obsessive-compulsive disorder using adjunctive olanzapine: a placebo-controlled trial. J Clin Psychiatry 2004; 65:565–568.
227. Cora-Locatelli G, Greenberg BD, Martin J, et al. Gabapentin augmentation for fluoxetine-treated patients with obsessive-compulsive disorder. J Clin Psychiatry 1998; 59:480–481.
228. Cora-Locatelli G, Greenberg BD, Martin JD, et al. Rebound psychiatric and physical symptoms after gabapentin discontinuation. J Clin Psychiatry 1998; 59:131.
229. Deltito JA. Valproate pretreatment for the difficult-to-treat patient with OCD. J Clin Psychiatry 1994; 55:500.
230. Cora-Locatelli G, Greenberg BD, Martin JD, et al. Valproate monotherapy in an SRI-intolerant OCD patient. J Clin Psychiatry 1998; 59:82.
231. Iwata Y, Kotani Y, Hoshino R, et al. Carbamazepine augmentation of clomipramine in the treatment of refractory obsessive-compulsive disorder. J Clin Psychiatry 2000; 61: 528–529.
232. Jenike MA, Brotman AW. The EEG in obsessive-compulsive disorder. J Clin Psychiatry 1984; 45:122–124.
233. Joffe RT, Swinson RP. Carbamazepine in obsessive-compulsive disorder. Biol Psychiatry 1987; 22:1169–1171.
234. Hollander E, Dell'Osso B. Topiramate plus paroxetine in treatment-resistant obsessive-compulsive disorder. Int Clin Psychopharmacol 2006; 21:189–191.
235. Van Ameringen M, Mancini C, Patterson B, et al. Topiramate augmentation in treatment-resistant obsessive-compulsive disorder: a retrospective, open-label case series. Depress Anxiety 2006; 23:1–5.
236. Rubio G, Jimenez-Arriero MA, Martinez-Gras I, et al. The effects of topiramate adjunctive treatment added to antidepressants in patients with resistant obsessive-compulsive disorder. J Clin Psychopharmacol 2006; 26:341–344.
237. Kumar TC, Khanna S. Lamotrigine augmentation of serotonin re-uptake inhibitors in obsessive-compulsive disorder. Aust N Z J Psychiatry 2000; 34:527–528.
238. Bowden CL, Calabrese JR, Sachs G, et al. A placebo-controlled 18-month trial of lamotrigine and lithium maintenance treatment in recently manic or hypomanic patients with bipolar I disorder. Arch Gen Psychiatry 2003; 60:392–400.
239. Crane D. Tiagabine for the treatment of anxiety. Depress Anxiety 2003; 18:51–52.
240. Schwartz TL, Azhar N, Husain J, et al. An open-label study of tiagabine as augmentation therapy for anxiety. Ann Clin Psychiatry 2005; 17:167–172.
241. Canadian Psychiatric Association. Clinical practice guidelines management of anxiety disorders. Can J Psychiatry 2006; 51(suppl 2):7S.

Antiepileptics in the Treatment of Alcohol Withdrawal and Alcohol Use Relapse Prevention

Mark A. Frye, Victor M. Karpyak, and Daniel Hall-Flavin
Department of Psychiatry and Psychology, Mayo Clinic, Rochester, Minnesota, U.S.A.

Ihsan M. Salloum
Department of Psychiatry, University of Miami, Miller School of Medicine, Miami, Florida, U.S.A.

Andrew McKeon
Department of Neurology, Mayo Clinic, Rochester, Minnesota, U.S.A.

Doo-Sup Choi
Departments of Psychiatry and Psychology and Molecular Pharmacology, Mayo Clinic, Rochester, Minnesota, U.S.A.

INTRODUCTION

In the World Health Organization's Global Burden of Disease Study (1), alcohol use disorders (abuse and dependence) ranked fifth in the undeveloped world and second in the developed world (ages 15–44 years) in disability-adjusted life years (DALYs); this measure is a composite of time lost because of premature mortality and time lived with a disability. In the United States alone, approximately 18 million people, or 7% of the population, suffer from alcohol abuse or dependence. The direct and indirect economic burden ascribed to alcohol use is estimated to be $185 billion (2). Clearly, more effective prevention and treatment of this major public health problem is needed.

For years, treatment for alcohol dependence predominantly focused on behavioral approaches or negative-reinforcement drug therapy such as disulfiram. Novel drug development over the last 10 to 15 years, as noted by the U.S. Food and Drug Administration (FDA) indications of naltrexone (1995), acamprosate (2004), and naltrexone extended-release injectable suspension (2006), has resulted in an increasing pharmacopoeia for the treatment of alcohol use disorders.

Over the course of the last 50 years, the language of an FDA alcoholism indication has evolved substantially from the 1951 indication of disulfiram ("management of selected chronic alcohol patients who want to remain in a state of enforced sobriety so that supportive and psychotherapeutic treatment may be applied to best advantage") to the 1995 naltrexone label ("an adjunct to other measures, including psychological and social counseling, in the treatment of alcohol dependence") and finally to the acamprosate 2004 label ("for the maintenance of sobriety in patients with alcohol dependence who are abstinent at treatment initiation as a part of a comprehensive management program, including psychosocial support") (3,4). This evolution in labeling not only reflects an increased understanding of the neurobiological underpinnings of addiction but also a conceptual change on how to integrate psychosocial, psychotherapeutic, and biologic treatments to maximize outcome measures such as complete abstinence and, more recently, reduction of hazardous drinking. Despite these advances, many alcoholics do not optimally respond to these current treatments. There remains an unmet need for pharmacological treatment options for both alcohol withdrawal and relapse prevention.

As recently reviewed by Mckeon et al. (5), the neurobiology of alcohol withdrawal is a complex set of voltage-dependent calcium channel, neuro-transmitter, and receptor-mediated interactions. Several neuromodulatory changes are potentially relevant when reviewing the mechanism of action of antiepileptic drugs (AEDs) and their potential utility in the treatment of alcohol withdrawal and relapse prevention. Acute alcohol ingestion has an inhibitory effect at N-methyl-D-aspartate (NMDA) receptors, reducing excitatory glutamatergic transmission (6,7), and an agonistic effect at gamma-aminobutyric acid type-A (GABA$_A$) receptors, which promotes inhibitory transmission. There is a subsequent NMDA receptor upregulation and GABA$_A$ receptor downregulation associated with chronic exposure to alcohol leading to tolerance (8). The roles are reversed during early abstinence, with enhanced NMDA receptor function, reduced GABAergic trans-mission, and dysregulation of the noradrenergic and dopaminergic systems, leading to many of the symptoms and signs of the alcohol withdrawal syndrome (9,10). Also, voltage-dependent calcium influx modulates neurotransmitter release and expression of genes that regulate production of NMDA and GABA receptor proteins; the continued presence of alcohol increases voltage-operated calcium channel expression and contributes to alcohol tolerance and the alcohol withdrawal syndrome (11).

The alcohol withdrawal syndrome is defined by two or more of the following after cessation or reduction of heavy or prolonged alcohol use: autonomic hyperactivity (sweating, tachycardia); psychomotor activation; anxiety/agitation; increased hand tremor; insomnia; nausea or vomiting; transient visual, tactile, or auditory illusions or hallucinations; and tonic-clonic seizures. While some alcohol withdrawal syndromes are mild and do not require treatment, if severe, it may be complicated by alcohol withdrawal seizures and delirium tremens (12). The chronic heavy user of alcohol is the typical patient who develops alcohol with-drawal seizures and is thought to occur secondary to a kindling effect of recurrent detoxifications (13).

Relapse prevention is the treatment intervention employed when a patient has been safely detoxified from alcohol and is now sober. This is often a time of great psychiatric instability as patients will commonly suffer from insomnia and have symptoms of anxiety, depression, or mania/hypomania at a subsyndromal or syndromal level. There may also be continued cravings for alcohol and anticipatory anxiety regarding psychosocial adjustments that need to be established in a new sober environment. By the *Diagnostic and Statistical Manual of Mental Disorders* (DSM-IV) criteria, most patients who start relapse prevention treatment have yet to meet or have just met criteria for abuse or dependence in early partial or full remission (14).

The AEDs have increasingly been identified as efficacious and effective compounds for treatment of both alcohol withdrawal and relapse prevention (15–17). The kindling model, well known in epilepsy and preclinical testing of AEDs, has also been proposed to be the neurophysiological mechanism by which alcohol withdrawal symptoms become more progressive with repeated episodes (18). This has been confirmed in retrospective and prospective clinical studies.

Brown et al. (19) studied male alcoholics with ($N = 25$) and without ($N = 25$) alcohol withdrawal–related seizures at the time of index admission for alcohol detoxification. In this study, 48% of the seizure group and only 12% of the non-seizure group had a history of greater than five prior detoxification admissions. Booth and Blow (20) reported that men with delirium tremens, alcoholic hallucinations, and withdrawal seizures at index detoxification were more likely than men without these symptoms to have subsequent readmissions for alcoholism, withdrawal symptoms, and withdrawal seizures.

Although the intermediate (oxazepam, lorazepam) and longer-acting benzodiazepines (diazepam, clonazepam) are the established agents for treating alcohol detoxification, there has been interest in developing other compounds with less addiction potential and a reduced sedative side-effect burden. In fact, comparative studies in alcohol withdrawal have shown that the AED carbamazepine decreases global distress and anxiety more than the benzodiazepines oxazepam and lorazepam, respectively. As anxiety and depressive symptoms can increase the likelihood of relapse, these limitations to the standard of benzodiazepine treatment are relevant. Other possible advantages of AEDs over benzodiazepines include the absence of potentiation of alcohol intoxication and their long-term use for seizure prevention in epilepsy. With this background, the AEDs carbamazepine, divalproex, topiramate, lamotrigine, and gabapentin would appear to be promising treatments for alcohol withdrawal or relapse prevention.

CARBAMAZEPINE/OXCARBAZEPINE

Carbamazepine (Tegretol®) is approved for use in the United States for the treatment of trigeminal neuralgia and for temporal lobe epilepsy (complex partial seizures). Carbamazepine was synthesized as a potential antidepressant, but its atypical profile in a number of animal models led to its initial development for pain control and seizure disorders. It is now recognized in most guidelines as a second-line mood stabilizer useful in the treatment and prevention of both phases of bipolar disorder. A long-acting sustained-release formulation (Carbatrol®) has been approved by the FDA for partial seizures, generalized seizures, and trigeminal neuralgia. Under an alternate name (Equetro®), the long-acting formulation has been FDA approved for the treatment of acute mania. The structure and chemistry of carbamazepine are closely related to the more recently introduced anticonvulsant oxcarbazepine (Trileptal®).

Carbamazepine inhibits voltage-dependent sodium channels, activates voltage-dependent potassium channels, and suppresses withdrawal-induced kindling in limbic structures (21). Animal studies have shown that carbamazepine is able to prevent alcohol withdrawal seizures and reduce withdrawal symptoms (22,23). A recent retrospective pooled analysis (24) encompassing 540 patients with alcohol withdrawal reported that carbamazepine (mean dose 540 mg/day) in combination with tiapride, a benzamide D2/D3-receptor antagonist, was safe and effective in reducing quantified signs and symptoms of alcohol withdrawal. In total, 103 (19%) had a history of alcohol withdrawal delirium and 151 (28%) of an epileptic seizure during withdrawal; these rates were reduced to 0.9% and 1.5%, respectively, while on carbamazepine-tiapride treatment. Keck et al. (25) reviewed six studies that evaluated carbamazepine's efficacy for treatment of withdrawal symptoms. In a seven-day trial comparing carbamazepine ($N = 32$; 800 mg/day) to oxazepam ($N = 34$; 120 mg/day) in the treatment of acute alcohol withdrawal, both drugs were effective; however, carbamazepine was more effective than oxazepam in decreasing global distress as measured by the Clinical Institute Withdrawal Assessment for Alcohol-Revised (CIWA-Ar) score (26). More recently, Malcolm et al. compared the effects of carbamazepine (600–800 mg/day) and lorazepam (6–8 mg/day) in divided doses in a randomized double-blind controlled trial (27). The CIWA-Ar was used to assess alcohol withdrawal symptoms on days 1 through 5 and then post medication on days 7 and 12. Both drugs were equally efficacious at treating the symptoms of alcohol withdrawal, but carbamazepine had greater efficacy than lorazepam in preventing posttreatment relapses to drinking over the 12 days of follow-up in those with multiple alcohol withdrawals. Furthermore, carbamazepine was associated with a greater reduction in anxiety symptoms, as measured by the Zung Anxiety Scale.

A Cochrane database systematic review (28) demonstrated that carbamazepine had a small but statistically significant protective effect over benzodiazepines. There was also a nonsignificant reduction in seizures and side effects favoring patients treated with AEDs over patients treated with other drugs in that review.

More direct evidence for the use of carbamazepine in the treatment of alcohol dependence comes from a placebo-controlled pilot study of 29 alcohol-dependent patients. Carbamazepine increased time to first drink and time to first heavy drinking within the first 120 days of the study. There was no difference between carbamazepine and placebo after one year, but low patient compliance complicates this finding (29). Complimentary to this work is the study of Bjorkqvist et al. (30), where alcohol-dependent patients randomized to carbamazepine returned to vocational functioning faster than alcohol-dependent patients randomized to placebo.

Oxcarbazepine (Trileptal®) is currently FDA approved for the treatment of partial seizures in children and adults. It is the 10-keto-analog of carbamazepine with no epoxide metabolite, less hepatic metabolism, and fewer drug-drug interactions. These advantages may explain the overall greater tolerability of oxcarbazepine over carbamazepine (31–33). Oxcarbazepine is a prodrug and is rapidly metabolized to a pharmacologically active monohydroxyderivative, which has been shown to reduce high voltage-dependent calcium channels and subsequent NMDA glutamatergic transmission (34).

Oxcarbazepine has shown comparable effects to carbamazepine in the treatment of the alcohol withdrawal syndrome in one randomized, single-blind study (35). However, a recent multisite, six-day, double-blind, detoxification trial of 50 inpatients reported that oxcarbazepine was no different than placebo in the primary outcome measure of clomethiazole (a GABA-mediated sedative hypnotic) rescue medication use (36). The authors highlighted that the study was underpowered and that the protocol-driven threshold for trigger-based clomethiazole use may have been lower than what is done clinically, thereby reducing the potential to demonstrate a drug-placebo difference.

The data for oxcarbazepine in relapse prevention are more promising, as there are two small proof-of-concept studies comparing the AED to two standard antidipsotropic drugs (37,38). In a 24-week randomized, parallel-group, open-label clinical trial of 30 acutely detoxified alcohol-dependent patients, oxcarbazepine (1200 mg/day) was compared with acamprosate (1998 mg/day) by survival analysis with time to first severe relapse (defined as ethanol consumptions of greater than 60 g/day for males and 48 g/day for females) as the primary outcome measure (37). While the effect size for survival analysis favored oxcarbazepine, the primary outcome measure was not significantly different between groups. In a

12-week randomized, open-label, comparison study of naltrexone 50 mg/day ($N = 27$), oxcarbazepine 1500 to 1800 mg/day ($N = 29$), and oxcarbazepine 600 to 900 mg/day ($N = 28$), a significantly larger number of subjects remained completely abstinent with high-dose oxcarbazepine (59%) compared with low-dose oxcarbazepine (43%) or naltrexone (41%). High-dose oxcarbazepine was also associated with a greater reduction in hostility-aggression subscores of the SCL-90-R and an overall better response rate in dual-diagnosis patients compared with the other two treatments (38).

DIVALPROEX

Valproic acid (*N*-dipropylacetic acid) is a simple branched chain carboxylic acid with a number of formulation derivatives, including divalproex sodium (Depakote$^®$), divalproex sodium extended release (Depakote ER$^®$), and valproate sodium injection (Depacon$^®$). Divalproex is approved by the FDA for (*i*) monotherapy or adjunctive therapy of complex partial seizures that occur in isolation or in conjunction with other types of seizures, (*ii*) monotherapy and adjunctive therapy of simple and complex absence seizures, (*iii*) adjunctive therapy for patients with multiple seizures that include absence seizures, (*iv*) acute manic and mixed episodes associated with bipolar disorder with or without psychosis, and (*v*) prophylaxis of migraine. Intravenous valproate sodium is currently FDA approved as an alternative in patients for whom oral administration is temporarily not feasible [i.e., those who are unresponsive or otherwise on nothing-by-mouth (NPO) status]. The drug has been shown to enhance GABA activity and suppress glutamate function via NDMA receptors (39,40).

Divalproex has been studied in the treatment of alcohol withdrawal in both open and randomized trials. In a one-week open-label study, inpatients with alcohol dependence were randomized to valproate (1200 mg/day) or control treatment with chlormethiazole or other tranquilizers, multivitamins, and fluid replacements. Five seizures occurred during the study (all in the control group) and withdrawal symptoms resolved more quickly with valproate, even though fewer valproate-treated patients received chlormethiazole (41). In a second study of 23 inpatients hospitalized for dysphoric mania, complicated by substance use (primarily alcohol), treatment with divalproex resulted not only in dysphoric symptom reduction [as measured by the Young Mania Rating Scale (YMRS) and the Hamilton Rating Scale for Depression (HAM-D)], but also in effective alcohol withdrawal symptom reduction and abstinence over the subsequent 20-week prospective follow-up (42). Mild hepatocellular enzyme elevation (not >3 times normal) at the time of admission, presumably related to alcohol ingestion, decreased over the study period. In a one-week double-blind, placebo-controlled study of nonbipolar subjects ($N = 36$) with alcohol withdrawal, subjects randomized to divalproex (1500 mg/day) required less rescue oxazepam than the placebo group (43). Furthermore, only 6% of patients in the divalproex group had an increase in withdrawal symptoms (as measured by CIWA-Ar) over time, whereas 40% of patients in the placebo group experienced an increase in CIWA-Ar scores. The ability to reduce benzodiazepine use in patients undergoing detoxification with divalproex without further significant hepatocellular risk (i.e., liver function tests decreased during detoxification) is a benefit clinically.

An open randomized trial pilot study by Longo et al. (44) evaluated divalproex in the treatment of both alcohol withdrawal and sustained abstinence in patients with alcohol dependence. Divalproex (mean dose 1500 mg/day) was as effective as standard chlordiazepoxide treatment in reducing alcohol withdrawal symptoms. Further benefit (i.e., increasing rate of abstinence) was observed at six weeks follow-up in those subjects who were maintained on divalproex compared with subjects who received either the benzodiazepine or divalproex only in the acute detoxification phase.

Alcohol relapse prevention has also been evaluated with divalproex (45). Twenty-nine outpatients with alcohol dependence participated in a 12-week, double-blind, placebo-controlled, pilot trial of divalproex. Mean valproic acid level at week 12 was 88.2 µg/mL. All patients received weekly cognitive behavioral therapy during the trial. There was a greater reduction in irritability in the divalproex treatment group, and a smaller percentage of divalproex-treated patients relapsed to heavy drinking (37%) compared with placebo-treated patients (63%; $p \leq 0.05$). There were no significant differences in reported side effects or abnormal laboratory values; in both treatment groups, a reduction in hepatocellular enzymes [alanine aminotransferase (ALT), aspartate aminotransferase (AST), and gamma-glutamyltransferase (GGT)] was observed during the course of the study. Given the extensive comorbidity of alcoholism with other Axis I disorders, particularly bipolar disorders, treatment with divalproex may stabilize mood and help treat components of alcoholism (withdrawal and relapse prevention). These results have now been replicated and extended.

In a 24-week, double-blind, placebo-controlled study of bipolar patients with comorbid active alcoholism maintained on lithium and psychosocial treatment as usual, divalproex showed greater effects than placebo on several measures of drinking (46). Of the 25 patients randomized to placebo, 68% returned to heavy drinking (defined as ≥ 4 drinks/day in women; ≥ 5 drinks/day in men) compared with 44% of the 27 randomized to divalproex ($p = 0.02$). Liver function tests ALT and AST did not differ between treatment groups, but gamma-glutamyltranspeptidase (GTP) was higher in those on placebo and was correlated with the amount of alcohol consumed per week. Of patients who did return to heavy drinking, time to relapse was significantly delayed for those on divalproex (93 days) compared with those on placebo (62 days; $p = 0.02$). Of note, this was one of the first studies to address the treatment of both drinking behavior and acute mood symptoms, which is an important situation regularly encountered in clinical practice.

TOPIRAMATE

Topiramate (Topomax®) is a sulfamate fructopyranose derivative that is FDA approved for the treatment of complex partial epilepsy, primary generalized epilepsy, seizures associated with Lennox-Gastaut syndrome, and prevention of migraine headache. Although five placebo-controlled studies of topiramate monotherapy in acute mania failed to show any demonstrable difference compared with placebo, topiramate shows promise as a treatment for alcohol dependence (47). First, topiramate has several mechanisms of action that theoretically are important in relation to treating alcoholism. Topiramate facilitates GABAergic neurotransmission through a nonbenzodiazepine site on the $GABA_A$ receptor; this action decreases extracellular release of midbrain dopamine, which is thought to mediate the craving and reward related to alcohol. In addition, topiramate antagonizes glutamate activity at AMPA and kainate receptors (48).

Second, mounting clinical trial data indicate topiramate is an effective treatment for alcohol dependence. In a prospective, open-label, 70-day study of 24 patients with alcohol dependence, adjunctive topiramate (mean dose 261 mg/day) significantly reduced alcohol consumption and craving as measured by a visual analog scale (49). A subsequent placebo-controlled study reported similar results. In addition to a brief weekly behavioral therapy to enhance medication compliance, 150 subjects with alcohol dependence were randomized to placebo or topiramate (50). The groups were matched on age, baseline drinking, and age of onset of problem drinking. The Timeline Follow Back (TLFB) method was the primary drinking outcome measure. There were no baseline differences between groups in TLFB measures of drinking outcome. At study endpoint, there were no group differences in dropout or completion rates or attrition from adverse events. However, topiramate (mean daily dose 120 ±38 mg/day) was statistically superior to placebo on all drinking and craving measures. This study was recently replicated in a 14-week, double-blind, randomized, placebo-controlled trial in 371 patients with alcohol dependence who also received a weekly compliance enhancement intervention (51). Subjects randomized to topiramate (mean dose 170 mg/day), compared with those receiving placebo, had a significantly reduced percentage of heavy drinking days. The percentage of heavy drinking days for the topiramate group was reduced from 82% at baseline to 44% at study endpoint; the placebo group's drinking was reduced from 82% at baseline to 52% at study endpoint. Topiramate was also associated with significant reductions in plasma GGT, AST, ALT, and body mass index (BMI). There was no correlation between topiramate dose and percent reduction of heavy drinking days.

GABAPENTIN

Gabapentin (Neurontin®) is approved for the adjunctive treatment of complex partial epilepsy with and without secondary generalization and postherpetic neuralgia. Calcium channel blockade and enhanced synthesis of brain GABA have been suggested as the potential antiepileptic mechanisms of action of this agent (52). Gabapentin has been shown to decrease excitability and convulsions in animal models of alcohol withdrawal (53). The lack of hepatic metabolism, cytochrome P450 enzyme induction, protein-binding, and addictive properties make gabapentin a potentially useful compound in this patient population.

Interest in gabapentin for treating the alcohol withdrawal syndrome grew after several positive reports emerged, using various doses of the drug, including starting at 400 mg three times daily and tapering over five days (54). One study demonstrated an efficacy similar to phenobarbital in treating the alcohol withdrawal syndrome (55). Another controlled trial, however, did not substantiate a benefit over placebo (56). This latter study included 61 inpatients admitted for a one-week alcohol detoxification who were randomized to gabapentin (400 mg q.i.d.) versus placebo with a protocol-driven trigger for the rescue medication clomethiazole (1 capsule = 192 mg). The primary outcome was the amount of rescue medication received in the first 24 hours, which was 6.2 capsules for the gabapentin group and 6.1 capsules for the placebo group. During the withdrawal study, there was a significant increase in the Profile of Mood State (POMS) vigor subscore in the gabapentin compared with the placebo group; this finding was particularly robust in the group with comorbid depression.

Despite the conflicting results for gabapentin in alcohol withdrawal, there is increasing recognition of its therapeutic benefit for the sleep disturbance component of the alcohol withdrawal syndrome. In an open-label pilot study, low-dose gabapentin (mean dose 900 mg/day) in the treatment of alcohol withdrawal, in comparison with trazodone, was associated with greater improvement in sleep problems, as assessed with the Sleep Problems Questionnaire (57). In a controlled trial in patients with a history of multiple previous alcohol withdrawals, gabapentin, in comparison with lorazepam, was associated with significant reductions in self-report sleep disturbances and sleepiness (58).

There is one four-week placebo-controlled, randomized, double-blind study evaluating gabapentin in alcohol abuse relapse prevention (59). After detoxification, 60 male alcohol-dependent subjects who had been drinking on average 17 drinks/day for the preceding three months were randomized to gabapentin (300 mg b.i.d.) versus placebo. The gabapentin group showed a significant reduction in the number of drinks per day, the percent heavy drinking days, and in craving for alcohol, specifically automaticity of drinking. In addition, gabapentin-treated patients showed an increase in percentage of abstinent days.

LAMOTRIGINE

Lamotrigine (Lamictal®) is currently FDA approved for simple and complex partial seizures, primary generalized tonic clonic seizures, the difficult-to-treat generalized seizures of Lennox-Gastaut syndrome, and the maintenance phase of bipolar I disorder. Lamotrigine inhibits presynaptic glutamate release through inhibition of sodium and calcium channels (60,61). Additionally, lamotrigine has been shown to modulate basal extracellular levels of serotonin and dopamine (62). Recent animal work has shown that pretreatment with lamotrigine was associated with significant reductions in both cue-induced reinstatement of alcohol-seeking behavior and voluntary alcohol intake after alcohol deprivation (63); both of these animal models have become widely used in examining the efficacy of drug therapy in preventing alcohol seeking and relapse.

Like other antiglutamatergic AEDs, lamotrigine may have some effectiveness in alcohol withdrawal. A recent double-blind study found lamotrigine 25 mg q.i.d. superior to placebo and equivalent to diazepam in the treatment of alcohol withdrawal in individuals with alcohol dependence (64).

While there are no clinical trials of lamotrigine in alcohol relapse prevention, lamotrigine has been reported to reduce drinking in alcoholics with bipolar disorder (65). In this open-label study, alcohol-dependent subjects with bipolar disorder received lamotrigine either as monotherapy or add-on therapy to other mood stabilizing medications for 12 weeks. Significant reductions in drinks per week, craving for alcohol, and carbohydrate-deficient transferrin were reported. Improved alcohol outcomes were paralleled by reductions in both mania and depression ratings. This study has a number of limitations, including small sample size and no control group for comparison. Moreover, it is unclear whether improved drinking outcomes were a cause or consequence of improved mood stability.

CONCLUSION

Studies completed to date suggest that nonbenzodiazepine, GABAergic, or antiglutamatergic AEDs may be effective treatments for the alcohol withdrawal syndrome and for preventing alcohol abuse relapse. Carbamazepine has the largest amount of evidence-based data for short-term efficacy for alcohol withdrawal followed by divalproex, with single studies providing support for topiramate and lamotrigine. For alcohol abuse relapse prevention or reduction in hazardous drinking, topiramate, divalproex, and to a lesser degree (because of sample size or study design), carbamazepine, oxcarbazepine, and gabapentin appear to be promising. Further controlled study is encouraged.

Generally, in studies of alcohol withdrawal and relapse prevention, AEDs were well tolerated with few serious adverse events. However, these agents are not without serious side effects (15,17,25,31). Carbamazepine, in addition to the difficulty of establishing stable blood levels due to its cytochrome P450 autoinduction properties, may produce significant hyponatremia and rare severe skin reactions. The hyponatremia risk is greater with oxcarbazepine (32,33). There are black box warning labels for serious dermatological conditions for carbamazepine, oxcarbazepine, and lamotrigine. One of the major concerns with the use of valproate in actively drinking or recovering alcoholics is the potential for hepatic and/or pancreatic compromise. Valproate has black box warnings for the rare but serious side effects, hepatic failure and pancreatitis. Thus far, most studies of divalproex in patients with alcohol abuse or dependence have reported a decrease, rather than increase, in liver function tests, presumably because of a decrease in alcohol use. Topiramate may produce cognitive deficits such as word-finding difficulties with prevalence rates varying from 7% in patients with epilepsy (66) to 27% in patients with migraine (67). Another concern with AEDs is their reproductive and teratogenic effects. Thus, careful reproductive history taking and education are essential before initiating treatment, as are ongoing monitoring and counseling, when using these medications in women of childbearing potential (68).

Many of the reviewed AEDs are conventional mood stabilizers (carbamazepine, divalproex, lamotrigine), and thus, in comparison with disulfiram, acamprosate, or naltrexone, may be preferred treatments in active dually diagnosed bipolar patients. Clinically, this is not an insignificant group as women and men with bipolar disorder are 7.4 and 2.8 times more likely than their counterparts in the general population to meet criteria for alcohol abuse or dependence (69). In one study, greater amounts of depression and anxiety were correlates in bipolar women with abuse alcohol, suggesting that alcohol abuse was a form of self-medication and that earlier and more effective intervention of these target symptoms could lessen the incidence of alcohol comorbidity (70).

The use of combined medications to decrease alcohol use among these patients may also be a viable option (71). In a randomized, open-label, pilot study, the combined pharmacotherapy of valproate plus naltrexone was compared with valproate alone in acutely ill, actively drinking bipolar alcoholics over an eight-week period. Those receiving the combination of valproate plus naltrexone versus valproate alone had a better outcome on avoiding relapse to alcohol use and on improvement in alcohol craving and mood symptoms. As always, careful consideration of the risk-benefit ratio of using adjunctive medications must be undertaken as polypharmacy, while prevalent, does pose some clinical challenges in the treatment of bipolar disorder (72).

It is very encouraging that interest and efforts at evaluating pharmacotherapeutic compounds for alcohol use disorders has substantially increased over the past few years. Antiepileptic mood stabilizers such as carbamazepine, divalproex, and lamotrigine, as well as the AEDs oxcarbazepine, gabapentin, and topiramate, appear to be promising agents for the treatment of alcohol withdrawal and relapse prevention. With such a diverse group of treatments potentially available (AEDs and antidipsotropics), it will be valuable to better understand how both withdrawal symptom management and relapse prevention management are achieved.

REFERENCES

1. Murray CJ, Lopez AD. Global mortality, disability, and the contribution of risk factors. Global Burden of Disease Study. Lancet 1997; 349(9063):1436–1442.
2. Li T, Hewitt B, Grant B. Alcohol use disorders and mood disorders: a National Institute on Alcohol Abuse and Alcoholism perspective. Biol Psychiatry 2004; 56:718–720.
3. USP DI® Drug Information for the Health Care Professional and PDR, 2006.
4. Physicians Desk Reference. 60th ed. Montvale, NJ: Thomson PDR, 2006.
5. McKeon A, Frye MA, Delanty N. The alcohol withdrawal syndrome. J Neurol Neurosurg Psychiatry 2008 (In press).
6. Tsai G, Gastfriend DR, Coyle JT. The glutamatergic basis of human alcoholism. Am J Psychiatry 1995; 152:332–340.
7. Tsai G, Coyle JT. The role of glutamatergic neurotransmission in the pathophysiology of alcoholism. Annu Rev Med 1998; 49:173–184.
8. Sanna E, Mostallino MC, Busonero F, et al. Changes in GABA(A) receptor gene expression associated with selective alterations in receptor function and pharmacology after ethanol withdrawal. J Neurosci 2003; 23:11711–11724.
9. Nutt D. Alcohol and the brain. Pharmacological insights for psychiatrists. Br J Psychiatry 1999; 175:114–119.
10. Lingford-Hughes A, Nutt D. Neurobiology of addiction and implications for treatment. Br J Psychiatry 2003; 182:97–100.
11. Kovacs GL. Natriuretic peptides in alcohol withdrawal: central and peripheral mechanisms. Curr Med Chem 2003; 10:2559–2576.
12. Seitz PF. The sensorium in delirium tremens and alcoholic hallucinosis. Am J Psychiatry 1951; 108:145.
13. Lechtenberg R, Worner TM. Total ethanol consumption as a seizure risk factor in alcoholics. Acta Neurol Scand 1992; 85:90–94
14. American Psychiatric Association, American Psychiatric Association Task Force on DSM-IV, Teton Data Systems (firm). Diagnostic and Statistical Manual of Mental Disorders DSM-IV-TR. 4th ed. Washington, DC: American Psychiatric Association, 2000.
15. Ait-Saoud N, Malcolm RJ, Johnson BA. An overview of medications for the treatment of alcohol withdrawal and alcohol dependence with an emphasis on the use of older and newer anticonvulsants. Addict Behav 2006; 31:1628–1649.
16. Leggio L, Kenna GA, Swift RM. New developments for the pharmacological treatment of alcohol withdrawal syndrome. A focus on non-benzodiazepine GABAergic medications. Prog Neuro-Psychopharmacol Biol Psychiatry 2008 (In press).
17. Malcolm R, Myrick H, Brady KT, et al. Update on anticonvulsants for the treatment of alcohol withdrawal. Am J Addict 2001; 10(S):16–23.
18. Ballenger JC, Post RM. Kindling as a model for alcohol withdrawal syndromes. Br J Psychiatry 1978; 133:1–14.
19. Brown ME, Anton RE, Malcom R, et al. Alcohol detoxification and withdrawal seizures clinical support for a kindling hypothesis. Biol Psychiatry 1988; 23:507–514.
20. Booth BM, Blow FC. The kindling hypothesis: further evidence from a U.S. national study of alcoholic men. Alcohol Alcohol 1993; 28:593–598.
21. Armijo JA, Shushtarian M, Valdizan EM, et al. Ion channels and epilepsy. Curr Pharm Des 2005; 11:1975–2003.
22. Chu NS. Carbamazepine: prevention of alcohol withdrawal seizures. Neurology 1979; 29:1397–1401.
23. Strzelec JS, Czarnecka E. Influence of clonazepam and carbamazepine on alcohol withdrawal syndrome, preference and development of tolerance to ethanol in rats. Pol J Pharmacol 2001; 53:117–124.
24. Soyka M, Schmidt P, Franz M, et al. Treatment of alcohol withdrawal syndrome with a combination of tiapride/carbamazepine: results of a pooled analysis in 540 patients. Eur Arch Psychiatry Clin Neurosci 2006; 256:395–401.

25. Keck PE Jr., McElroy SL, Friedman LM. Valproate and carbamazepine in the treatment of panic and posttraumatic stress disorders, withdrawal states, and behavioral dyscontrol syndromes. J Clin Psychopharmacol 1992; 12:36S–41S.
26. Malcolm R, Ballenger JC, Sturgis ET, et al. Double-blind controlled trial comparing carbamazepine to oxazepam treatment of alcohol withdrawal. Am J Psychiatry 1989; 146:617–621.
27. Malcolm R, Myrick H, Roberts J, et al. The effects of carbamazepine and lorazepam on single versus multiple previous alcohol withdrawals in an outpatient randomized trial. J Gen Intern Med 2002; 17:349–355.
28. Polycarpou A, Papanikolaou P, Ioannidis JP, et al. Anticonvulsants for alcohol withdrawal. Cochrane Database Syst Rev 2005; 3:CD005064.
29. Mueller TI, Stout RL, Rudden S, et al. A double-blind, placebo-controlled pilot study of carbamazepine for the treatment of alcohol dependence. Alcohol Clin Exp Res 1997; 21:86–92.
30. Bjorkqvist SE, Isohanni M, Makela R, et al. Ambulant treatment of alcohol withdrawal symptoms with carbamazepine: a formal multicentre double-blind comparison with placebo. Acta Psychiatr Scand 1976; 53:333–342.
31. Keck PE, McElroy SL. Clinical pharmacodynamics and pharmacokinetics of antimanic and mood stabilizing medications. J Clin Psychiatry 2002; 63:(suppl 4):3–122.
32. Glauser TA. Oxcarbazepine in the treatment of epilepsy. Pharmacotherapy 2001; 21: 904–919.
33. Beydoun A, Kutluay E. Oxcarbazepine. Expert Opin Pharmacother 2002; 3:59–71.
34. Wellington K, Goa KL. Oxcarbazepine: an update on its efficacy in the management of epilepsy. CNS Drugs 2001; 15:137–163.
35. Schik G, Wedegaertner FR, Liersch J, et al. Oxcarbazepine versus carbamazepine in the treatment of alcohol withdrawal. Addict Biol 2005; 10:283–288.
36. Koethe D, Juelicher A, Nolden BM, et al. Oxcarbazepine: efficacy and tolerability during treatment of alcohol withdrawal: a double-blind, randomized, placebo-controlled multicenter pilot study. Alcohol Clin Exp Res 2007; 31:1188–1194.
37. Croissant B, Diehl A, Klein O, et al. A pilot study of oxcarbazepine versus acamprosate in alcohol-dependent patients. Alcohol Clin Exp Res 2006; 4:630–635.
38. Martinotti G, Di Nicola M, Romanelli R, et al. High and low dosage oxcarbazepine versus naltrexone for the prevention of relapse in alcohol dependent patients. Hum Psychopharmacol 2007; 22:149–156.
39. Keck PE, McElroy SL, Friedman LM. Valproate and carbamazepine in the treatment of panic and posttraumatic stress disorders, withdrawal states, and behavioural dyscontrol syndromes. J Clin Pscyhopharmacol 1992; 12(1 suppl):36S–41S.
40. Loscher W. Basic pharmacology of valproate: a review after 35 years of clinical use for the treatment of epilepsy CNS Drug 2002; 16:669–694.
41. Lambie D, Johnson RH, Vijayasenan ME, et al. Sodium valproate in the treatment of the alcohol withdrawal syndrome. Aust NZ J Psychiatry 1980; 14:213–215.
42. Brady KT, Sonne SC, Anton R, et al. Valproate in the treatment of acute bipolar affective episodes complicated by substance abuse: a pilot study. J Clin Psychiatry 1995; 56:118–121.
43. Reoux JP, Saxon AJ, Malte CA, et al. Divalproex sodium in alcohol withdrawal: a randomized double-blind placebo-controlled clinical trial. Alcohol Clin Exp Res 2001; 25: 1324–1329.
44. Longo LP, Campbell T, Hubatch S. Divalproex sodium (Depakote) for alcohol withdrawal and relapse prevention. J Addict Dis 2002; 21(2):55–64.
45. Brady KT, Myrick H, Henderson S, et al. The use of divalproex in alcohol relapse prevention: a pilot study. Drug Alcohol Depend 2002; 67(3):323–330.
46. Salloum IM, Cornelius JR, Daley DC, et al. Efficacy of valproate maintenance in patients with bipolar disorder and alcoholism: a double-blind placebo controlled study. Arch Gen Psychiatry 2005; 62(1):37–45.
47. Kushner SF, Khan A, Olson WH. Topiramate monotherapy in the management of acute mania: results of four double-blind placebo controlled trials. Bipolar Disord 2006; 8:15–27.
48. Moghaddam B, Bolinao ML. Glutamatergic antagonists attenuate ability of dopamine uptake blockers to increase extracellular levels of dopamine: implications for tonic influence of glutamate on dopamine release. Synapse 1994; 18:337–342.

49. Rubio G, Ponce G, Jimenez-Arriero MA, et al. Effectiveness of topiramate in control of alcohol craving. Eur Neuropsychoparmacol 2002; 12(suppl 3):S367.
50. Johnson BA, Ait-Daoud N, Bowden CL, et al. Oral topiramate for treatment of alcohol dependence: a randomised controlled trial. Lancet 2003; 361(9370):1677–1685.
51. Johnson BA, Rosenthal N, Capece JA, et al. Topiramate for treating alcohol depndence: a randomized controlled trial. JAMA 2007; 298:1641–1651.
52. McLean M. Clinical pharmacokinetics of gabapentin. Neurology 1994; 44:S17–S22.
53. Watson WP, Robinson E, Little HJ. The novel anticonsultant gabapentin protects against both convulsant and anxiogenic aspects of the ethanol withdrawal syndrome. Neuropharmacology 1997; 36:1369–1375.
54. Bozikas V, Petrikis P, Gamvrula K, et al. Treatment of alcohol withdrawal with gabapentin. Prog Neuropsychopharmacol Biol Psychiatry 2002; 26:197–199.
55. Mariani JJ, Rosenthal RN, Tross S, et al. A randomized, open-label, controlled trial of gabapentin and phenobarbital in the treatment of alcohol withdrawal. Am J Addict 2006; 15:76–84.
56. Bonnet U, Banger M, Leweke FM, et al. Treatment of acute alcohol withdrawal with gabapentin: results from a controlled two-center trial. J Clin Psychopharmacol 2003; 23:514–519.
57. Karam-Hage M, Brower KJ. Open pilot study of gabapentin versus trazodone to treatment insomnia in alcoholic outpatients. Psychiatry Clin Neurosci 2003; 57:542–544.
58. Malcolm R, Myrick LH, Veatch LM, et al. Self-reported sleep, sleepiness, and repeated alcohol withdrawals: a randomized, double blind, controlled comparison of lorazepam vs. gabapentin. J Clin Sleep Med 2007; 15:24–32.
59. Furieri FA, Nakamura-Palacios EM. Gabapentin reduces alcohol consumption and craving: a randomized, double-blind, placebo-controlled trial. J Clin Psychiatry 2007; 11:1691–1700.
60. Lees G, Leach MJ. Studies on the mechanism of action of the novel anticonvulsant lamotrigine using primary neurological cultures from rat cortex. Brain Res 1993; 612:190–199.
61. Wang SJ, Sibra TS, Gean PW. Lamotrigine inhibition of glutamate release from isolated cerebrocortical nerve terminals by suppression of voltage activated calcium channel activity. Neuroreport 2001; 12:2255–2258.
62. Ahmad S, Fowler LJ, Whitton PS. Effects of acute and chronic lamotrigine treatment on basal and stimulated extracellular amino acids in the hippocampus of freely moving rats. Brain Res 2004; 1029:41–47.
63. Vengelien V, Heidbreder CA, Spanagel R. The effects of lamotrigine on alcohol seeking and relapse. Neuropharmacology 2007; 53:951–957.
64. Krupitsky EM, Rudenko AA, Burakov AM, et al. Antiglutamatergic strategies for ethanol detoxification: comparison with placebo and diazepam. Alcohol Clin Exp Res 2007; 31:604–611.
65. Rubio G, Lopez-Munoz F, Alamo C. Effects of lamotrigine in patients with bipolar disorder. Bipolar Disord 2006; 8:289–293.
66. Mula M, Trimble MR, Thompson P, et al. Topiramate and word-finding difficulties in patients with epilepsy. Neurology 2003; 60(7):1104–1107
67. Coppola F, Rossi C, Mancini ML, et al. Language disturbances as a side effect of prophylactic treatment of migraine. Headache 2008; 48(1):86–94.
68. Altshuler LL, Cohen L, Szuba MP, et al. Pharmacologic management of psychiatric illness during pregnancy: dilemmas and guidelines. Am J Psychiatry 1996; 154(5):592–606.
69. Frye MA, Altshuler LL, McElroy SL, et al. Gender differences in prevalence, risk, and clinical correlates of alcoholism comorbidity in bipolar disorder. Am J Psychiatry 2003; 160:883–889.
70. Salloum IM, Cornelius JR, Mezzich JE, et al. Characterizing female bipolar alcoholic patients presenting for initial evaluation. Addict Behav 2001; 26:341–348.
71. Salloum IM, Cornelius JR, Daley DC, et al. Efficacy of valproate in bipolar alcoholics: a double blind, placebo-controlled study. Presented at: the Fifth International Conference on Bipolar Disorder; June 12–14, 2003; Pittsburgh, PA.
72. Frye MA, Ketter TA, Leverich GS, et al. The increasing use of polypharmacotherapy for refractory mood disorders: 22 years of study. J Clin Psychiatry 2000; 61(1):9–15.

9 Antiepileptic Drugs in the Treatment of Drug Use Disorders

Kyle M. Kampman

University of Pennsylvania School of Medicine, Philadelphia, Pennsylvania, U.S.A.

INTRODUCTION

Antiepileptic drugs (AEDs) such as phenobarbital have been traditionally used in the treatment of sedative-hypnotic dependence to help patients withdraw safely from sedatives, including benzodiazepines. More recently, newer AEDs, including carbamazepine and valproate, have also shown some potential in treating benzodiazepine withdrawal. AEDs such as GVG [gamma-vinyl gamma-aminobutyric acid (GABA)], topiramate, and tiagabine may be promising for the treatment of stimulant dependence, primarily as relapse-prevention medications. Finally, AEDs such as carbamazepine and lamotrigine may be particularly beneficial in helping drug-addicted patients with comorbid mood disorders achieve and maintain abstinence from drugs of abuse, including from stimulants.

ANTIEPILEPTIC DRUGS FOR THE TREATMENT OF SEDATIVE-HYPNOTIC WITHDRAWAL

For many years, phenobarbital has been used to facilitate withdrawal from sedative hypnotics (1). Its usefulness as a detoxification medication is related to its cross-tolerance with other sedatives including benzodiazepines (2). Phenobarbital acts primarily by facilitating transmission at the $GABA_A$ receptor, as do sedatives, including benzodiazepines (3). Although patients addicted to benzodiazepines could be treated by gradually tapering the dose of the benzodiazepine or other sedative to which they are already addicted, phenobarbital is favored by many clinicians because of its long half-life and because many clinicians believe that it is better not to administer the drug of abuse during treatment.

Withdrawal from high doses of benzodiazepines (doses much higher than recommended therapeutic doses) is usually done in a hospital setting. The starting dose of phenobarbital can be calculated on the basis of the patient's history of benzodiazepine use over the past month. A dose of 30 mg of phenobarbital is roughly equivalent to 10 mg of diazepam, 25 mg of chlordiazepoxide, 1 mg of alprazolam, or 2 mg of clonazepam (4). The calculated phenobarbital-equivalent dose is given in three divided doses each day. Because patients often cannot give an accurate estimate of the type or dose of sedative they have been abusing, they need to be closely observed after the first few doses of phenobarbital and the dose adjusted on the basis of clinical response. The maximum starting dose of phenobarbital is 500 mg daily. After two days of stabilization, the dose is decreased by 30 mg daily (4). Patients addicted to lower doses of benzodiazepines (i.e., those within the therapeutic range) can also be detoxified using phenobarbital replacement, but the rate of the taper is usually much longer, i.e., many weeks to months in an outpatient setting.

More recently, other AEDs such as carbamazepine and valproate have been tested with some success for the treatment of benzodiazepine withdrawal. Carbamazepine's mechanism of action is unique. It has no effect on benzodiazepine receptors or on the GABA receptor complex in general. Carbamazepine limits the repetitive firing of action potentials by slowing the rate of recovery of voltage-activated sodium channels from inactivation (2). Its ability to inhibit electrical activation in the limbic system is thought to be a possible mechanism of action for the treatment of sedative withdrawal. It has been hypothesized that repeated withdrawal from alcohol or other sedatives induces long-lasting neuronal changes that alter the organism's response to sedatives, resulting in more severe withdrawal symptoms (5). Carbamazepine has been shown to be effective in blocking the progression of disorders on the basis of the kindling model, such as bipolar disorder, alcohol withdrawal, and electrically induced kindling in rats (6–8). Thus, it was hypothesized that carbamazepine would be effective as a treatment for sedative-hypnotic withdrawal based on its effects on kindling (5).

There have been several case series and open trials reported in the literature, supporting the use of carbamazepine for the treatment of benzodiazepine withdrawal (9–14). In most cases, carbamazepine was added to a tapering dose of benzodiazepine, although in at least one open trial, the benzodiazepines were abruptly stopped when carbamazepine was started (11).

There has been only one double-blind, controlled trial of carbamazepine as an adjunct to a tapering dose of benzodiazepine to treat benzodiazepine withdrawal (15). In this trial, 40 benzodiazepine-dependent patients were randomized to carbamazepine 200 to 800 mg daily or placebo. After starting study medication, patients' benzodiazepine doses were tapered 25% per week. Patients assigned to carbamazepine were significantly more likely to be abstinent from benzodiazepines five weeks after the taper was complete compared with placebo-treated patients (15). However, the difference between carbamazepine- and placebo-treated patients was no longer statistically significant at 12 weeks after taper completion. Carbamazepine-treated patients reported less severe withdrawal symptoms compared with placebo-treated patients, but this effect was significant only at a trend level. Carbamazepine was reasonably well tolerated. The most commonly experienced side effects included headache, nausea, and mental impairment (15).

Valproate has also been used for benzodiazepine withdrawal. Its anti-convulsant effects appear to be mediated by a prolonged recovery of voltage-activated sodium ion channels from inactivation (2). In addition, valproate may increase brain GABA levels. It stimulates the activity of the GABA synthetic enzyme glutamic acid decarboxylase and inhibits the GABA degradative enzymes GABA transaminase and succinic semialdehyde dehydrogenase (2). Valproate's usefulness in the treatment of benzodiazepine withdrawal is thought to be related to its ability to increase GABAergic neurotransmission.

The evidence supporting the usefulness of valproate for the treatment of benzodiazepine withdrawal consists of two small case studies and one double-blind trial. In one case, valproate treatment appeared to facilitate benzodiazepine tapering (16). In the other, therapy with valproate appeared to reduce protracted abstinence symptoms in four patients recently detoxified from benzodiazepines (17). In the only double-blind, controlled trial of valproate for benzodiazepine withdrawal, Rickels and colleagues compared the serotonergic antidepressant trazodone with valproate and to placebo in 78 benzodiazepine-dependent patients (18). Patients were stabilized on a dose of benzodiazepine and then pretreated for two weeks with either trazodone 100 to 500 mg daily, valproate 500 to 2500 mg daily, or placebo. After two weeks, patients' benzodiazepines were tapered 25% each week. All treatments were continued for five weeks post taper. Follow-up evaluations were conducted 5 and 12 weeks after completion of the taper. At the five-week follow-up, both the trazodone- and valproate-treated patients were significantly more likely to be free from benzodiazepines than the placebo-treated patients. At the 12-week follow-up, however, there were no statistically significant differences in benzodiazepine use between the three groups. Additionally, neither trazodone nor valproate was effective in reducing benzodiazepine withdrawal symptom severity (18).

In sum, the evidence supporting the usefulness of carbamazepine and valproate for the treatment of benzodiazepine withdrawal is not overwhelming. While several open trials and case series suggest carbamazepine may be useful, the one double-blind trial did not completely support carbamazepine's efficacy. Carbamazepine was associated with a higher rate of abstinence from benzodiazepines five weeks after completing a benzodiazepine taper, but this effect was not seen at 12-week follow-up. In addition, carbamazepine had no effect on benzodiazepine withdrawal symptom severity. The data supporting the efficacy of valproate for benzodiazepine detoxification are even weaker, with only two very small case series suggesting the drug's utility in this area. No open trials have been published, and the results of the one double-blind trial of valproate for benzodiazepine detoxification are similar to those obtained for carbamazepine. Valproate was associated with a higher rate of benzodiazepine abstinence five weeks after completing a benzodiazepine taper compared with placebo, but this effect was not seen at 12-week follow-up.

ANTIEPILEPTIC DRUGS FOR THE TREATMENT OF STIMULANT DEPENDENCE

AEDs have received a great deal of study for the treatment of cocaine dependence where they have been mainly viewed as potentially helpful for the prevention of relapse. None are FDA approved for the treatment of cocaine dependence, and most of the data supporting their usefulness in this area come from small, pilot clinical trials that have not yet been replicated in large well-controlled trials. Initially, it was believed that AEDs that were useful in the control of kindled seizures, such as carbamazepine, would be useful for the treatment of cocaine dependence. However, in three separate double-blind, placebo-controlled trials, carbamazepine was not found to be better than placebo for the treatment of cocaine dependence (19–21). More recently, attention has shifted to AEDs that have GABAergic properties, and these medications appear to hold more promise. These GABAergic AEDs may be able to affect the mesocortical dopaminergic reward center in a way that reduces craving and prevents relapse in cocaine-dependent patients.

The mesocortical dopamine system plays a central role in the reinforcing effects of cocaine (22–25). Mesocortical dopaminergic neurons receive modulatory inputs from both GABergic and glutamatergic neurons. GABA is primarily an inhibitory neurotransmitter in the central nervous system, and activation of GABAergic neurons tends to decrease activity in the dopaminergic reward system. Preclinical trials of AEDs that enhance GABAergic neurotransmission have suggested that these compounds reduce the dopamine response to both cocaine administration and to conditioned reminders of prior cocaine use (26–28).

GABAergic medications also reduce self-administration of cocaine in animal models (29,30). Therefore, GABAergic medications could prevent relapse either by blocking cocaine-induced euphoria or by reducing craving caused by exposure to conditioned reminders of prior cocaine use. Some promising GABAergic AEDs include GVG, tiagabine, and topiramate.

GVG is an AED that has been in use in many countries throughout the world for a number of years, but not the United States. It is an irreversible inhibitor of GABA transaminase and thus elevates brain GABA concentrations. Preclinical trials of GVG have been promising. GVG has been shown to block cocaine- and cocaine cue–induced increases in nucleus accumbens dopamine (27,31). It has also been shown to block cocaine self-administration in rodents (29). Similar results have been shown for GVG with both amphetamine and methamphetamine (28).

There has been only one clinical trial of GVG for the treatment of stimulant dependence. This was a small open-label trial involving 20 patients with either cocaine or amphetamine dependence. In this trial, GVG treatment was well tolerated and was associated with significant reductions in stimulant use in 40% of patients (32).

GVG has not been approved for use in the United States because of an association with visual field defects. However, available data suggest that such visual field defects occur after relatively long-term exposure to GVG and that brief treatment with GVG may be safely conducted (33,34). Large-scale, well-controlled trials of GVG for both cocaine and amphetamine dependence have, therefore, been planned.

Tiagabine is another GABAergic AED that may be promising for the treatment of cocaine dependence. Currently approved for the treatment of seizures, it is a selective blocker of the presynaptic GABA reuptake transporter type 1 (35). Tiagabine was found to be well tolerated and moderately effective for improving abstinence in a pilot study that included 45 cocaine- and opiate-dependent patients participating in a methadone maintenance program. In this 10-week trial, the number of cocaine metabolite–free urine samples increased by 33% in the group treated with tiagabine (24 mg/day) and decreased by 14% in the placebo-treated group (36). The results of this trial were recently replicated in another 10-week trial also conducted in cocaine- and opiate-dependent patients stabilized on methadone. Patients treated with tiagabine (24 mg/day; $N = 25$) significantly reduced their cocaine use compared with placebo-treated patients ($N = 25$). At the end of the trial, tiagabine-treated patients submitted 48% cocaine-free urine samples compared with 24% cocaine-free samples for the placebo group (37).

Topiramate may be an excellent medication for relapse prevention based on its effects on both GABA and glutamate neurotransmission. Topiramate facilitates GABA neurotransmission and increases cerebral levels of GABA (38,39). It also inhibits glutamate neurotransmission through blockade of α-amino-3 hydroxy-5-methyl-4-isoxazole propionic acid (AMPA)/kainate receptors (40). In animal models of cocaine relapse, blockade of AMPA receptors in the nucleus accumbens has been shown to prevent reinstatement of cocaine self-administration (41).

In a 13-week, double-blind, placebo-controlled pilot trial of topiramate involving 40 cocaine-dependent patients, topiramate-treated patients were significantly more likely to be abstinent during the last five weeks of treatment compared with placebo-treated patients (42). In addition, among patients who returned for at least one visit after receiving medication, topiramate-treated patients were significantly more likely to achieve at least three weeks of continuous abstinence from cocaine compared with placebo-treated patients (59% vs. 26%). Topiramate-treated patients were also significantly more likely than placebo-treated patients to be rated very much improved on their last visit (71% vs. 32%) (42). Topiramate is currently undergoing large-scale confirmatory trials for the treatment of cocaine dependence as well as for the treatment of combined cocaine and alcohol dependence.

AEDs are among the most promising medications for the treatment of cocaine dependence. Medications such as GVG and topiramate may be efficacious for many drugs of abuse in addition to cocaine, including nicotine and alcohol. However, at this time there are no large-scale, well-controlled trials that have shown any AED to be efficacious for the treatment of cocaine or amphetamine dependence. More research is needed before any AED can be recommended for the treatment of cocaine or amphetamine dependence.

ANTIEPILEPTIC DRUGS FOR THE TREATMENT OF DRUG DEPENDENCE AND COMORBID MOOD DISORDERS

AEDs have been shown to be effective for the treatment of bipolar disorder (43). Mood disorders, in general, and bipolar disorder, in particular, are commonly seen in patients with substance use disorders (44). For the treatment of drug-dependent patients with comorbid mood disorders, at least two AEDs have shown some promise: carbamazepine and lamotrigine.

Carbamazepine was not found to be effective for the treatment of cocaine dependence in three separate double-blind, placebo-controlled trials (19–21). However, it is an effective medication for the treatment of bipolar disorder and its mood-stabilizing properties may help cocaine-dependent patients with comorbid mood disorders reduce their cocaine use. In one double-blind, placebo-controlled trial, Brady and colleagues found that, among cocaine-dependent patients with comorbid mood disorders, those treated with carbamazepine were less likely to relapse to cocaine use (45). This trial involved 139 cocaine-dependent patients, 57 with a comorbid mood disorder. Of those with mood disorders, 33 had major depression or dysthymia and 24 had bipolar disorder or cyclothymia. Patients were treated with carbamazepine 800 mg daily or placebo. Among patients with a comorbid mood disorder, carbamazepine treatment was associated with a significantly longer time to relapse to cocaine use. By contrast, among patients without a comorbid mood disorder, carbamazepine had no effect on cocaine use.

There is some evidence from two open trials that lamotrigine may be effective for the treatment of cocaine dependence in patients with bipolar disorder. Brown and colleagues conducted two open trials of lamotrigine that included a total of 62 cocaine-dependent patients with comorbid bipolar disorder (bipolar I, II, or bipolar disorder NOS) (46,47). In the most recent trial, lamotrigine was added to the patient's ongoing regimen and titrated up to a maximum dose of 300 mg/day (average dose 155 mg/day). Over the 36-week trial, mood symptoms declined, as did cocaine craving and dollars spent for cocaine. In addition, there was a significant correlation between improvement in mood symptoms and reductions in cocaine craving and cocaine use (47).

In sum, among bipolar patients with comorbid cocaine dependence, there is preliminary evidence that AEDs may be effective for the treatment of both mood and drug dependence symptoms. In a double-blind trial, carbamazepine reduced relapse to cocaine in patients with co-occurring bipolar and unipolar mood disorders. In two open trials in bipolar patients, lamotrigine treatment was associated with less cocaine craving and less cocaine use. These data need to be replicated in larger, well-controlled clinical trials before either medication can be recommended for the treatment of cocaine dependent patients with comorbid mood disorders.

REFERENCES

1. Smith DE, Wesson DR. Phenobarbital technique for treatment of barbiturate dependence. Arch Gen Psychiatry 1971; 24(1):56–60.
2. McNamara JO. Drugs effective in the therapy of the epilepsies. In: Hardman JG, Limbard LE, eds. Goodman and Gillman's The Pharmacological Basis of Therapeutics. 10th ed. New York, NY: McGraw Hill, 2001:521–547.
3. Charney D, Mihic S, Harris R. Hypnotics and sedatives. In: Hardman J, Limbird L, Goodman Gilman A, eds. Goodman and Gillman's The Pharmacological Basis of Therapeutics. 10th ed. New York, NY: McGraw Hill, 2001:399–427.
4. Wesson D, Smith D, Seymore M. Sedative-hypnotics and tricyclics. In: Lowinson J, Ruiz P, Millman R, et al. eds. Substance Abuse, A Comprehensive Textbook. 2nd ed. Philadelphia, PA: Williams and Wilkins, 1992:217–279.
5. Mueller TI, Stout RL, Rudden S, et al. A double-blind, placebo-controlled pilot study of carbamazepine for the treatment of alcohol dependence. Alcohol Clin Exp Res 1997; 21(1): 86–92.
6. Post RM, Weiss SR, Chuang DM. Mechanisms of action of anticonvulsants in affective disorders: comparisons with lithium. J Clin Psychopharmacol 1992; 12(suppl 1):S23–S35.
7. Ballenger JC, Post RM. Kindling as a model for alcohol withdrawal syndromes. Br J Psychiatry 1978; 133:1–14.
8. Silver JM, Shin C, McNamara JO. Antiepileptogenic effects of conventional anticonvulsants in the kindling model of epilespy. Ann Neurol 1991; 29(4):356–363.
9. Klein E, Uhde TW, Post RM. Preliminary evidence for the utility of carbamazepine in alprazolam withdrawal. Am J Psychiatry 1986; 143(2):235–236.
10. Ries RK, Roy-Byrne PP, Ward NG, et al. Carbamazepine treatment for benzodiazepine withdrawal. Am J Psychiatry 1989; 146(4):536–537.
11. Ries R, Cullison S, Horn R, et al. Benzodiazepine withdrawal: clinicians' ratings of carbamazepine treatment versus traditional taper methods. J Psychoactive Drugs 1991; 23(1):73–76.
12. Swantek SS, Grossberg GT, Neppe VM, et al. The use of carbamazepine to treat benzodiazepine withdrawal in a geriatric population. J Geriatr Psychiatry Neurol 1991; 4(2): 106–109.
13. Garcia-Borreguero D, Bronisch T, Apelt S, et al. Treatment of benzodiazepine withdrawal symptoms with carbamazepine. Eur Arch Psychiatry ClinNeurosci 1991; 241(3): 145–150.
14. Klein E, Colin V, Stolk J, et al. Alprazolam withdrawal in patients with panic disorder and generalized anxiety disorder: vulnerability and effect of carbamazepine. Am J Psychiatry 1994; 151(12):1760–1766.
15. Schweizer E, Rickels K, Case WG, et al. Carbamazepine treatment in patients discontinuing long-term benzodiazepine therapy. Effects on withdrawal severity and outcome. Arch Gen Psychiatry 1991; 48(5):448–452.
16. McElroy SL, Keck PE Jr., Lawrence JM. Treatment of panic disorder and benzodiazepine withdrawal with valproate. J Neuropsychiatry Clin Neurosci 1991; 3(2):232–233.
17. Apelt S, Emrich HM. Sodium valproate in benzodiazepine withdrawal. Am J Psychiatry 1990; 147(7):950–951.
18. Rickels K, Schweizer E, Garcia Espana F, et al. Trazodone and valproate in patients discontinuing long-term benzodiazepine therapy: effects on withdrawal symptoms and taper outcome. Psychopharmacology 1999; 141(1):1–5.

19. Montoya ID, Levin FR, Fudala PJ, et al. Double-blind comparison of carbamazepine and placebo for treatment of cocaine dependence. Drug Alcohol Depend 1995; 38(3):213–219 (comment).
20. Cornish JW, Maany I, Fudala PJ, et al. Carbamazepine treatment for cocaine dependence. Drug Alcohol Depend 1995; 38(3):221–227 (comment).
21. Kranzler HR, Bauer LO, Hersh D, et al. Carbamazepine treatment of cocaine dependence: a placebo-controlled trial. Drug Alcohol Depend 1995; 38(3):203–211 (comment).
22. Roberts DCS, Koob GF, Klonoff P, et al. Extinction and recovery of cocaine self-administration following 6-hydroxydopamine lesions of the nucleus accumbens. Pharmacol Biochem Behav 1980; 12:781–787.
23. Koob G, Vaccarino F, Amalric M, et al. Positive reinforcement properties of drugs: search for neural substrates. In: Engel J, Oreland L, eds. Brain Reward Systems and Abuse. New York, NY: Raven Press, 1987:35–50.
24. Goeders NE, Dworkin SI, Smith JE. Neuropharmacological assessment of cocaine self-administration into the medial prefrontal cortex. Pharmacol Biochem Behav 1986; 24: 1429–1440.
25. Dworkin SI, Smith JE. Neurobehavioral pharmacology of cocaine. In: Clouet D, Ashgar K, Brown R, eds. Mechanisms of Cocaine Abuse and Toxicity. National Institute on Drug Abuse Research Monograph Number 88. Washington, DC: U.S. Government Printing Office, 1988:185–198.
26. Dewey S, Smith G, Logan J, et al. GABAergic inhibition of endogenous dopamine release measured in vivo with 11c- raclopride and positron emission tomography. J Neurosci 1992; 12(10):3773–3780.
27. Dewey SL, Chaurasia CS, Chen CE, et al. GABAergic attenuation of cocaine-induced dopamine release and locomotor activity. Synapse 1997; 25(4):393–398.
28. Gerasimov MR, Ashby CR Jr., Gardner EL, et al. Gamma-vinyl GABA inhibits methamphetamine, heroin, or ethanol-induced increases in nucleus accumbens dopamine. Synapse 1999; 34(1):11–19.
29. Kushner SA, Dewey SL, Kornetsky C. The irreversible gamma-aminobutyric acid (GABA) transaminase inhibitor gamma-vinyl-GABA blocks cocaine self-administration in rats. J Pharmacol Exp Ther 1999; 290(2):797–802.
30. Roberts DC, Andrews MM, Vickers GJ. Baclofen attenuates the reinforcing effects of cocaine in rats. Neuropsychopharmacology 1996; 15(4):417–423.
31. Morgan AE, Dewey SL. Effects of pharmacologic increases in brain GABA levels on cocaine-induced changes in extracellular dopamine. Synapse 1998; 28(1):60–65.
32. Brodie JD, Figueroa E, Laska EM, et al. Safety and efficacy of gamma-vinyl GABA (GVG) for the treatment of methamphetamine and/or cocaine addiction. Synapse 2005; 55(2):122–125.
33. Manuchehri K, Goodman S, Siviter L, et al. A controlled study of vigabatrin and visual abnormalities. Br J Ophthalmol 2000; 84(5):499–505.
34. Schmitz B, Schmidt T, Jokiel B, et al. Visual field constriction in epilepsy patients treated with vigabatrin and other antiepileptic drugs: a prospective study. J Neurol 2002; 249 (4):469–475.
35. Schachter S. Tiagabine. Epilepsia 1999; 40:S17–S22.
36. Gonzalez G, Sevarino K, Sofuoglu M, et al. Tiagabine increases cocaine-free urines in cocaine-dependent methadone-treated patients: results of a randomized pilot study. Addiction 2003; 98(11):1625–1632.
37. Gonzalez G, Desai R, Sofuoglu M, et al. Clinical efficacy of gabapentin versus tiagabine for reducing cocaine use among cocaine dependent methadone-treated patients. Drug Alcohol Depend 2007; 87:1–9.
38. Kuzn[iecky R, Hetherington H, Ho S, et al. Topiramate increases cerebral GABA in healthy humans. Neurology 1998; 51(2):627–629.
39. Petroff OA, Hyder F, Mattson RH, et al. Topiramate increases brain GABA, homocarnasine, and pyrrolidinone in patients with epilepsy. Neurology 1999; 52(3):473–478.
40. Gibbs J, Sombati S, DeLorenzo R, et al. Cellular actions of topiramate: blockade of kainate-evoked inward currents in cultured hippocampal neurons. Epilepsia 2000; (suppl 1):S10–S16.

41. Cornish JL, Kalivas PW. Glutamate transmission in the nucleus accumbens mediates relapse in cocaine addiction. J Neurosci 2000; 20(RC89):1–5 (rapid communication).
42. Kampman KM, Pettinati H, Lynch KG, et al. A pilot trial of topiramate for the treatment of cocaine dependence. Drug Alcohol Depend 2004; 75(3):233–240.
43. McElroy SL, Keck PE Jr. Pharmacologic agents for the treatment of acute bipolar mania. Biol Psychiatry 2000; 48(6):539–557.
44. Regier DA, Farmer ME, Rae DS, et al. Comorbidity of mental disorders with alcohol and other drug abuse. Results from the Epidemiologic Catchment Area (ECA) Study. JAMA 1990; 264(19):2511–2518 (comment).
45. Brady KT, Sonne SC, Malcolm RJ, et al. Carbamazepine in the treatment of cocaine dependence: subtyping by affective disorder. Exp Clin Psychopharmacol 2002; 10(3):276–285.
46. Brown ES, Nejtek VA, Perantie DC, et al. Lamotrigine in patients with bipolar disorder and cocaine dependence. J Clin Psychiatry 2003; 64(2):197–201.
47. Brown ES, Perantie DC, Dhanani N, et al. Lamotrigine for bipolar disorder and comorbid cocaine dependence: a replication and extension study. J Affect Disord 2006; 93(1–3):219–222.

Antiepileptic Drugs in the Treatment of
Impulsivity and Aggression and Impulse
Control and Cluster B Personality Disorders

Heather A. Berlin and Eric Hollander
*Department of Psychiatry, Mount Sinai School of Medicine,
New York, New York, U.S.A.*

INTRODUCTION

We review here evidence that suggest that antiepileptic drugs (AEDs) (a.k.a. anti-convulsants) may be effective for the treatment of impulsivity and aggression across a range of psychiatric disorders. AEDs are increasingly used as primary or adjunctive treatments for impulse control disorders (ICDs) and cluster B personality disorders [in particular borderline personality disorder (BPD)]. Thus, in addition to the reviewing the effects of AEDS on the symptoms of impulsivity and aggression across a variety of diagnoses, we will focus on ICDs and BPD. The AEDs valproate (e.g., divalproex sodium), carbamazepine, and lamotrigine have U.S. Food and Drug Administration (FDA) indications for the treatment of bipolar disorder. Other AEDs, like oxcarbazepine, gabapentin, topiramate, levetiracetam, phenytoin, and tiagabine, are often used as mood stabilizers but do not have FDA indication for bipolar disorder. Use of off-label AEDs requires careful monitoring and publication of all significant results, including adverse effects. The choice of specific AED is often dependent on drug-drug interactions and side-effect profile (1). Side effects from AEDs are typically mild to moderate. Although data regarding longer-term safety of the newer AEDs are limited, they may have more desirable side-effect profiles.

Impulsivity and Aggression

Impulsivity and aggression are natural behaviors controlled by brain mechanisms, which are essential for survival in all species. Understanding those mechanisms may lead to targeted treatment strategies for this symptom domain when these behaviors become dysfunctional. The concept of impulsivity covers a wide range of "actions that are poorly conceived, prematurely expressed, unduly risky, or inappropriate to the situation and that often result in undesirable outcomes" (2). Moeller et al. (3) defined impulsivity as: "a predisposition toward rapid, unplanned reactions to internal or external stimuli without regard to the negative consequences of these reactions to the impulsive individual or to others." Aggressive behavior has been defined as a verbal or physical act directed against a person or object that can potentially cause physical or emotional harm that occurs in a premeditated or impulsive manner (3,4). The symptoms of impulsivity and aggression are a significant public health problem and can be manifested by self-injurious behavior (SIB), suicide, suicide attempts, substance abuse, accidents (e.g., motor vehicle), domestic violence, assault, and destruction of property (5–10). Intervention can occur at the symptom, syndrome, or behavioral level.

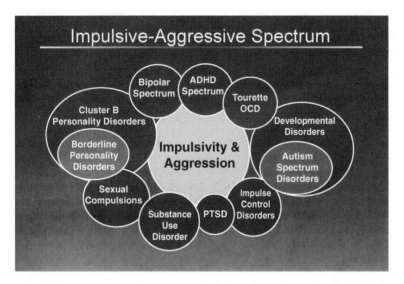

FIGURE 1 Impulsive-aggressive spectrum. *Abbreviations*: ADHD, attention deficit hyperactivity disorder; OCD, obsessive-compulsive disorder; PTSD, posttraumatic stress disorder.

Impulsive and aggressive behaviors can be conceptualized as existing on a spectrum where they are the core symptoms of a broad range of psychiatric disorders that are often comorbid with one another, like cluster B personality disorders, ICDs, autism spectrum disorders, and bipolar disorder (Fig. 1). This is based on similarities in associated clinical features (e.g., age of onset, clinical course, comorbidity) and response to pharmacological treatment [e.g., selective serotonin reuptake inhibitors (SSRIs)], suggesting a high degree of overlap among disorders (11). Further, impulsivity can be thought of as part of a compulsive-impulsive dimensional model, where impulsivity and compulsivity represent polar opposite complexes that can be viewed along a continuum of compulsive and impulsive disorders (Fig. 2). One endpoint marks compulsive or risk-aversive behaviors characterized by overestimation of the probability of future harm, exemplified by obsessive-compulsive disorder (OCD). The other endpoint designates impulsive action characterized by the lack of complete consideration of the negative results of such behavior, exemplified by borderline disorder and antisocial personality disorder (ASPD). Anti-impulsive medication classes include SSRIs, serotonin (5-HT)1A agonists, 5-HT2 antagonists (Table 1), lithium, AEDs, atypical and typical antipsychotics, β blockers, α2-agonists (e.g., clonidine, guanfacine), opiate antagonists (e.g., naltrexone), and dopamine agonists (e.g., stimulants, bupropion).

There are many contributing factors to impulsivity and aggression such as genes, gender, environment, psychiatric disorders, and substance abuse. Early environment can alter a person's neurochemistry related to impulsivity and aggression (12). The neurochemistry of aggression and impulsivity may involve serotonin, gamma-aminobutyric acid (GABA), glutamate, norepinephrine, dopamine, androgens, vasopressin, and nitric oxide.

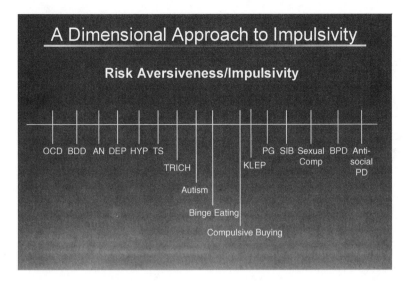

FIGURE 2 A dimensional approach to impulsivity. *Abbreviations*: OCD, obsessive-compulsive disorder; BDD, body dysmorphic disorder; AN, anorexia; DEP, depression; HYP, hypochondriasis; TS, Tourette's syndrome; TRICH, trichotillomania; KLEP, kleptomania; PG, pathological gambling; SIB, self-injurious behavior; Comp, compulsion; BPD, borderline personality disorder; PD, personality disorder.

TABLE 1 Mechanisms of Impulsive Behavioral Disturbances

Serotonin-sensitive	Serotonin-resistant
Low serotonin	Severe arousal
Impulsive aggression	Multiple disturbances
Trait dependent	Mixed-state trait
Increased serotonin function would ameliorate disturbance	Decreased arousal would ameliorate disturbance

Neural Substrates

The orbitofrontal cortex (OFC), with its extensive reciprocal connections with the amygdala (which is implicated in emotional behavior) (13,14), may play a role in correcting or regulating emotional and behavioral responses (15–19). Limbic-orbitofrontal circuit dysfunction may be involved in impulsivity and aggression, at least in a subgroup of patients (20). Impulsivity and aggression may conceivably involve increased limbic discharge, decreased OFC function, and/or hypoactive frontolimbic circuitry (21). Studies suggest that the amygdala and OFC act as part of an integrated neural system, as well as alone, in guiding decision making and adaptive response selection on the basis of stimulus-reinforcement associations (13,22–25). Thus, underactivation of prefrontal areas involved in inhibiting behavior, overstimulation of the limbic regions involved in drive, or a combination of both may result in disinhibited and aggressive behaviors.

For example, in 15 healthy subjects, Pietrini et al. (26) found that compared with imagined scenarios involving emotionally neutral behavior, imagined scenarios involving aggressive behavior were associated with significant emotional reactivity and reductions in reginal cerebral blood flow (rCBF) in the ventromedial prefrontal cortex (PFC). These results in healthy subjects support previous animal and human studies, which suggest the involvement of the OFC in the expression of aggressive behavior. Reduced serotonergic activity has been associated with impulsive aggression in personality-disordered patients in metabolite, pharmacological challenge, and position emission tomography (PET) studies. In an [^{18}F] fluorodeoxyglucose PET study (27), six impulsive-aggressive patients with intermittent explosive disorder (IED) and five healthy volunteers were evaluated for changes in regional glucose metabolism after administration of d,l-fenfluramine (a serotonergic releasing agent) or placebo. Healthy controls showed increases in glucose metabolism in the orbitofrontal, ventral medial frontal, cingulate, and inferior parietal cortices, while impulsive-aggressive patients had no significant increases in glucose metabolism in any region after fenfluramine. Compared with controls, impulsive-aggressive patients also had significantly blunted metabolic responses in orbitofrontal, ventral medial, and cingulate cortices but not in inferior parietal lobe. These results suggest that impulsive-aggressive personality disorder patients have reduced serotonergic modulation of orbital frontal, ventral medial frontal, and cingulate cortices.

OFC [Brodmann area (BA) 10] and ventrolateral PFC (BA 47) activation are thought to exhibit top-down control over limbic pathways (28,29). The amygdala is known to receive major visual input from sensory areas of the cortex, which provide fast responses to simple perceptual and associative aspects of external stimuli (30). Thus, in addition to subcortical pathways of emotional processing, which are thought to act automatically even without awareness of stimuli (31), the OFC and ventrolateral PFC, with their strong interconnections with subcortical areas implicated in emotional behavior, may play a role in correcting emotional responses (15,18,19). In fact, using functional magnetic resonance imaging (FMRI), an abnormal elevation of CBF in the ventrolateral PFC in response to aversive emotional stimuli was found in four of six BPD subjects, but not in controls (29), and was also reported during induced aversive emotional states in patients with anxiety disorders or depression (28). This part of the PFC is directly connected with the basal nucleus of the amygdala, and has been regarded as a gateway for distinctive sensory information, and may modulate or inhibit amygdala-driven emotional responses and thus provide top-down control of the amygdala (28,32,33).

ANTIEPILEPTIC DRUGS AND IMPULSE CONTROL DISORDERS

IED, kleptomania, pyromania, pathological gambling, trichotillomania, and ICDs not otherwise specified (NOS) are the classic disorders of impulse control listed under "impulse-control disorders not elsewhere classified" in the Diagnostic and Statistical Manual of Mental Disorders IV-Text Revision (DSM-IV-TR) (34), in which impulsivity is a core and defining symptom. Further, currently categorized under ICDs-NOS, but proposed to be included as individual ICDs in the DSM-V, are impulsive-compulsive sexual behaviors, shopping, Internet addiction, and excoriation (skin picking). The essential feature of an ICD is the failure to resist an impulse, drive, or temptation to perform an act that is harmful to the person or to others. Additional features include increasing tension or arousal before the act; pleasure, gratification, or relief at the time of the act; and self-reproach or guilt following the act. Impulsivity also plays a significant role in a wide range of other psychiatric disorders, including mood disorders (particularly mania), personality disorders (borderline and antisocial), eating disorders [e.g., binge eating disorder (BED), bulimia nervosa], substance use disorders, schizophrenia, attention deficit hyperactivity disorder (ADHD), paraphilias, conduct disorder, and neurological disorders with disinhibition.

There is gender predominance for most of the ICDs. Pathological gambling, IED, pyromania, and sexual compulsions are more prevalent in males, whereas kleptomania, trichotillomania, SIB, compulsive shopping, and BED are more prevalent in females. This differential gender distribution indicates that both men and women express impulsivity but do so in different ways. The reasons for this differential gender distribution are unclear but may be related to genetic factors, differences in serotonin turnover, hormonal differences, or social/environmental pressures.

We review here treatment studies of ICDs with AEDs, focusing on pathological gambling as an ICD that may be successfully treated with AEDs.

Pathological Gambling

Pathological gambling has traits in common with many different psychiatric disorders (Fig. 3). The link between pathological gambling and antisocial disorders, including ASPD, conduct disorder, and adult antisocial behavior, is largely determined by genetic propensity. Slutske et al. (35) found that genetic factors account for 61% to 86% of the overlap between antisocial behaviors and pathological gambling and 16% to 22% of the variance for pathological gambling overall. Nonfamilial environmental factors also significantly contribute to pathological gambling and to ASPD and adult antisocial behavior. Antisocial behavior is not just a consequence of pathological gambling but also an independent psychiatric symptom. Further, the risk of alcohol abuse/dependence and adult antisocial behavior overlap, suggesting that impulsivity is a mediator in these conditions. In

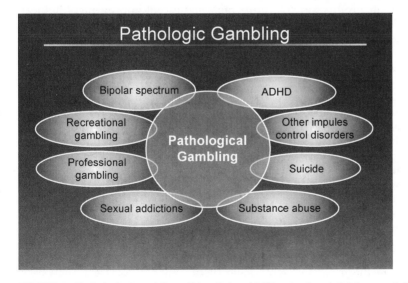

FIGURE 3 Pathological gambling. *Abbreviation*: ADHD, attention deficit hyperactivity disorder.

other words, impulsivity can be thought of as a common endophenotype, or nonobvious underlying trait, in these and related psychiatric disorders.

In FMRI studies, researchers observed that, compared with healthy subjects, pathological gamblers have decreased activity in their ventromedial PFC during presentation of gambling cues (36) and during a cognitive inhibition task (e.g., Stroop color-word) (37). The ventromedial PFC is associated with decision making (38), and the OFC plays a role in the processing of rewards during the expectancy and experiencing of monetary gains or losses (17,39–41). In a recent imaging study of pathological gamblers ($N = 7$), Hollander et al. (41) found that during a gambling task, monetary reward, as opposed to game points, was associated with significantly higher metabolic activity in the primary visual cortex (BA 17), cingulate gryus (BA 24), putamen, and OFC (BAs 47 and 10).

An understanding of the neurobiology of pathological gambling is beginning to emerge. Serotonin (5-HT) is linked to behavioral initiation and disinhibition, which are important in the onset of the gambling cycle and the difficulty in ceasing gambling behavior. Norepinephrine is associated with the arousal and risk taking in patients with pathological gambling. Dopamine is linked to positive and negative reward and the addictive component of pathological gambling (42). Studies suggest that potentially useful treatments for pathological gambling include the SSRIs clomipramine (43) and fluvoxamine (44–46), the opioid antagonist naltrexone (which may reduce the "high" associated with gambling) (47), the mood stabilizer lithium (48–50), and the AEDs carbamazepine (51), valproate (49), and topiramate (46).

While SSRIs may be effective for some patients with pathological gambling (43–46), those with comorbid conditions, like bipolar spectrum disorders, may relapse during such treatment. Thus treatment with AEDs for pathological gambling has been suggested, especially when bipolar mood symptoms are present. In the first controlled trial of mood stabilizers in pathological gambling, Pallanti et al. (49) compared the efficacy and safety of lithium and valproate in nonbipolar pathological gamblers. At the end of the 14-week trial, both the lithium and valproate groups showed comparable significant improvement in mean score on the Yale-Brown Obsessive-Compulsive Scale Modified for Pathological Gambling (YBOCS-PG). Thirteen (68.4%) of the nineteen patients taking valproate and 14 (60.9%) of the 23 patients taking lithium were responders based on a Clinical Global Impressions-Improvement Scale (CGI-I) score of much or very much improved.

Dannon et al. (46) compared the effectiveness of randomly assigned topiramate versus fluvoxamine in the treatment of male pathological gamblers. After 12 weeks, 9 of the 12 topiramate completers reported full remission of gambling behavior, and three completers had a partial remission. The CGI-I score was significantly better for the topiramate group at the 12-week visit as compared with baseline. Six of the eight fluvoxamine completers reported a full remission and the remaining two completers reported a partial remission. The fluvoxamine group showed improvement in the CGI-I score at week 12 but the change was not significant. Hollander (personal communication, 2007) recently completed a randomized, 14-week, double-blind, placebo-controlled, multicenter trial of topiramate (flexibly dosed to 300 mg or the maximum tolerated dose) in 50 subjects with pathological gambling. The primary endpoint was the change from baseline in the obsession component of the YBOCS-PG. Data analysis is presently ongoing.

Other ICDs

Topiramate has been reported to be effective in the treatment of a number of ICDs other than pathological gambling (46), including kleptomania (52), skin picking (53,54), trichtillomania (55), and IED (56,57). For example, topiramate augmentation of clomipramine/fluvoxamine was reported useful in a case of trichotillomania (58). In an open-label pilot study, Lochner et al. (55) evaluated topiramate monotherapy in 14 adults with trichtillomania. Patients received 16 weeks of flexible-dose treatment (50–250 mg/day), followed by a flexible-dose taper over two to four weeks. Severity of hair pulling in those who completed the 16-week trial ($N = 9$) decreased significantly from baseline to endpoint according to the Massachusetts General Hospital Hair Pulling Scale. Although CGI-I scores (a secondary outcome measure) suggested that hair pulling was not significantly reduced, six of nine completers were classified as responders. Five patients dropped out because of adverse effects. These results suggest that topiramate may be useful in the treatment of some patients with trichtillomania.

Prader-Willi syndrome (PWS) is a multisystem neurogenetic obesity disorder with behavioral manifestations, including hyperphagia, compulsive behaviors, mild to moderate mental retardation, and SIBs in the form of skin picking, nail biting, and rectal gouging. In the first published study of topiramate for the treatment of PWS or SIB, Shapira et al. (53) reported attenuation of SIBs resulting in lesion healing in three PWS adults treated with topiramate in an eight-week open-label trial. In another eight-week open-label study, Shapira et al. (54) evaluated adjunctive therapy with topiramate in eight adults with PWS. Topiramate did not significantly change compulsions, calories consumed, body mass index (BMI), or increased self-reported appetite. However, there was a clinically significant improvement in the self-injury characteristics (i.e., skin picking) of this syndrome. Double-blind or crossover studies are needed to establish the role of topiramate in attenuating SIB in PWS and other disorders involving SIB.

Regarding other ICDs, Dannon (52) reported three kleptomaniac patients who responded well to topiramate given either alone or in combination with SSRIs. Kaufman et al. (59) described two patients with ICDs with aggressive features and postencephalitic epilepsy where adjunctive tiagabine, a novel GABA reuptake inhibitor AED, was effective in the management of both epilepsy and severe impulsive and aggressive behaviors. This is consistent with observations that GABAergic modulation is important in impulsive aggression. De Dios Perrino et al. (56) reported three IED patients in whom good control of aggressive behavior was achieved using SSRIs in combination with carbamazepine. Indeed, in a survey completed by 2543 psychiatrists in the United States in 1988, carbamazepine was reported to be moderately to markedly effective in 65.2% of IED patients and 43.0% of BPD patients (57). In sum, AEDs may be effective treatments for ICDs, but more appropriately powered randomized, double-blind, placebo-controlled trials are needed.

ANTIEPILEPTIC DRUGS AND CLUSTER B PERSONALITY DISORDERS

Borderline Personality Disorder

We review here AED treatment studies across cluster B personality disorders. Since the majority of studies focus specifically on BPD, we will also discuss BPD in this section.

Personality disorders are characterized by interpersonal styles that are rigid and constant over time with onset before adulthood. BPD has been the most extensively studied among the current personality disorders. The DSM-IV-TR (34) classifies BPD as an axis II cluster B personality disorder with criteria that include affective instability, impulsive risk-taking behavior, inappropriate and intense anger, fear of abandonment, unstable relationships that rapidly shift between idealization and devaluation, unstable self-image, feelings of emptiness, dissociative experiences, SIB like superficial skin cutting or burning, and multiple suicide attempts. The designation of BPD as an axis II disorder reflects the historical conceptualization that personality disorders are psychologically and developmentally rooted, rather than biologically based and genetically determined like axis I disorders. Recently, alternative conceptualizations of BPD in particular and personality disorders in general have arisen, providing a theoretical rationale for the investigation into their neurobiology.

BPD is characterized by the core features of affective instability (possibly related to increased responsivity of the cholinergic system) and impulsivity and aggression (both thought to be related to reduced serotonergic brain activity). A typical symptom for BPD is the tendency to have outbursts of aggressive impulsivity (60). BPD is associated with high levels of functional impairment, treatment utilization, and mortality by suicide (61,62). Approximately 10% of patients with BPD commit suicide (63). BPD has an estimated prevalence of 1% to 2% of the U.S. population (34,64–67), with men constituting only about 25% of patients (67). The disorder accounts for approximately 10% of all psychiatric outpatients and 20% of acute inpatient hospitalizations (34,68,69). There are several psychotherapies for the treatment of BPD, like dialectic behavior therapy, but they are very time consuming, therapists must be specially trained, and patients must be highly motivated, as many are resistant to treatment. Thus, pharmacotherapy may serve as a useful adjunct to psychotherapeutic interventions in BPD, and a combination of these approaches may be most effective (70,71).

In evaluating the use of medications for treating personality disorders, one can (*i*) treat the disorder itself, (*ii*) treat associated axis I disorders, or (*iii*) treat symptom clusters/psychobiological dimensions within and across disorders (72). Three symptom clusters that can be targeted in BPD are impulsivity and aggression, mood symptomatology, and psychotic-like symptoms. No single medication is thought to be effective for all three of these symptom clusters (73). New and old antipsychotics, monoamine oxidase inhibitors (MAOIs), SSRIs, and AEDs are all currently used for BPD (74). Tricyclics are used to decrease irritability and aggression, but are lethal in overdose; MAOIs are used for affective instability, but risks include hypertensive crisis; SSRIs are used to decrease anger, irritability, and aggression, but comorbid bipolar spectrum patients may develop rapid cycling; antipsychotics are used to improve psychosis, but side effects are common and controlled data are lacking; and benzodiazepines are used to decrease episodes of behavioral dyscontrol. In a review of the treatment of rapid-cycling bipolar disorder, which overlaps with BPD, Coryell (75) stated that placebo-controlled studies so far provided the most support for the use of lithium and lamotrigine as prophylactic agents. The combination of lithium and carbamazepine, valproate, or lamotrigine for maintenance has some support from controlled studies, as does the adjunctive use of olanzapine. However, it appears that AEDs are used more widely than lithium in treating BPD.

Valproate

Recently, AED trials have focused on valproate, a widely used mood stabilizer, and to a lesser extent on the newer anticonvulsants, for efficacy in BPD. Valproate has been shown to improve symptoms of irritability, agitation, aggression, and anxiety in patients with BPD (76–81). In an open-label study, eight BPD patients completed an eight-week trial of valproate (76). Half of the patients were rated as overall responders, with significant to modest decreases in depression, anxiety, anger, impulsivity, rejection sensitivity, and irritability, as measured by Overt Aggression Scale-Modified (OAS-M) and Symptom Checklist-90 (SCL-90) scores. Wilcox (77) treated 30 BPD inpatients in a naturalistic open study of valproate. Brief Psychiatric Rating Scale (BPRS) scores (particularly the anxiety subcomponents), aggressive outbursts, and time in seclusion significantly decreased during the six-week trial. In addition to treating the aggressive and impulsive symptoms of BPD patients, valproate may also be helpful in treating BPD patients who report changeable mood (i.e., those who have mood instability but who are subsyndromal for major depression or hypomania) (82). In one valproate treatment study, six of nine BPD patients with mood instability (defined by the BPD DSM-III-R diagnostic criterion "affective instability due to marked reactivity of mood"), without bipolar or current major depression, were responders in that their CGI score on their last visit was "much improved" or better (82). Responders showed a greater reduction in Hamilton Rating Scale for Depression (HAM-D) scores than nonresponders.

In a preliminary, double-blind trial, BPD outpatients were treated for 10 weeks with valproate ($N = 12$) or placebo ($N = 4$) (80). There was significant improvement from baseline in measures of global symptom severity (as assessed by the CGI-I) and functioning [as assessed by the Global Assessment of Function (GAF) scale], following treatment. A high dropout rate precluded finding significant differences between the treatment groups in the intent-to-treat (ITT) analyses. However, all results were in the predicted direction so that patients in the treatment group had decreases in scores on the Aggression Questionnaire and the Beck Depression Inventory (BDI) compared with placebo. In another controlled, double-blind study of valproate, efficacy was examined in 30 women with comorbid BPD and bipolar II disorder over six months of treatment (81). Valproate, at an average dose of 850 mg/day (blood levels between 50 and 100 mg/L), was well tolerated and superior to placebo in diminishing interpersonal sensitivity and anger/hostility as measured by the SCL-90 and overall aggression as measured by the OAS-M. Taken together, these studies suggest valproate may be more effective than placebo for global symptomatology, level of functioning, aggression, and depression in BPD.

Since valproate may improve impulsive aggression, irritability, and global severity in patients with cluster B personality disorders (9), Hollander et al. (83) examined clinical characteristics of BPD outpatients that might predict response of impulsive aggression to valproate. In this randomized, double-blind, 12-week study, valproate ($N = 20$) was superior to placebo ($N = 32$) in reducing impulsive aggression in BPD patients. Both pretreatment trait impulsivity and state aggression symptoms, independently of one another, predicted a favorable response to valproate relative to placebo. However, baseline affective instability did not affect differential treatment response. These may help identify BPD patient subgroups or baseline characteristics (e.g., those with high levels of trait impulsivity or state aggression) that could guide future trials of AEDs. These data also suggest that BPD may be characterized by independent symptom domains that are amenable to treatment (40,84).

Carbamazepine and Oxcarbazepine

Carbamazepine, an anticonvulsant with effects on subcortical limbic structures, is effective in the treatment of several psychiatric disorders, including bipolar mania. Because patients with BPD show prominent affective symptomatology and symptoms suggestive of an epileptoid disorder, carbamazepine might be useful in treating BPD. In fact, in a double-blind, crossover trial, carbamazepine decreased the severity of behavioral dyscontrol in 11 women with BPD significantly more than placebo (85). In another double-blind, placebo-controlled, crossover study, carbamazepine led to a dramatic, highly significant decrease in clinician-rated behavioral dyscontrol and had a modest effect on mood in female BPD outpatients with prominent behavioral dyscontrol and without current major depression (86). However, one carbamazepine study of 20 BPD inpatients without concurrent depression or concomitant medications yielded negative results (87). After four weeks of treatment at standard doses, carbamazepine was no better than placebo in treating depression, behavioral dyscontrol, or global symptomatology. In another study, 3 (18%) of 17 BPD patients developed melancholia during carbamazepine treatment, which remitted upon discontinuation of carbamazepine (88). Thus, while carbamazepine may be an effective medication for some BPD patients, clinicians should be alert for any worsening in depressive symptoms.

More recently, Bellino et al. (89) tested 17 DSM-IV-TR-diagnosed BPD outpatients with oxcarbazepine, an AED that is structurally related to carbamazepine and sometimes used for treating patients with bipolar disorders, substance abuse, schizoaffective disorder, and treatment-resistant psychosis. Patients were administered oxcarbazepine 1200 to 1500 mg/day and evaluated at baseline, and after 4 and 12 weeks of treatment. A statistically significant response to oxcarbazepine was observed according to change in mean scores on the CGI-S, BPRS, and Hamilton Rating Scale for Anxiety (HAM-A); in interpersonal relationships, impulsivity, affective instability, and outbursts of anger items; and in total score of the Borderline Personality Disorder Severity Index. Oxcarbazepine was well tolerated with no severe adverse effects; four patients discontinued treatment due to noncompliance. Thus, oxcarbazepine may be an effective and safe treatment for some BPD patients. However, controlled studies are needed.

Topiramate

In an eight-week, double-blind, placebo-controlled trial of topiramate to treat aggression in females with DSM-IV-diagnosed BPD, the topiramate group ($N = 19$) showed significantly more efficacy than the placebo group ($N = 10$) (90) as measured by four subscales (i.e., the state-anger, trait-anger, anger-out, and anger-control subscales) of the State Trate Anger Expression Inventory (STAXI) scale. Significant changes on the same four STAXI subscales were also observed in males with DSM-IV-diagnosed BPD treated with topiramate ($N = 22$) in a similarly designed eight-week, double-blind, placebo ($N = 20$) controlled study (91). In both studies, topiramate was well tolerated and significant weight loss was observed. These findings suggest topiramate may be a safe and effective treatment of anger in both men and women with BPD and correspond with other studies where topiramate therapy resulted in significantly decreased symptoms of aggression (92,93).

Recently, Loew et al. explored whether topiramate could influence BPD patients' borderline psychopathology, health-related quality of life, and interpersonal problems (94,95). DSM-IV SCID-II–diagnosed BPD women were randomly assigned in a 1:1 ratio to topiramate titrated from 25 to 200 mg/day ($N = 28$) or placebo ($N = 28$) for 10 weeks. Significant changes were observed on the somatization, interpersonal sensitivity, anxiety, hostility, phobic anxiety, and Global Severity Index scales of the SCL-90 in the topiramate-treated subjects after 10 weeks. In addition, significant differences were found on all eight scales of the SF-36 Health Survey and in the overly autocratic, competitive, introverted, and expressive scales of the Inventory of Interpersonal Problems. Significant weight loss was also observed.

Finally, do Prado-Lima et al. (96) reported a woman with BPD and a history of childhood trauma who showed a significant clinical response with a low dosage of topiramate. The authors suggested that topiramate might decrease emotional and behavioral reactivity by facilitating memory extinction.

Lamotrigine

In a small, open trial of lamotrigine in eight BPD patients without concurrent major depression, two subjects discontinued because of adverse events or noncompliance and three did not respond (97). However, the remaining three were robust responders with a marked increase in their overall level of functioning, a cessation of impulsive behaviors like promiscuity, substance abuse, and suicidality, and maintenance of response at one-year follow-up. In a retrospective study of borderline symptoms in bipolar patients, it was estimated that 43% of this subgroup experienced a reduction in such symptoms during lamotrigine treatment (98).

Tritt et al. (99) investigated the efficacy of lamotrigine in the treatment of aggression in 24 women meeting Structured Clinical Interview for DSM-IV (SCID) criteria for BPD. In this double-blind, placebo-controlled study, subjects were randomly assigned in a 2:1 ratio to lamotrigine ($N = 18$) or placebo ($N = 9$) for eight weeks. Compared with the placebo group, highly significant changes on four STAXI scales (e.g., state-anger, trait-anger, anger-out, anger-control) were observed in subjects treated with lamotrigine after eight weeks. All the patients tolerated lamotrigine relatively well, and it had no clinically significant effect on body weight.

Weinstein and Jamison (100) assessed lamotrigine treatment for affective instability symptoms of BPD patients. Charts of patients treated with lamotrigine in a private practice during 2003–2004 were reviewed. Patients were included in the analysis if they had been given a DSM-IV-R diagnosis of BPD; had continued to display affective instability while taking their previous medications before lamotrigine initiation; had received a CGI-S score before and after lamotrigine therapy; had been treated with lamotrigine, as monotherapy or adjunctive therapy, at a dose ranging from 50 to 200 mg/day; and continued to take lamotrigine for at least three months. The charts of 13 patients met inclusion criteria. All patients were female, 19 to 43 years of age, and had reported continuing symptoms of affective instability despite treatment with two to seven psychotropic drugs, including, but not limited to, fluoxetine, paroxetine, escitalopram, buproprion, and clonazepan. The duration of lamotrigine treatment ranged from 3 to 15 months. The patients had initial CGI-S scores of 5 or 6 and final scores of 1 or 2, except one patient with an initial score of 3 and a final score of 1 and another patient with an initial score of 6 and a final score of 7.

In sum, there is preliminary evidence that lamotrigine may have efficacy in treating BPD symptomatology, especially symptoms of anger, affective instability, and impulsivity.

Cluster B Personality Disorders

Many researchers have recommended AEDs for the treatment of the affective, impulsive, and aggressive symptoms of cluster B personality disorders in general. Stein (101) has suggested that carbamazepine and lithium may help some personality-disordered people with episodic behavioral dyscontrol and aggression, even in the absence of affective, organic, or epileptic features. Stone (63) has suggested that BPD patients with bipolar II may benefit from lithium or from carbamazepine if irritability is prominent. In a review of double-blind, placebo-controlled drug trials for personality disorders, Hori (102) concluded that patients with BPD and behavioral dyscontrol respond to carbamazepine, which reduces episodes of dyscontrol, and that patients with personality disorders with aggressive behavior respond to lithium. Coccaro and Kavoussi (103) concluded that affective instability in BPD, which may be related to abnormalities in the brain's adrenergic and cholinergic systems, appears to respond to lithium and carbamazepine. In another review, Pelissolo and Lepine (104) argued that for cluster B personality disorders, especially antisocial and BPD, positive results have been obtained using lithium, carbamazepine, and valproate for aggressive and impulsive behaviors.

In an eight-week open trial of valproate in patients with at least one personality disorder who had failed one SSRI trial, six of eight completers showed a significant decline in irritability and impulsive aggression on the OAS-M score (78). Hollander et al. (9) conducted a large, placebo-controlled, multicenter trial of valproate for the treatment of impulsive aggression in cluster B personality disorders, IED, or posttraumatic stress disorder (PTSD). These different diagnoses were included in the same study, as they have the symptom dimension of impulsivity and aggression, which could benefit from the same treatment. Entry criteria required evidence of current impulsive-aggressive behavior (e.g., two or more impulsive-aggressive outbursts per week on average for the previous month) and an OAS-M score of 15 or greater. Ninety-one (43 valproate; 48 placebo) of the 96 randomized cluster B personality disorder patients were included in the ITT data set (defined as subjects who received at least one dose of the study drug and had at least one postbaseline OAS-M rating). The most common primary diagnosis was BPD (55% of patients), followed by cluster B personality disorder NOS (21%), narcissistic (13%), antisocial (10%), and histrionic (1%) personality disorders. Subjects were randomized to 12 weeks of valproate or placebo, and OAS-M (aggression and irritability) and CGI scores were obtained weekly (except for weeks 5 and 7).

A treatment effect was not observed when all three diagnostic groups were combined, but valproate was superior to placebo in the treatment of impulsive aggression, irritability, and global severity in the subgroup of patients with cluster B personality disorders. A treatment effect was observed in both ITT and evaluable (defined as receiving at least 21 days of treatment with study drug) data sets for cluster B personality disorder patients in terms of average OAS-M Aggression scores over the last four weeks of treatment. In the cluster B evaluable data set, statistically significant treatment differences favoring valproate were also observed for component items of the OAS-M Aggression scale (including verbal assault and assault against objects), OAS-M Irritability scale, and CGI-S at multiple time points throughout the study. Across psychiatric diagnoses, 21 (17%) patients in the valproate group prematurely discontinued because of an adverse event, compared with four (3%) patients in the placebo group.

These results support previous findings of decreased impulsive-aggressive behavior and irritability in BPD patients treated with valproate (80), including in those who failed to respond to other agents with antiaggressive properties (i.e., SSRIs) (78). Unlike a previous pilot study where valproate was superior to placebo for the treatment of irritability and hostility in women with bipolar II and BPD (81), patients in the study by Hollander et al. (9) were excluded if they had bipolar disorder I or II with recent (i.e., past year) hypomania. This suggests that the effect of valproate in impulsive aggression may be unrelated to its effect in mania. However, the possibility that the impulsive aggression of cluster B personality disorders has an affective component or that valproate is treating a subclinical mood disorder in cluster B personality disorders cannot be excluded.

Gabapentin is an AED structurally similar to GABA, with unclear mechanisms of action and a good safety profile. Biancosino et al. (105) reported a case of successful gabapentin treatment of chronic impulsive-aggressive behavior in a patient with severe BPD. Morana et al. (106) treated 29 cluster B personality disorder outpatients (8 antisocial, 13 impulsive, 7 histrionic, and 1 narcissistic type) with gabapentin (1200 mg/day), alone or with other drugs (antipsychotics, mood stabilizers, and benzodiazepines). After six weeks of treatment, there was an improvement in 23 (79.9%) patients, with a decrease in aggressiveness, impulsivity, antisocial behavior, and drug abuse and an improvement in their concentration, introspection capabilities, and interest in productive activities, as reported by patients and their caregivers. Morana and Camara (107) found that after more than four years of study of personality disorder patients from the Personality Disorder Ambulatory of the Department of Psychiatry of Sao Paulo University Medical School, about 79.3% of the patients treated with gabapentin had reduced their antisocial behaviors, as reported by patient informers. The authors observed a decrease in aggressiveness, impulsiveness, offender behavior, and drug abuse, and a general improvement in tolerance, concentration, and introspective capacity, with a greater interest in productive activities. It has been suggested that gabapentin reduces reactivity and turbulent behavior perhaps because of its inhibitory effect in central neurotransmission (108). The authors concluded that, in their clinical experience, gabapentin was the most effective mood stabilizer for the treatment of personality disorders.

Summary

A symptom-specific method using current empirical evidence for drug efficacy in each symptom domain of BPD is proposed for treatment. Drugs in each medication class have some potential utility against specific symptoms of BPD (109). As there is no "drug of choice" to treat BPD, a more rational clinical approach might be to treat different symptom clusters (e.g., cognitive, affective, impulsive, and aggressive) rather than the disorder itself. On the basis of the above evidence, we suggest that selective AEDs may be effective in treating the affective, impulsive, and aggressive symptoms of BPD and other cluster B personality disorders.

ANTIEPILEPTIC DRUGS AND IMPULSIVITY AND AGGRESSION ACROSS DIAGNOSES

The antiaggressive effects of AEDs in patients with neurological disorders make them good candidates for the treatment of aggression in the context of psychopathology. AEDs are generally considered the treatment of choice for patients with abnormal EEG findings and outbursts of rage (110). In a retrospective chart review, Salpekar et al. (111) identified 38 children with bipolar spectrum disorders and epilepsy comorbidity. Common bipolar symptoms included impulsivity, psychomotor agitation, and explosive rage. Forty-two medication trials with 11 different AEDs were identified. Of the 30 cases in which AED monotherapy was attempted, carbamazepine, valproate, lamotrigine, and oxcarbazepine were associated with better CGI-I ratings than were other AEDs. In many cases, selected AEDs appeared to simultaneously treat both epilepsy and mood disorder. However, with the exception of cluster B personality disorders, AEDs have received only preliminary exploration in the treatment of impulse control and aggression in psychiatric disorders, without an associated seizure disorder.

Nonetheless, there is some evidence for the efficacy of valproate and carbamazepine for the treatment of pathological aggression in patients with organic brain syndromes, dementia, psychosis, and, as discussed, personality disorders (109,110). Firm evidence for the efficacy of valproate or carbamazepine in managing aggression and/or agitation following traumatic brain injury (TBI) is lacking (112). In a literature review of AEDs for migraine, neuropathic pain, movement disorders, pervasive developmental disorders, bipolar disorder, and aggressive behavior in children and adolescents, Golden et al. (113) concluded that valproate is "probably effective" in decreasing aggressive behavior, carbamazepine is "probably ineffective" in treating aggression, and lamotrigine is "possibly ineffective" for the core symptoms of pervasive developmental disorders. They also concluded that the data are insufficient to make recommendations about the efficacy of AEDs in these conditions in children and adolescents.

The likelihood of aggression may increase from stress or environmental overstimulation, problems related to impulsivity, or neurotransmitter balances, favoring dopamine and excitatory amino acid transmission over serotonin and inhibitory amino acid (GABA) transmission (114). AEDs may work by altering the inhibitory excitatory amino acid balance in favor of GABA, thereby protecting against overstimulation and raising the convulsive threshold when aggression is associated with a seizure disorder. Useful AEDs might also be those that combine dopaminergic and serotonergic actions (114).

Treatments for aggression should be based on the underlying causes. Barratt (115) proposed that aggression could be divided into three general categories: (i) medically related, where aggression is a symptom secondary to a neurological, psychiatric, or other medical disorder; (ii) premeditated, predatory, or planned, where the aggressive behavior is an instrumental response; and (iii) impulsive, where aggression is a trigger response in that information is not processed in an adaptive way during the temper outburst. Barratt hypothesized that certain anticonvulsants (e.g., phenytoin, carbamazepine) would be effective for treating impulsive aggression.

Valproate

Valproate, which enhances GABA neurotransmission, was first introduced as an AED in 1967. Its use in the treatment of aggressive and violent behaviors has been reported in the literature as far back as 1988. This literature, which includes several double-blind, placebo-controlled studies (9,80,81,83,116), supports the use of valproate in the treatment of hostility/aggression, impulsive aggression, and affective instability in patients in a variety of psychiatric and neuropsychiatric disorders.

Thus, valproate has been reported to be effective against impulsive aggression and/or hostility in subjects with bipolar disorder (9,74,77,80–83,117) and adolescents with aggression and labile mood (118,119). Improved behavioral dyscontrol and aggression with valproate treatment has also been noted in patients with PTSD (120–122), temper outbursts (118,119,123), TBI (124,125), dementia (116,126–129), and autism (130).

In a review of studies of nonbipolar subjects with aggressive and violent behaviors (the most frequent diagnoses were dementia, organic brain syndromes, and mental retardation), valproate was found to be effective in 77% of 164 subjects in 17 studies, though these were open studies that often included more than one treatment (131). Wroblewski et al. (125) described the effectiveness of VPA in reducing and improving destructive and aggressive behaviors in five patients with TBI. In all cases, valproate was effective after other pharmacological interventions had failed, and neurobehavioral improvement was fairly rapid, often within one to two weeks. Although AEDs may be best suited for subacute or chronic treatment (114), rapid stabilization of severe agitation has been reported with intravenous valproate (132). Buchalter and Lantz (127) described a patient with vascular dementia in whom valproate led to reduced overt aggression, diminished impulsivity, and improved functional status. In a retrospective study of a long-term care database of elderly nursing home residents with a history of dementia-related behavior problems, Meinhold et al. (133) found that valproate therapy had beneficial effects on various behavioral, mood, and cognitive indicators, as monotherapy with benzodiazepines, and with antipsychotics, and at both higher and lower doses. In general, the higher-dose valproate group had more favorable results.

In a retrospective study (130), 14 patients with DSM-IV-diagnosed autism, Asperger's disorder, or pervasive developmental disorder NOS, with or without a history of seizure disorders or EEG abnormalities, received open-label treatment with valproate. Ten (71%) patients had a sustained response to valproate, as assessed by the CGI-I scale. Improvement was noted in the core autistic symptoms of social interaction, speech/communication skills, and repetitive behaviors as well as the associated features of affective instability, impulsivity, and aggression. Valproate was generally well tolerated. By contrast, no treatment difference was observed between groups in a prospective, eight-week, randomized, double-blind, placebo-controlled study of 30 outpatient subjects ($N = 20$ boys) with pervasive developmental disorders (ages 6–20 years) with significant aggression (134). However, these negative findings should not be considered conclusive, partly because of the large placebo response, subject heterogeneity, and small sample size.

Evidence supporting the use of valproate in the treatment of juvenile bipolar disorder with reactive aggression has grown (135,136). In one study, three boys with ADHD associated with giant somatosensory evoked potentials (SEP) responded well to valproate extended-release (ER) in particular, showing reduced hyperactivity and impulsivity (137). In two patients, previous methylphenidate treatment had worsened symptoms, suggesting that they may have had bipolar spectrum conditions. Valproate was also effective in a randomized, controlled trial of adolescent males with conduct disorder openly treated with high-dose or low-dose VPA (138). There was significant improvement in the high-dose group on a number of outcome measures, including self-reported weekly impulse control. Donovan et al. (119) sought to replicate open-label findings where 10 adolescents with a disruptive behavior disorder, who met operationalized criteria for explosive temper and mood lability, showed improvement with valproate for five weeks (118).

In the double-blind, placebo-controlled crossover study (119,120), outpatient children and adolescents (ages 10–18 years) with a disruptive behavior disorder (oppositional defiant disorder or conduct disorder), who met the specific criteria for explosive temper and mood lability, were randomly assigned to receive six weeks of valproate or placebo. At the end of phase one, 8 of 10 subjects responded to valproate and 0 of 10 responded to placebo. Twelve of the 15 subjects who completed both phases had a superior response to valproate.

In a randomized, double-blind, 28-day study, valproate and quetiapine showed similar efficacy for the treatment of impulsivity and reactive aggression related to co-occurring bipolar and disruptive behavior disorders in adolescents ($N = 33$) (139). In a retrospective, case-controlled study, Gobbi et al. (140) compared the effects of topiramate, valproate, and their combination in 45 psychiatric inpatients with schizophrenia, schizoaffective, or bipolar disorder with marked aggression and agitation. Topiramate-treated patients showed a decrease in mean OAS scores, episodes of agitation, and strict surveillance interventions. The effect was similar in the valproate-alone and combination valproate-topiramate treatment groups. However, valproate alone, but not topiramate alone, decreased the intensity of agitation episodes; and valproate alone and the valproate-topiramate combination decreased the number of psychotic disorganization episodes. MacMillan et al. (141) reviewed medical records of 31 pediatric bipolar disorder patients (age < 18 years) with severe aggression who received valproate ($N = 20$) or oxcarbazepine ($N = 11$). Overall CGI-S scores and CGI-S scores specific to aggression significantly improved from baseline to the four-month time point with valproate but not oxcarbazepine. Discontinuation rates from adverse events were similar. However, more discontinuations due to worsening aggression occurred with oxcarbazepine (27.3% vs. none for valproate). In a medical records review of 42 patients (ages 12–19 years) hospitalized for acute mania and discharged with a diagnosis of DSM-III-R or DSM-IV bipolar disorder, a history of ADHD was associated with a significantly diminished acute response to both valproate and lithium as a treatment for their bipolar manic phase (142). Response rates for lithium versus valproate in subjects with and without ADHD did not differ.

Barzman et al. (143) retrospectively reviewed the charts of 46 children and adolescents admitted to a crisis stabilization center with prominent impulsive aggression and irritability who met criteria for a potential pediatric bipolar phenotype and who responded to valproate. Significant improvements were obtained on the Children's Global Assessment Scale, with significant decreases on the OAS and the Anger-Hostility Subscale of the SCL-90 at discharge, following a maximal 14-day stay. No severe side effects were reported. The above data are in line with valproate response in children and adolescents with explosive temper and mood instability (118,119) and suggest that such symptoms, together with impulsive aggression, irritability, and other manic symptoms, may constitute a pediatric valproate-responsive bipolar spectrum disorder. In a 12-week, open-label trial of valproate in 24 bipolar offspring, ages 6 to 18 years (17 boys), with mixed diagnoses of major depression, cyclothymia, ADHD, and oppositional defiant disorder, 71% of subjects were considered valproate responders by the OAS (144). Thus, youths who were at high risk for bipolar disorder experienced an overall decrease in aggressive behavior in response to valproate.

Prospective, randomized, double-blind, placebo-controlled trials are needed to further assess valproate's optimal usage for the treatment of aggression and impulsivity across psychiatric disorders.

Carbamazepine and Oxcarbazepine

In the 1980s, carbamazepine became an AED of primary interest in treating impulsive aggression because it was the drug of choice for treating temporal lobe epilepsy patients with aggressive outbursts and irritability (145). Several reviews have since then concluded that carbamazepine reduces aggressive and associated behaviors across a wide range of diagnoses (146–149). Carbamazepine has been reported effective in treating pathological aggression in dementia (150) and in decreasing combativeness, agitated behavior, irritability, and disinhibition in subjects with head injuries (151,152). Freymann et al. (153) described the successful use of carbamazepine in a 78-year-old Alzheimer's disease patient with hypersexual behavior. The efficacy of carbamazepine in this case is in parallel to its effects on aggression and agitation in dementia (150). One open-label study of inpatient children with conduct disorder found statistically and clinically significant declines of explosiveness and aggression (154). A double-blind, placebo-controlled trial, however, found no difference between carbamazepine and placebo, and side effects were common (146). Indeed, the few placebo-controlled trials with carbamazepine have been small and in diverse patient populations (147,148). For example, Mattes (155) randomly assigned propranolol or carbamazepine treatment for temper outbursts to 80 patients with diverse diagnoses. Both medications were beneficial, but a diagnosis of ADHD predicted better response to propranolol, and a diagnosis of IED predicted better response to carbamazepine.

The ICD-10 diagnosis "Organic Personality Disorder," listed under "Personality Change Due to a General Medical Condition" in the DSM-IV, may involve aggression and impulsivity. Many different treatments have been proposed for this condition, including carbamazepine. Munoz and Gonzalez Torres (156) described a 28-year-old male who had aggressive episodes along with an intensification of previous personality traits, sexual exhibitionism, promiscuity, suspiciousness, and low impulse control after a severe brain injury sustained in a car accident. Antipsychotics, benzodiazepines, and antidepressants had no effect. After two months of carbamazepine treatment, the patient had marked improvement with the absence of aggressive episodes and exhibitionistic behavior, a tendency toward normalization of mood and anxiety, stabilization of his social and family relationships, and employment. Morikawa et al. (157) reported a 19-year-old male who had a personality change, marked by irritability, aggression, labile mood, childishness, irresponsibility, and lack of motivation, six months after a mild injury to his left frontotemporal cortex from a motorbike accident. He was diagnosed with posttraumatic personality disorder and treated with clonazepam, which moderately improved his symptoms but caused drowsiness. Within a few days of the addition of carbamazepine, he improved to his preinjury personality. After clonazepam was discontinued, he maintained good mental status and at two-year follow-up continued to be well. Lewin and Sumners (158) described an 18-year-old man who, following a traffic accident, developed episodic dyscontrol. Two years post injury, carbamazepine treatment was started and his aggressive outbursts subsided.

Oxcarbazepine, like carbamazepine, is effective for complex partial seizures and may have mood-stabilizing effects (159). In a double-blind, placebo-controlled, 10-week study, adult outpatients with clinically significant impulsive aggression were randomized to placebo ($N = 24$) or oxcarbazepine ($N = 24$) (160). Nine patients dropped out because of adverse events, but 45 completed at least four weeks of treatment. Results showed a benefit from oxcarbazepine compared with placebo on OAS-M scores and patient-rated global improvement. Guadino et al. (161) described an adolescent with treatment-resistant aggression (and a mood disorder and ADHD), which improved with oxcarbazepine, the only side effect being sedation. Cordas et al. (162) presented two cases of severe bulimia and BPD, in which self-mutilating behavior was successfully controlled with oxcarbazepine treatment.

Topiramate
Topiramate, a newer AED, which acts on voltage-activated sodium channels and glutamate and GABA receptors, has also been reported to be effective in a variety of aggressive patients (92). In a retrospective chart review study, Janowsky et al. (93) examined topiramate treatment in 22 severely or profoundly intellectually disabled, institutionalized adults, most with a concurrent mood disorder. Patients were treated for aggression, SIBs, destructive/disruptive behaviors, and/or other challenging and maladaptive behaviors. Significant decreases in global severity scores, cumulative aggression, and worst behavior rates occurred, especially when comparing the three months before and the three to six months after starting topiramate. In a randomized, double-blind, placebo-controlled, 10-week study of topiramate in 64 females diagnosed with recurrent major depressive disorder, topiramate significantly reduced anger and depressive symptoms compared with placebo (163). There was also significant weight loss in the topiramate group and topiramate was relatively well tolerated. In seven patients with PWS, topiramate reduced aggressive and SIB, improved mood, and stabilized weight (164). These reports correspond with other studies in which topiramate resulted in significantly decreased aggressive symptoms (90,91).

Impulsivity plays a significant role in a wide range of psychiatric disorders including eating disorders like BED. Topiramate has also shown efficacy in the treatment of a number of disorders involving impulsivity including BED (165,166). BED is characterized by recurrent episodes of binge eating that are not followed by the regular use of inappropriate compensatory weight loss behaviors. It is often associated with overweight or obesity and psychopathology. The literature offers support, including from double-blind, placebo-controlled trials, for the use of antidepressants, appetite suppressants (e.g., sibutramine), and AEDs in the treatment of BED (167–169). Topiramate, in particular, appears to be promising for the treatment of BED because of its beneficial effects on body weight as well as impulsivity.

In a preliminary naturalistic, open-label study with topiramate, 9 of 13 BED outpatients showed a moderate or better response of binge eating symptoms after beginning treatment that was maintained for 3 to 30 months (165). Two other patients had moderate or marked responses that subsequently diminished and the remaining two patients had a mild or no response. In another preliminary study, treatment with topiramate (150 mg daily) was administered over 16 weeks to eight obese patients with BED and no medical or psychiatric comorbidity (170). All six of the trial completers showed reduced binge eating. Four patients had a complete remission, and two had a marked reduction in binge eating frequency. Patients also had significant weight loss. In a 14-week, double-blind, flexible-dose topiramate trial, 61 BED outpatients with obesity were randomly assigned to receive topiramate ($N = 30$) or placebo ($N = 31$) (166). Compared with placebo, topiramate resulted in a significantly greater rate of reduction in binge frequency, binge day frequency, BMI, weight, and scores on the CGI-S and the Y-BOCS modified for binge eating (Y-BOCS-BE) (166). Topiramate was also found to have positive effects for the long-term treatment of BED in a 42-week, open-label extension trial (171) of the acute study (166). For all patients ($N = 43$) receiving topiramate during either the double-blind or open-label extension study, there was a significant decline from baseline to final visit in weekly binge frequency, CGI-Score, Y-BOCS-BE total, and compulsion, and obsession subscale scores, weight, and BMI.

Zilberstein et al. (172) analyzed 16 patients with binge eating and inadequate weight loss after adjustable gastric banding while receiving topiramate for three months (12.5–50 mg/day). There was a mean increase in excess weight loss from 20.4% to 34.1% without the need for band readjustment. Two patients, however, could not tolerate topiramate. Dolberg et al. (173) reported the effects of adjunctive topiramate on eating patterns and weight in 17 patients with TBI, posttraumatic epilepsy, and weight gain of various etiologies. The six patients with BED had the most pronounced effects, with marked decreases in binges and a normalization of BMI. In another study, three obese BED patients, who had recurrent binge eating and weight gain after initially successful bariatric surgery, reported complete improvement of their binge eating and displayed weight loss after receiving top-iramate for 10 months on average (174). De Bernardi et al. (175) reported a BED patient who was unresponsive to several treatments but was successfully treated with topiramate. In a 10-week double-blind, placebo-controlled study, topiramate was also effective in reducing the frequency of binging/purging and body weight in bulimic patients (176).

Topiramate may also be effective in treating self-mutilating behavior. Top-iramate improved self-mutilation and manic symptoms in two patients with bipolar disorder and BPD (177). Further, topiramate (200 mg/day) administered in an on-off-on design to a 24-year-old woman with bipolar II depression and BPD led to long-term remission of self-mutilation despite the persistence of depression (178). No self-injurious acts occurred over nine months, and mood was sufficiently stabilized.

Dolengevich et al. (179) evaluated 11 child and adolescent outpatients with impulsive behavioral disorders by DSM-IV criteria at one and three months after starting topiramate treatment. There were significant differences in the cognitive impulsivity subscale and total score of the Barratt Impulsivity scale after one month and the motor impulsivity subscale after three months. Thus, topiramate may be an effective treatment for impulsivity in children and adolescents as well as in adults with some psychiatric disorders. More studies with larger samples and control groups are needed to confirm the efficacy of topiramate for the treatment of aggression and impulsivity in all age groups.

Levetiracetam

There is preliminary evidence that levetiracetam, FDA approved as an adjunctive treatment for partial-complex seizures, may be effective in some psychiatric disorders characterized by affective lability, impulsivity, and anxiety (180–183). In an open-label prospective study of 10 autistic boys aged 4 to 10 years, levetiracetam significantly reduced hyperactivity, impulsivity, mood instability, and disruptive outbursts (180). Aggressive behavior showed significant improvement only in subjects who were not recently weaned from medications that reduced aggression (e.g., risperidone, carbamazepine, desipramine). However, in a 10-week, double-blind, placebo-controlled trial of levetiracetam in 20 autistic children aged 5 to 17 years, no significant difference was found between drug and placebo groups in terms of change in CGI-I, Aberrant Behavior Checklist, Children's Y-BOCS, or Conners' scales (184). These findings suggest that levetiracetam may not improve the behavioral disturbances of autism, but are limited by the small sample size and lack of stratification of the autistic sample at baseline.

In some studies, levetiracetam has actually increased aggression as a side effect. Dinkelacker et al. (185) reported 33 patients with long-standing histories of epilepsy who experienced aggressive episodes during levetiracetam therapy (3.5% of levetiracetam-treated patients vs. <1% of patients not receiving levetiracetam). Among these cases, 24 showed only moderate, transient irritability, with 10 patients requiring reduction or discontinuation of levetiracetam; but nine patients had severe aggressive symptoms with physical violence, two of whom needed psychiatric emergency treatment. Weber et al. (186) gave levetiracetam to 10 generalized epilepsy patients, and one patient with Lennox-Gastaut syndrome discontinued the drug because of aggression. In an observational survey, 128 (44.9%) of 285 pediatric patients (mean age 9.9 years) with refractory generalized and focal epilepsy reported mild to moderate side effects after receiving levetiracetam as an add-on open-label treatment (187). Behavioral changes were the second most frequent side effect after somnolence, included aggressive behavior in 44 patients (15.4%) and prompted discontinuation of the drug in 23 cases (8.1%). The most common behavioral adverse event was aggression, which was seen in 30 patients (10.5%) and was often severe. Two patients violently attacked others, which they had never done before. In another study (188), 11 (13%) of 85 pediatric patients (mean age 10.5 years) with refractory generalized and focal epilepsy, who received levetiracetam as add-on treatment, reported mild to moderate side effects, consisting most frequently of general behavioral changes, aggression, and sleep disturbances, which ceased after decreasing the levetiracetam dosage.

In sum, levetiracetam may reduce impulsivity, mood instability, and aggression in some populations, but studies in other patient populations, including BPD, are warranted. Morever, because of reports of increased aggression, the behavioral tolerability of levetiracetam should be monitored carefully, especially in patients with histories of aggression.

Gabapentin

Gabapentin increases CNS GABA, a neurotransmitter important for the control of aggressive behavior and has been reported to have antiaggressive effects across several disorders (189). Thus, several studies have reported significant improvement with gabapentin of aggressive behavior in dementia patients (190,191). In a retrospective chart review, Hawkins et al. (192) examined the use of gabapentin for the treatment of aggressive and agitated behaviors in 24 nursing home patients with DSM-IV-diagnosed dementia. On the CGR-I, 17 of 22 patients were rated as much or greatly improved, four were minimally improved, and one remained unchanged. Two patients discontinued the medication because of excessive sedation. No other significant side effects were noted after treatment for up to two years. Alkhalil et al. (193) described three dementia nursing home residents whose sexual disinhibition was effectively treated with gabapentin.

McManaman and Tan (194) described a patient with Lesch-Nyhan syndrome (an X-linked disorder of purine metabolism) whose SIB was effectively treated with gabapentin. Gupta et al. (195) described a patient with aggression and violent behavior due to DSM-IV-diagnosed conduct disorder whose symptoms were controlled with gabapentin after he failed a trial of valproate. In another case (196), gabapentin treatment resulted in a decrease in the frequency and intensity of violent episodes in a young patient with IED, ADHD, organic mood disorder secondary to a TBI, and a simple partial seizure disorder. Cherek et al. (189) measured aggression in 20 adult parolees with a pattern of antisocial behavior ($N = 2$ females), using the Point Subtraction Aggression Paradigm, which provided subjects aggressive, escape, and monetary reinforced response options. Ten subjects had a history of conduct disorder (CD^+) and 10 had no history of conduct disorder (non-CD). Acute doses (200, 400, and 800 mg) of gabapentin had similar effects on aggressive responses among both CD^+ and non-CD control subjects. Aggressive responses of CD^+ and non-CD subjects increased at lower gabapentin doses and decreased at the highest dose (800 mg). Specifically, gabapentin increased escape responses for both groups at the lowest dose, but then produced dose-related decreases at the two higher doses in both groups. No changes in monetary reinforced responses were observed, suggesting an absence of CNS stimulation or sedation.

Phenytoin

Although phenytoin did not improve aggressive behavior in children with temper tantrums in one early study (197), it has been reported to reduce the frequency of impulsive-aggressive behavior in a variety of conditions (115,198), to alter mid-latency-evoked potentials (199), and to significantly reduce violent outbursts in psychiatric patients with episodic dyscontrol syndrome (200,201). Thus, incarcerated inmates with impulsive-aggressive behavior showed significant reductions in the frequency and intensity of aggressive acts, normalization of event-related potentials (ERPs) (i.e., increased P300 amplitude), and improved mood state measures during a six-week, double-blind, placebo-controlled trial of phenytoin (300 mg/day) (202,203). Further, inmates whose aggressive behavior was considered premeditated did not show improvement (203). Stanford et al. (199) corroborated and extended these findings in a double-blind, placebo-controlled, crossover study of a noninmate population. Individuals meeting previously established criteria for impulsive aggression were given phenytoin and placebo during separate six-week conditions. Compared with baseline and placebo, the frequency of impulsive-aggressive outbursts significantly decreased during phenytoin treatment. Phenytoin also affected sensory/attentional processing (measured by ERPs) as indicated by increased P1 amplitude, longer-evoked potential latencies, and the suggestion of reduced N1 amplitude. In a double-blind, placebo-controlled, parallel group design, impulsive-aggressive men were randomly assigned to one of four six-week treatments: phenytoin ($N = 7$), carbamazepine ($N = 7$), valproate ($N = 7$), or placebo ($N = 8$) (199). A significant reduction in impulsive aggression (as measured by the OAS global severity index) was found during all three AED conditions compared with placebo. Compared with phenytoin and valproate, there was a slightly delayed effect during carbamazepine treatment.

In sum, these findings suggest that phenytoin could have a significant impact in the control of impulsive aggression in mental health and criminal populations. Further, because the antiaggressive properties of phenytoin appear selective for impulsive aggression, it suggests that biological mechanisms may distinguish impulsive from premeditated aggression (204).

DISCUSSION

Effective treatment of impulsivity and aggression depends on determining the cause(s) of these behaviors and selecting treatments accordingly. Pharmacological treatments may reduce impulsivity or aggression and normalize arousal by reducing dopaminergic activity, enhancing serotonergic activity, shifting the balance of amino acid neurotransmitter from excitatory (glutamatergic) toward inhibitory (GABAergic) transmission, and/or reducing or stabilizing nonadrenergic effects. Pharmacological and nonpharmacological treatment, like behavioral strategies aimed at reducing aggressive or impulsive behavior, may be most effective for the long-term treatment of the underlying chronic or recurrent illness (114). In general, there is no treatment of choice for impulse control and cluster B personality disorders. Many drugs from different classes seem to offer some benefit to selected individuals depending on their symptom presentations. For example, BPD patients with prominent cognitive and/or perceptual distortion may respond to antipsychotics, while those with depressed mood may respond best to antidepressants. Biological and behavioral dimensions may underlie treatment response in personality disorder patients (4,21). There may be several developmental trajectories to impulsivity and aggression (e.g., ADHD, bipolar spectrum, and trait impulsivity) and various routes to altering motivational circuitry, like modulating of corticostriatal-limbic circuits. We suggest that core symptoms within disorders should be treated and appropriate outcome measures should be used to determine targeted treatment response.

On the basis of the evidence presented here, AEDs appear to be effective for treating the symptom domains of impulsivity and aggression across a wide range of psychiatric disorders and for impulse control and cluster B personality disorders in particular. It is suggested that interventions should be directed at the brain circuitry, which modulates core symptoms that may be shared across disorders rather than DSM diagnoses. In addition to core symptom domains like impulsivity, affective instability, and aggression, clinicians should identify comorbid conditions and associated symptoms related to brain systems as they can also influence overall treatment response. AEDs may be effective for the treatment of the brain circuitry related to impulsivity, aggression, comorbid affective instability, and traumatic arousal, by modulating GABA, glutamate, serotonin, and norepinephrine.

Since ICDs and cluster B personality disorders have been found to be highly comorbid with other psychiatric disorders, the most effective and best-tolerated medication may vary depending on the comorbidity (101). Thus, AEDs, traditionally used to treat bipolar disorder, can also be effective for ICDs and cluster B personality disorders when there are associated bipolar symptoms. When treating the core symptoms of impulsivity and aggression, the associated bipolar and mood lability symptoms may improve as well. Clinicians should treat target symptoms like impulsivity and aggression regardless of their overall diagnosis, while taking into account comorbid disorders (e.g., bipolar disorder, ADHD), associated symptoms, developmental trajectory, and family history. For example, while SSRIs may be effective in treating pathological gambling with a comorbid obsessive-compulsive spectrum disorder or obsessive-compulsive features, they may not be the optimal treatment of pathological gambling with comorbid ADHD or a bipolar spectrum disorder (205,206). Clinicians must be careful when treating patients at risk for bipolar disorder, as SSRI-induced manic behaviors could emerge in those with a history of, or at risk for, mania or hypomania (44). Thus, a mood-stabilizing

AED like valproate may be a better treatment option for ICD patients with a comorbid bipolar disorder.

Accordingly, BPD patients with comorbid bipolar II disorder or subclinical bipolar symptomology may benefit from mood-stabilizing AEDs, like carbamazepine, if irritability is pronounced (63). Preliminary data indicate personality disorders with aggressive behavior, and emotionally unstable character disorder with mood swings, respond to AEDs. A variety of personality factors and comorbid conditions overrepresented in BPD patients, like premenstrual syndrome, bulimia, agoraphobia, major affective disorder (e.g., bipolar II), and hypersomnia, often complicate the clinical picture. Depending on the mix of these factors, certain drugs may need to be avoided, nonstandard drug combinations may need to be used, and safer drugs may need to be used in place of more effective drugs (102).

The growing experience of psychiatrists in treating ICDs, cluster B personality disorders, and impulsivity and aggression across disorders should compliment the knowledge obtained from research. This will lead to a better understanding of the brain mechanisms underlying impulsive and aggressive symptom domains within DSM disorders and to more targeted treatments with improved outcomes.

REFERENCES

1. Asconape JJ. Some common issues in the use of antiepileptic drugs. Semin Neurol 2002; 22:27–39.
2. Evenden JL. Varieties of impulsivity. Psychopharmacology 1999; 146:348–361.
3. Moeller G, Barratt ES, Dougherty DM, et al. Psychiatric aspects of impulsivity. Am J Psychiatry 2001; 158:1783–1793.
4. Coccaro EF. Impulsive aggression: a behavior in search of clinical definition. Harv Res Psychiatry 1998; 5:336–339.
5. Virkkunen M. Reactive hypoglycemic tendency among habitually violent offenders. Nutr Rev 1975; 44:94–103.
6. Pattison E, Kahan J. The deliberate self-harm syndrome. Am J Psychiatry 1983; 140: 867–872.
7. Cold JW. Axis II disorders and motivation for serious criminal behavior. In: Skodal AE, ed. Psychopathology and Violent Crime. Washington, DC: American Psychiatric Press, 1998.
8. Hollander E, Berlin HA. Neuropsychiatric aspects of aggression and impulse control disorders. In: Yudofsky SC, Hales RE, eds. American Psychiatric Press Textbook of Neuropsychiatry and Clinical Neurosciences. Washington, DC: American Psychiatric Press, (in press).
9. Hollander E, Tracy KA, Swann AC, et al. Divalproex in the treatment of impulsive aggression: efficacy in cluster B personality disorders. Neuropsychopharmacology 2003; 28: 1186–97.
10. Critchfield KL, Levy KN, Clarkin JF. The relationship between impulsivity, aggression, and impulsive-aggression in borderline personality disorder: an empirical analysis of self-report measures. J Personal Disord 2004; 18:555–570.
11. Hollander E, Rosen J. Impulsivity. J Psychopharmacol 2000; 14:S39–S44.
12. Delville Y, Melloni RH Jr., Ferris CF. Behavioral and neurobiological consequences of social subjugation during puberty in golden hamsters. J Neurosci 1998; 18:2667–2672.
13. Davidson JR. Anxiety and affective style: role of prefrontal cortex and amygdala. Biol Psychiatry 2002; 51:68–80.
14. Davis M, Whalen PJ. The amygdala: vigilance and emotion. Mol Psychiatry 2001; 6:13–34.
15. Rolls ET, Hornak J, Wade D, et al. Emotion-related learning in patients with social and emotional changes associated with frontal lobe damage. J Neurol Neurosurg Psychiatry 1994; 57:1518–1524.

16. Hornak J, Bramham J, Rolls ET, et al. Changes in emotion after circumscribed surgical lesions of the orbitofrontal and cingulate cortices. Brain 2003; 126:1691–1712.
17. Hornak J, O'Doherty J, Bramham J, et al. Reward-related reversal learning after surgical excisions in orbitofrontal and dorsolateral prefrontal cortex in humans. J Cogn Neurosci 2004; 16:463–478.
18. Hornak J, Rolls ET, Wade D. Face and voice expression identification in patients with emotional and behavioural changes following ventral frontal lobe damage. Neuropsychologia 1996; 34:247–261.
19. Drevets WC. Functional neuroimaging studies of depression: the anatomy of melancholia. Annu Rev Med 1998; 49:341–361.
20. Van Reekum R. Acquired and developmental brain dysfunction in borderline personality disorder. Can J Psychiatry 1993; 38:S4–S10.
21. Berlin HA, Rolls ET, Iversen SD. Borderline personality disorder, impulsivity, and the orbitofrontal cortex. Am J Psychiatry 162:2360–2373.
22. Rolls ET. The Brain and Emotion. Oxford, UK: Oxford University Press, 1999.
23. Baxter MG, Parker A, Lindner CC, et al. Control of response selection by reinforcer value requires interaction of amygdala and orbital prefrontal cortex. J Neurosci 2000; 20:4311–4319.
24. Herpertz SC, Dietrich TM, Wenning B, et al. Evidence of abnormal amygdala functioning in borderline personality disorder: a functional MRI study. Biol Psychiatry 2001; 50: 292–298.
25. Tebartz van Elst L, Hesslinger B, Thiel T, et al. Frontolimbic brain abnormalities in patients with borderline personality disorder: a volumetric magnetic resonance imaging study. Biol Psychiatry 2003; 54:163–171.
26. Pietrini P, Guazzelli M, Basso G. Neural correlates of imaginal aggressive behavior assessed by positron emission tomography in healthy subjects. Am J Psychiatry 2000; 157:1772–1781.
27. Siever LJ, Buchsbaum MS, New AS, et al. d,l-fenfluramine response in impulsive personality disorder assessed with [18F]fluorodeoxyglucose positron emission tomography. Neuropsychopharmacology 1999; 20:413–423.
28. Drevets WC. Prefrontal cortical-amygdalar metabolism in major depression. Ann N Y Acad Sci 1999; 877:614–637.
29. Herpertz SC, Dietrich TM, Wenning B, et al. Evidence of abnormal amygdala functioning in borderline personality disorder: a functional MRI study. Biol Psychiatry 2001; 50: 292–298.
30. LeDoux JE. The Emotional Brain. New York: Simon and Schuster, 1996.
31. Whalen PJ, Rauch SL, Etcoff NL, et al. Masked presentations of emotional facial expressions modulate amygdala activity without explicit knowledge. J Neurosci 1998; 18: 411–418.
32. Morgan MA, Romanski LM, LeDoux JE. Extinction of emotional learning: contribution of medial prefrontal cortex. Neuroscience 1993; 163:109–113 (letter).
33. Rauch SL, Shin LM, Whalen PJ. Neuroimaging and the neuroanatomy of posttraumatic stress disorder. CNS Spectrums 1998; 3(suppl 2):30–41.
34. American Psychiatric Association (APA). Diagnostic and Statistical Manual of Mental Disorders IV-TR. Washington, DC: APA, 2000.
35. Slutske WS, Eisen S, Xian H, et al. A twin study of the association between pathological gambling and antisocial personality disorder. J Abnorm Psychol 2001; 110:297–308.
36. Potenza MN, Steinberg MA, Skudlarski P, et al. Gambling urges in pathological gambling: a functional magnetic resonance imaging study. Arch Gen Psychiatry 2003; 60: 828–836.
37. Potenza MN, Leung HC, Blumberg HP, et al. An FMRI Stroop task study of ventromedial prefrontal cortical function in pathological gamblers. Am J Psychiatry 2003; 160: 1990–1994.
38. Bechara A, Damasio H, Damasio AR, et al. Different contributions of the human amygdala and ventromedial prefrontal cortex to decision-making. J Neurosci 1999; 19:5473–5481.
39. O'Doherty J, Kringelbach ML, Rolls ET, et al. Abstract reward and punishment representations in the human orbitofrontal cortex. Nat Neurosci 2001; 4:95–102.

40. Berlin HA, Rolls ET, Kischka U. Impulsivity, time perception, emotion, and reinforcement sensitivity in patients with orbitofrontal cortex lesions. Brain 2004; 127:1108–1126.
41. Hollander E, Pallanti S, Rossi NB, et al. Imaging monetary reward in pathological gamblers. World J Biol Psychiatry 2005; 6(2):113–120.
42. Hollander E, Buchalter AJ, DeCaria CM. Pathological gambling. Psychiatr Clin North Am 2000; 23:629–642.
43. Hollander E, Frenkel M, DeCaria C, et al. Treatment of pathological gambling with clomipramine. Am J Psychiatry 1992; 149:710–711 (letter).
44. Hollander E, DeCaria CM, Mari E, et al. Short-term single-blind fluvoxamine treatment of pathological gambling. Am J Psychiatry 1998; 155:1781–1783.
45. Hollander E, DeCaria CM, Finkell JN, et al. A randomized double-blind fluvoxamine/ placebo crossover trial in pathologic gambling. Biol Psychiatry 2000; 47:813–817.
46. Dannon PN, Lowengrub K, Gonopolski Y, et al. Topiramate versus fluvoxamine in the treatment of pathological gambling: a randomized, blind-rater comparison study. Clin Neuropharmacol 2005; 28:6–10.
47. Kim SW. Opioid antagonists in the treatment of impulse-control disorders. J Clin Psychiatry 1998; 59:159–164.
48. Moskowitz JA. Lithium and lady luck: use of lithium carbonate in compulsive gambling. N Y State J Med 1980; 80:785–788.
49. Pallanti S, Quercioli L, Sood E, et al. Lithium and valproate treatment of pathological gambling: a randomized single-blind study. J Clin Psychiatry 2002; 63:559–64.
50. Hollander E, Pallanti S, Allen A, et al. Does sustained-release lithium reduce impulsive gambling and affective instability versus placebo in pathological gamblers with bipolar spectrum disorders? Am J Psychiatry 2005; 162:137–145.
51. Haller R, Hinterhuber H. Treatment of pathological gambling with carbamazepine. Pharmacopsychiatry 1994; 27:129.
52. Dannon PN. Topiramate for the treatment of kleptomania: a case series and review of the literature. Clin Neuropharmacol 2003; 26:1–4.
53. Shapira NA, Lessig MC, Murphy TK, et al. Topiramate attenuates self-injurious behaviour in Prader–Willi Syndrome. Int J Neuropsychopharmacol 2002; 5:141–145.
54. Shapira NA, Lessig MC, Lewis MH, et al. Effects of topiramate in adults with Prader–Willi syndrome. Am J Ment Retard 2004; 109:301–309.
55. Lochner C, Seedat S, Niehaus DJ, et al. Topiramate in the treatment of trichotillomania: an open-label pilot study. Int Clin Psychopharmacol 2006; 21:255–259.
56. De Dios Perrino C, Santo-Domingo Carrasco J, Lozano Suarez M. Pharmacological treatment of the intermittent explosive disorder. Report of three cases and literature review. Actas Luso Esp Neurol Psiquiatr Cienc Afines 1995; 23:74–77.
57. Denicoff KD, Meglathery SB, Post RM, et al. Efficacy of carbamazepine compared with other agents: a clinical practice survey. J Clin Psychiatry 1994; 55:70–76.
58. Adu L, Lessig M, Shapira N. Topiramate in the treatment of trichotillomania. Presented at: The Southern Association for Research in Psychiatry 14th Annual Meeting, Gainesville, Florida, 2001.
59. Kaufman KR, Kugler SL, Sachdeo RC. Tiagabine in the management of postencephalitic epilepsy and impulse control disorder. Epilepsy Behav 2002; 3:190–194.
60. Nickel M, Nickel C, Leiberich P, et al. Psychosocial characteristics in people who often change their psychotherapists. Wien Med Wochenschr 2004; 154:163–169.
61. Skodol AE, Gunderson JG, Pfohl B, et al. The borderline diagnosis I: psychopathology, comorbidity, and personality structure. Biol Psychiatry 2002; 51:936–950.
62. Skodol AE, Siever LJ, Livesley WJ, et al. The borderline diagnosis II: biology, genetics, and clinical course. Biol Psychiatry 2002; 51:951–963.
63. Stone MH. The role of pharmacotherapy in the treatment of patients with borderline personality disorder. Psychopharmacol Bull 1989; 25:564–571.
64. Swartz M, Blazer D, George L, et al. Estimating the prevalence of borderline personality disorder in the community. J Personality Dis 1990; 4:257–272.
65. Maier W, Lichtermann D, Klinger T, et al. Prevalences of personality disorders (DSM-III-R) in the community. J Personality Dis 1992; 6:187–196.

66. Hollander E. Managing aggressive behavior in patients with obsessive-compulsive disorder and borderline personality disorder. J Clin Psychiatry 1999; 60:38–44.
67. Skodol AE, Bender DS. Why are women diagnosed borderline more than men? Psychiatr Q 2003; 74:349–360.
68. Kass F, Skodol A, Spitzer CE, et al. Scaled ratings of DSM-III personality disorders. Am J Psychiatry 1985; 142:627–630.
69. Piersma HL. The MCMI as a measure of DSM-Ill axis II diagnoses: an empirical comparison. J Clin Psychol 1987; 43:478–483.
70. Gunderson JG. Pharmacotherapy for patients with borderline personality disorder. Arch Gen Psychiatry 1986; 43:698–700.
71. Cowdry R, Gardner DL. Pharmacotherapy of borderline personality disorder. Alprazolam, carbamazepine, trifluoperazine, and tranylcypromine. Arch Gen Psychiatry 1988; 45: 111–9.
72. Gitlin MJ. Pharmacotherapy of personality disorders: conceptual framework and clinical strategies. J Clin Psychopharmacol 1993; 13:343–353.
73. New AS, Trestman RL, Siever LJ. The pharmacotherapy of borderline personality disorder. CNS Drugs 1994; 5:347–354.
74. Zanarini MC. Update on pharmacotherapy of borderline personality disorder, Curr Psychiatry Rep 2004; 6:66–70.
75. Coryell W. Rapid cycling bipolar disorder: clinical characteristics and treatment options. CNS Drugs 2005; 19:557–569.
76. Stein DJ, Simeon D, Frenkel M, et al. An open trial of valproate in borderline personality disorder. J Clin Psychiatry 1995; 56:506–510.
77. Wilcox JA. Divalproex sodium as a treatment for borderline personality disorder. Ann Clin Psychiatry 1995; 7:33–37.
78. Kavoussi RJ, Coccaro EF. Divalproex sodium for impulsive aggressive behavior in patients with personality disorder. J Clin Psychiatry 1998; 59:676–680.
79. Davis LL, Ryan W, Adinoff B, et al. Comprehensive review of the psychiatric uses of valproate. J Clin Psychopharmacol 2000; 20(suppl 1):S1–S17.
80. Hollander E, Allen A, Lopez RP, et al. A preliminary double-blind, placebo-controlled trial of divalproex sodium in borderline personality disorder. J Clin Psychiatry 2001; 62: 199–203.
81. Frankenburg FR, Zanarini MC. Divalproex sodium treatment of women with borderline personality disorder and bipolar II disorder: a double-blind placebo-controlled pilot study. J Clin Psychiatry 2002; 63:442–446.
82. Townsend MH, Cambre KM, Barbee JG. Treatment of borderline personality disorder with mood instability with divalproex sodium: series of ten cases. J Clin Psychopharmacol 2001; 21:249–251.
83. Hollander E, Swann AC, Coccaro EF, et al. Impact of trait impulsivity and state aggression on divalproex versus placebo response in borderline personality disorder. Am J Psychiatry 2005; 162:621–624.
84. Berlin HA, Rolls ET. Time perception, impulsivity, emotionality, and personality in self-harming borderline personality disorder patients. J Personal Disord 2004; 18:358–378.
85. Gardner DL, Cowdry RW. Positive effects of carbamazepine on behavioral dyscontrol in borderline personality disorder. Am J Psychiatry 1986; 143:519–522.
86. Cowdry RW, Gardner DL. Pharmacotherapy of borderline personality disorder. Alprazolam, carbamazepine, trifluoperazine, and tranylcypromine. Arch Gen Psychiatry 1988; 45:111–119.
87. De la Fuente JM, Lotstra F. A trial of carbamazepine in borderline personality disorder. Eur Neuropsychopharmacol 1994; 4:479–486.
88. Gardner DL, Cowdry RW. Development of melancholia during carbamazepine treatment in borderline personality disorder. J Clin Psychopharmacol 1986; 6:236–239.
89. Bellino S, Paradiso E, Bogetto F. Oxcarbazepine in the treatment of borderline personality disorder: a pilot study. J Clin Psychiatry 2005; 66:1111–1115.
90. Nickel MK, Nickel C, Mitterlehner FO, et al. Topiramate treatment of aggression in female borderline personality disorder patients: a double-blind, placebo-controlled study. J Clin Psychiatry 2004; 65:1515–1519.

91. Nickel MK, Nickel C, Kaplan P, et al. Treatment of aggression with topiramate in male borderline patients: a double-blind, placebo-controlled study. Biol Psychiatry 2005; 57:495–499.

92. Teter CJ, Early JJ, Gibbs CM. Treatment of affective disorder and obesity with topiramate, Ann Pharmacother 2000; 34:1262–1265.

93. Janowsky DS, Kraus JE, Barnhill J, et al. Effects of topiramate on aggressive, self-injurious, and disruptive/destructive behaviors in the intellectually disabled: an open-label retrospective study. J Clin Psychopharmacol 2003; 23:500–504.

94. Loew TH, Nickel MK, Muehlbacher M, et al. Topiramate treatment for women with borderline personality disorder: a double-blind, placebo-controlled study. J Clin Psychopharmacol 2006; 26:61–66.

95. Killaspy H. Topiramate improves psychopathological symptoms and quality of life in women with borderline personality disorder. Evid Based Ment Health 2006; 9:74.

96. do Prado-Lima PA, Kristensen CH, Bacaltchuck J. Can childhood trauma predict response to topiramate in borderline personality disorder? J Clin Pharm Ther 2006; 31: 193–196.

97. Pinto OC, Akiskal HS. Lamotrigine as a promising approach to borderline personality: an open case series without concurrent DSM-IV major mood disorder. J Affect Disord 1998; 51:333–343.

98. Preston GA, Marchant BK, Reimherr FW, et al. Borderline personality disorder in patients with bipolar disorder and response to lamotrigine. J Affect Disord 2004; 79: 297–303.

99. Tritt K, Nickel C, Lahmann C, et al. Lamotrigine treatment of aggression in female borderline-patients: a randomized, double-blind, placebo-controlled study. J Psychopharmacol 2005; 19:287–291.

100. Weinstein W, Jamison KL. Retrospective case review of lamotrigine use for affective instability of borderline personality disorder. CNS Spectr 2007; 12:207–210.

101. Stein G. Drug treatment of the personality disorders. Br J Psychiatry 1992; 161:167–184.

102. Hori A. Pharmacotherapy for personality disorders. Psychiatry Clin Neurosci 1998; 52: 13–19.

103. Coccaro EF, Kavoussi RJ. Biological and pharmacological aspects of borderline personality disorder. Hosp Community Psychiatry 1991; 42:1029–1033.

104. Pelissolo A, Lepine JP. Pharmacotherapy in personality disorders: methodological issues and results. Encephale 1999; 25:496–507.

105. Biancosino B, Facchi A, Marmai L, et al. Gabapentin treatment of impulsive-aggressive behaviour. Can J Psychiatry 2002; 47:483–484.

106. Morana HC, Olivi ML, Daltio CS. Use of gabapentin in group B – DSM-IV personality disorders. Rev Bras Psiquiatr 2004; 26:136–137.

107. Morana HC, Camara FP. International guidelines for the management of personality disorders. Curr Opin Psychia 2006; 19:539–543

108. Herranz JL. Gabapentin: its mechanisms of action in the year 2003. Rev Neurol 2003; 12: 1159–1165.

109. Soloff PH. Psychopharmacology of borderline personality disorder. Psychiatr Clin North Am 2000; 23:169–192.

110. Fava M. Psychopharmacologic treatment of pathologic aggression. Psychiatr Clin North Am 1997; 20:427–451.

111. Salpekar JA, Conry JA, Doss W, et al. Clinical experience with anticonvulsant medication in pediatric epilepsy and comorbid bipolar spectrum disorder. Epilepsy Behav 2006; 9:327–334.

112. Fleminger S, Greenwood RJ, Oliver DL. Pharmacological management for agitation and aggression in people with acquired brain injury. Cochrane Database Syst Rev 2006; 18(4): CD003299.

113. Golden AS, Haut SR, Moshe SL. Nonepileptic uses of antiepileptic drugs in children and adolescents. Pediatr Neurol 2006; 34:421–432.

114. Swann AC. Neuroreceptor mechanisms of aggression and its treatment. J Clin Psychiatry 2003; 64(suppl 4):26–35.

115. Barratt ES. The use of anticonvulsants in aggression and violence. Psychopharmacol Bull 1993; 29:75–81.
116. Tariot PN, Schneider LS, Mintzer JE, et al. Safety and tolerability of divalproex sodium in the treatment of signs and symptoms of mania in elderly patients with dementia: results of a double-blind, placebo-controlled trial. Curr Ther Res 2001; 62:51–67.
117. Wulsin L, Bachop M, Hoffman D. Group therapy in manic-depressive illness. Am J Psychother 1988; 42:263–271.
118. Donovan SJ, Susser ES, Nunes EV, et al. Divalproex treatment of disruptive adolescents: a report of 10 cases. J Clin Psychiatry 1997; 58:12–15.
119. Donovan SJ, Stewart JW, Nunes EV, et al. Divalproex treatment for youth with explosive temper and mood lability: a double-blind, placebo-controlled crossover design. Am J Psychiatry 2000; 157:818–820.
120. Fesler FA. Valproate in combat-related posttraumatic stress disorder. J Clin Psychiatry 1991; 52:361–364.
121. Szymanski HV, Olympia J. Divalproex in posttraumatic stress disorder. Am J Psychiatry 1991; 148:1086–1087.
122. Petty F, Davis LL, Nugent AL, et al. Valproate therapy for chronic combat-induced posttraumatic stress disorder. J Clin Psychopharmacol 2002; 22:100–101.
123. Giakas WJ, Seibyl JP, Mazure CM. Valproate in the treatment of temper outbursts. J Clin Psychiatry 1990; 51:525.
124. Horne M, Lindley SE. Divalproex sodium in the treatment of aggressive behavior and dysphoria in patients with organic brain syndromes. J Clin Psychiatry 1995; 56:430–431.
125. Wroblewski BA, Joseph AB, Kupfer J, et al. Effectiveness of valproic acid on destructive and aggressive behaviours in patients with acquired brain injury. Brain Inj 1997; 11:37–47.
126. Haas S, Vincent K, Holt J, et al. Divalproex: a possible treatment alternative for demented elderly aggressive patients. Ann Clin Psychiatry 1997; 9:145–147.
127. Buchalter EN, Lantz MS. Treatment of impulsivity and aggression in a patient with vascular dementia. Geriatrics 2001; 56:53–54.
128. Porsteinsson AP, Tariot PN, Erb R, et al. Placebo-controlled study of divalproex sodium for agitation in dementia. Am J Geriatr Psychiatry 2001; 9:58–66.
129. Porsteinsson AP, Tariot PN, Jakimovich LJ, et al. Valproate therapy for agitation in dementia: open-label extension of a double-blind trial. Am J Geriatr Psychiatry 2003; 11: 434–440.
130. Hollander E, Dolgoff-Kaspar R, Cartwright C, et al. An open trial of divalproex sodium in autism spectrum disorders. J Clin Psychiatry 2001; 62:530–534.
131. Lindenmayer JP, Kotsaftis A. Use of sodium valproate in violent and aggressive behaviors: a critical review. J Clin Psychiatry 2000; 61:123–128.
132. Vitiello B, Behar D, Hunt J, et al. Subtyping aggression in children and adolescents. J Neuropsychiatry Clin Neurosci 1990; 2:189–192.
133. Meinhold JM, Blake LM, Mini LJ, et al. Effect of divalproex sodium on behavioural and cognitive problems in elderly dementia. Drugs Aging 2005; 22:615–626.
134. Hellings JA, Nickel EJ, Weckbaugh M, et al. The overt aggression scale for rating aggression in outpatient youth with autistic disorder: preliminary findings. J Neuropsychiatry Clin Neurosci 2005; 17:29–35.
135. Lopez-Larson M, Frazier JA. Empirical evidence for the use of lithium and anticonvulsants in children with psychiatric disorders. Harv Rev Psychiatry 2006; 14:285–304.
136. Connor DF, Carlson GA, Chang KD, et al. Stanford/Howard/AACAP workgroup on juvenile impulsivity and aggression. Juvenile maladaptive aggression: a review of prevention, treatment, and service configuration and a proposed research agenda. J Clin Psychiatry 2006; 67:808–820.
137. Miyazaki M, Ito H, Saijo T, et al. Favorable response of ADHD with giant SEP to extended-release valproate. Brain Dev 2006; 28:470–472
138. Steiner H, Petersen ML, Saxena K, et al. Divalproex sodium for the treatment of conduct disorder a randomized controlled clinical trial. J Clin Psychiatry 2003; 64:936–942.
139. Barzman DH, DelBello MP, Adler CM, et al. efficacy and tolerability of quetiapine versus divalproex for the treatment of impulsivity and reactive aggression in adolescents with co-occurring bipolar disorder and disruptive behavior disorder(s). J Child Adolesc Psychopharmacol 2006; 16:665–670.

140. Gobbi G, Gaudreau PO, Leblanc N. Efficacy of topiramate, valproate, and their combination on aggression/agitation behavior in patients with psychosis. J Clin Psychopharmacol 2006; 26:467–473.
141. MacMillan CM, Korndorfer SR, Rao S, et al. A comparison of divalproex and oxcarbazepine in aggressive youth with bipolar disorder. J Psychiatr Pract 2006; 12:214–222.
142. State RC, Frye MA, Altshuler LL, et al. Chart review of the impact of attention-deficit/hyperactivity disorder comorbidity on response to lithium or divalproex sodium in adolescent mania. J Clin Psychiatry 2004; 65:1057–1063.
143. Barzman DH, McConville BJ, Masterson B, et al. Impulsive aggression with irritability and responsive to divalproex: a pediatric bipolar spectrum disorder phenotype? J Affect Disord 2005; 88:279–285.
144. Saxena K, Howe M, Simeonova D, et al. Divalproex sodium reduces overall aggression in youth at high risk for bipolar disorder. J Child Adolesc Psychopharmacol 2006; 16: 252–259.
145. Mattes JA. Psychopharmacology of temper outbursts: a review. J Nerv Ment Dis 1986; 174:464–470.
146. Cueva JE, Overall JE, Small AM, et al. Carbamazepine in aggressive children with conduct disorder: a double-blind and placebo-controlled study. J Am Acad Child Adolesc Psychiatry 1996; 35:480–90.
147. De Vogelaer J. Carbamazepine in the treatment of psychotic and behavioral disorders: a pilot study. ACTA Psychiatr Belg 1981; 81:532–541.
148. Thibaut F, Colonna L. Carbamazepine and aggressive behavior: a review. Encephale 1993; 19:651–656.
149. Young AL, Hillbrand M. Carbamazepine lowers aggression: a review. Bull Am Acad Psychiatry Law 1994; 22:52–61
150. Tariot PN, Erb R, Podgorski CA, et al. Efficacy and tolerability of carbamazepine for agitation and aggression in dementia. Am J Psychiatry 1998; 155:54–61.
151. Chatham-Showalter PE. Carbamazepine for combativeness in acute traumatic brain injury. J Neuropsychiatry Clin Neurosci 1996; 8:96–969.
152. Azouvi P, Jokic C, Attal N, et al. Carbamazepine in agitation and aggressive behaviour following severe closed-head injury: results of an open trial. Brain Inj 1999; 13:797–804.
153. Freymann N, Michael R, Dodel R, Jessen F. Successful treatment of sexual disinhibition in dementia with carbamazepine – a case report. Pharmacopsychiatry 2005; 38:144–145.
154. Kafantaris V, Campbell M, Padron-Gayol MV, et al. Carbamazepine in hospitalized aggressive conduct disorder children An open pilot study. Psychopharmacol Bull 1992; 28: 193–199.
155. Mattes JA. Comparative effectiveness of carbamazepine and propranolol for rage outbursts. J Neuropsychiatry Clin Neurosci 1990; 2:159–64.
156. Munoz P, Gonzalez Torres MA. Organic personality disorder: response to carbamazepine. Actas Luso Esp Neurol Psiquiatr Cienc Afines 1997; 25:197–200.
157. Morikawa M, Iida J, Tokuyama A, et al. Successful treatment using low-dose carbamazepine for a patient of personality change after mild diffuse brain injury. Nihon Shinkei Seishin Yakurigaku Zasshi 2000; 20:149–53.
158. Lewin J, Sumners D. Successful treatment of episodic dyscontrol with carbamazepine. Br J Psychiatry 1992; 161:261–2.
159. American Psychiatric Association. Practice guideline for the treatment of patients with bipolar disorder. Am J Psychiatry 2002; 159:4–5, 9–10, 24 (revision).
160. Mattes JA. Oxcarbazepine in patients with impulsive aggression: a double-blind, placebo-controlled trial. J Clin Psychopharmacol 2005; 25:575–9.
161. Gaudino MP, Smith MJ, Matthews DT. Use of oxcarbazepine for treatment-resistant aggression. Psychiatr Serv 2003; 54:1166–7.
162. Cordas TA, Tavares H, Calderoni DM, et al. Oxcarbazepine for self-mutilating bulimic patients. Int J Neuropsychopharmacol 2006; 9:769–71.
163. Nickel C, Lahmann C, Tritt K, et al. Topiramate in treatment of depressive and anger symptoms in female depressive patients: a randomized, double-blind, placebo-controlled study. J Affect Disord 2005; 87:243–52.
164. Smathers SA, Wilson JG, Nigro MA, Topiramate effectiveness in Prader-Willi Syndrome. Pediatr Neurol 2003; 28:130–133.

165. Shapira NA, Goldsmith TD, McElroy SL. Treatment of binge-eating disorder with topiramate: a clinical case series. J Clin Psychiatry 2000; 61:368–372.
166. McElroy SL, Arnold LM, Shapira NA, et al. Topiramate in the treatment of binge eating disorder associated with obesity: a randomized, placebo-controlled trial. Am J Psychiatry 2003; 160:255–261.
167. Pederson KJ, Roerig JL, Mitchell JE. Towards the pharmacotherapy of eating disorders. Expert Opin Pharmacother 2003; 4:1659–1678.
168. Appolinario JC, McElroy SL. Pharmacological approaches in the treatment of binge eating disorder. Curr Drug Targets 2004; 5:301–7.
169. Carter WP, Hudson JI, Lalonde JK, et al. Pharmacologic treatment of binge eating disorder. Int J Eat Disord 2003; 34:S74–S88.
170. Appolinario JC, Fontenelle LF, Papelbaum M, et al. Topiramate use in obese patients with binge eating disorder: an open study. Can J Psychiatry 2002; 47:271–273.
171. McElroy SL, Shapira NA, Arnold LM, et al. Topiramate in the long-term treatment of binge-eating disorder associated with obesity. J Clin Psychiatry 2004; 65:1463–1469.
172. Zilberstein B, Pajecki D, Garcia de Brito AC, et al. Topiramate after adjustable gastric banding in patients with binge eating and difficulty losing weight. Obes Surg 2004; 14:802–805.
173. Dolberg OT, Barkai G, Gross Y, et al. Differential effects of topiramate in patients with traumatic brain injury and obesity–a case series. Psychopharmacology (Berl) 2005; 179: 838–845.
174. Guerdjikova AI, Kotwal R, McElroy SL. Response of recurrent binge eating and weight gain to topiramate in patients with binge eating disorder after bariatric surgery. Obes Surg 2005; 15:273–277.
175. De Bernardi C, Ferraris S, D'Innella P, et al. Topiramate for binge eating disorder. Prog Neuropsychopharmacol Biol Psychiatry 2005; 29:339–41.
176. Nickel C, Lahmann C, Tritt K, et al. Topiramate in treatment of depressive and anger symptoms in female depressive patients: a randomized, double-blind, placebo-controlled study. J Affect Disord 2005; 87:243–252.
177. Chengappa KNR, Rathore D, Levine J, et al. Topiramate as add-on treatment for patients with bipolar mania. Bipolar Dis 1999; 1:42–53.
178. Cassano P, Lattanzi L, Pini S, et al. Topiramate for self-mutilation in a patient with borderline personality disorder. Bipolar Disord 2001; 3:161.
179. Dolengevich Segal H, Rodriguez Salgado B, Conejo Garcia A, et al. Efficacy of topiramate in children and adolescent with problems in impulse control: preliminary results. Actas Esp Psiquiatr 2006; 34:280–282.
180. Rugino TA, Samsock TC. Levetiracetam in autistic children: an open-label study. J Dev Behav Pediatr 2002; 23:225–30.
181. Grunze H, Langosch J, Born C, et al. Levetiracem in the treatment of acute mania: an open add-on study with an on-off-on design. J Clin Psychiatry 2003; 64:781–784.
182. Kaufman KR. Monotherapy treatment of bipolar disorder with levetiracetam. Epilepsy Behav 2004; 5:1017–1020.
183. Simon NM, Worthington JJ, Doyle AC, et al. An open-label study of levetiracetam for the treatment of social anxiety disorder. J Clin Psychiatry 2004; 65:1219–22.
184. Wasserman S, Iyengar R, Chaplin WF, et al. Levetiracetam versus placebo in childhood and adolescent autism: a double-blind placebo-controlled study. Int Clin Psychopharmacol 2006; 21:363–367.
185. Dinkelacker V, Dietl T, Widman G, et al. Aggressive behavior of epilepsy patients in the course of levetiracetam add-on therapy: report of 33 mild to severe cases. Epilepsy Behav 2003; 4:537–547.
186. Weber S, Beran RG. A pilot study of compassionate use of Levetiracetam in patients with generalised epilepsy. J Clin Neurosci 2004; 11:728–731.
187. Opp J, Tuxhorn I, May T, et al. Levetiracetam in children with refractory epilepsy: a multicenter open label study in Germany. Seizure 2005; 14:476–484.
188. Neuwirth M, Saracz J, Hegyi M, et al. Experience with levetiracetam in childhood epilepsy. Ideggyogy Sz 2006; 59:179–82.

189. Cherek DR, Tcheremissine OV, Lane SD, et al. Acute effects of gabapentin on laboratory measures of aggressive and escape responses of adult parolees with and without a history of conduct disorder. Psychopharmacology (Berl) 2004; 171:405–412.
190. Herrmann N, Lanctôt K, Myszak M. Effectiveness of gabapentin for the treatment of behavioral disorders in dementia. J Clin Psychopharmacol 2000; 20:90–93.
191. Miller LJ. Gabapentin for treatment of behavioral and psychological symptoms of dementia. Ann Pharmacother 2001; 35:427–431.
192. Hawkins JW, Tinklenberg JR, Sheikh JI, et al. A retrospective chart review of gabapentin for the treatment of aggressive and agitated behavior in patients with dementias. Am J Geriatr Psychiatry 2000; 8:221–5.
193. Alkhalil C, Tanvir F, Alkhalil B, et al. Treatment of sexual disinhibition in dementia: case reports and review of the literature. Am J Ther 2004; 11:231–235.
194. McManaman J, Tam DA. Gabapentin for self-injurious behavior in Lesch-Nyhan Syndrome. Pediatr Neurol 1999; 20:381–382.
195. Gupta S, Frank BL, Masand PS. Gabapentin in the treatment of aggression associated with conduct disorder, primary care companion. J Clin Psychiatry 2000; 2:60–61.
196. Ryback R, Ryback L. Gabapentin for behavioral dyscontrol. Am J Psychiatry 1995; 152: 1399 (letter).
197. Looker A, Conners CK. Diphenylhydantoin in children with severe temper tantrums. Arch Gen Psychiatry 1970; 23:80–9.
198. Stanford MS, Helfritz LE, Conklin SM, et al. A comparison of anticonvulsants in the treatment of impulsive aggression. Exp Clin Psychopharmacol 2005; 13:72–77.
199. Stanford MS, Houston RJ, Mathias CW, et al. A double-blind placebo-controlled crossover study of phenytoin in individuals with impulsive aggression. Psychiatry Res 2001; 103:193–203.
200. Maletzky BM. The episodic dyscontrol syndrome. Dis Nerv Syst 1973; 34:178–185.
201. Maletzky BM, Klotter J. Episodic dyscontrol: a controlled replication. Dis Nerv Syst 1974; 35:175–179.
202. Barratt ES, Kent TA, Bryant SG, et al. A controlled trial of phenytoin in impulsive aggression. J Clin Psychopharmacol 1991; 6:388–389.
203. Barratt ES, Stanford MS, Felthous AR, et al. The effects of phenytoin on impulsive and premeditated aggression: a controlled study. J Clin Psychopharmacol 1997; 17:341–9.
204. Keele NB. The role of serotonin in impulsive and aggressive behaviors associated with epilepsy-like neuronal hyperexcitability in the amygdala. Epilepsy Behav 2005; 7:325–35.
205. Hollander E, Begaz T, DeCaria CM. Pharmacological approaches in the treatment of pathological gambling. CNS Spectrums 1998; 3:72–80.
206. Hollander E, Sood E, Pallanti S, et al. Pharmacological treatments of pathological gambling. J Gambl Stud 2005; 21:99–108.

Antiepileptic Drugs and Borderline Personality Disorder

Mary C. Zanarini

Laboratory for the Study of Adult Development, McLean Hospital, Belmont and the Department of Psychiatry, Harvard Medical School, Boston, Massachusetts, U.S.A.

INTRODUCTION

Several cross-sectional studies have documented the high percentage of patients with borderline personality disorder (BPD) who have a lifetime history of taking anticonvulsant mood stabilizers (1,2). More recently, a study of the longitudinal course of BPD (3) documented high rates of the use of anticonvulsant mood stabilizers throughout six years of prospective follow-up. More specifically, about a quarter of the patients with BPD studied took such a mood stabilizer during the first two years after their index admission, 22% took such a mood stabilizer during the third and fourth years after their entry into the study, and 18% during their fifth and sixth years of study participation.

This high rate of use is probably due to two factors. The first is the overlap of some of the symptoms of BPD (particularly pronounced mood lability and impulsivity) and some of the symptoms of bipolar disorder. The second is the belief of some mental health professionals (4) that BPD is actually an attenuated form of bipolar disorder—a belief that is not consistent with the results of longitudinal studies that have found that most borderline patients do not develop a bipolar disorder over time (5,6).

Despite the high rate of use mentioned above, surprisingly few open-label or controlled medication trials of anticonvulsant mood stabilizers in particular or antiepileptic drugs (AEDs) in general in the treatment of patients with BPD have been conducted. Below is a careful review of first-generation and second-generation studies. Only published studies will be described, and only studies limited to patients with BPD have been included.

FIRST-GENERATION STUDIES

Gardner and Cowdry (7) conducted a six-week, placebo-controlled crossover study. They found that carbamazepine was superior to placebo in the treatment of behavior dyscontrol in a sample of 11 women with BPD and histories of severe impulsivity. The average daily dose of carbamazepine was 820 mg. Somewhat later, De la Fuente and Lotstra (8) conducted a double-blind, placebo-controlled trial of carbamazepine in a sample of inpatients with BPD ($N = 20$) and no co-occurring axis I disorders. They failed to find any significant differences in any sector of borderline psychopathology between those treated with carbamazepine and those treated with placebo.

This between-study difference in outcome may be due to the fact that Gardner and Cowdry were studying women with BPD plus a history of severe problems with behavior dyscontrol. However, the subjects in the study of De la Fuente and Lotstra were inpatients and thus were acutely ill.

SECOND-GENERATION STUDIES

Divalproex Sodium

Two open-label studies of *Diagnostic and Statistical Manual of Mental Disorders-Third Edition, Revised* (DSM-III-R) borderline patients treated with divalproex sodium have been conducted. Stein et al. (9) studied 11 outpatients in an eight-week trial. All subjects were in psychotherapy and none had a current major depression or a history of bipolarity or a psychotic disorder. Eight of the eleven subjects (73%) completed the trial and half of them were responders. However, when the scores of all 11 subjects were examined, significant decreases in psychopathology were found for only two of the study's five main outcomes: subjective irritability as measured by the Modified Overt Aggression Scale (also called the Overt Aggression Scale-Modified; OAS-M) (10) and general psychopathology as assessed by the Symptom Checklist-90 (SCL-90) (11).

Wilcox (12) also conducted an open-label trial of divalproex sodium. He studied 30 inpatients without comorbid disorders meeting DSM-III-R criteria for BPD. The trial lasted for six weeks, and seven of the subjects were on a concurrent medication. Wilcox found significant decreases in the study's outcome measures— general psychopathology as measured by the Brief Psychiatric Rating Scale (BPRS) (13)— and number of minutes in seclusion (which was viewed as a measure of agitation). The author concluded that the medication had its greatest effect on anxiety (as rated by the BPRS) and that reduced anxiety led to reduced agitation.

Hollander et al. (14) completed the first placebo-controlled, double-blind study of the efficacy of divalproex sodium in criteria-defined patients with BPD. They conducted a 10-week trial and studied 16 patients with DSM-IV BPD, 12 randomized to divalproex sodium and 4 to placebo. Fifty percent of the subjects on active medication dropped out of the study, and 100% of those taking placebo dropped out before completing the study. No significant between-group differences were found. However, 42% of subjects taking divalproex sodium were judged to be responders, while none of the subjects being treated with placebo were judged to be responders. In addition, substantial reductions in aggression and depression were found for subjects treated with divalproex sodium.

Hollander et al. (15) conducted a second double-blind, placebo-controlled trial of divalproex sodium versus placebo in a sample of 50 patients meeting DSM-IV criteria for BPD. Exclusion criteria included lifetime bipolar I disorder and bipolar II disorder within the past year. In this 12-week study, data were analyzed for 18 subjects assigned to the active group and 32 subjects assigned to the placebo group. The mean modal dose of divalproex sodium was 1325 mg/day. Borderline patients treated with divalproex had a significantly greater decrease in their impulsive aggression as measured by the OAS-M. In addition, those borderline patients taking divalproex who were high in state impulsivity and trait aggression at baseline had a significantly greater decrease in impulsive aggression than similar subjects taking placebo.

Frankenburg and Zanarini (16) also conducted a double-blind, placebo-controlled trial of divalproex sodium in the treatment of symptomatic volunteers meeting rigorous criteria for BPD. However, these investigators conducted a six-month long trial of 30 women meeting the revised Diagnostic Interview for Borderlines (DIB-R) (17) and DSM-IV criteria for BPD and DSM-IV criteria for comorbid bipolar II disorder. Twenty of these subjects were randomized to divalproex sodium and 10 were randomized to placebo; most had histories of outpatient treatment.

Those on active treatment were found to have experienced significantly greater reductions in three of the study's outcome measures: interpersonal sensitivity, anger, and hostility as measured by the SCL-90 and the total score of the OAS-M. However, depression as assessed by the SCL-90 did not show a significant between-group difference. The average dose of divalproex sodium was 850 mg (SD = 249). The groups gained, on average, a small but not significantly different amount of weight [2.6 pounds (SD = 5.6) vs. 0.3 pounds (SD = 4.0)]. Retention was quite good through the first eight weeks of the study (70% of those treated with active compound and 60% of those treated with placebo). However, only 35% of the subjects treated with divalproex sodium and 40% of the subjects treated with placebo remained in the study all 24 weeks. Given the design of the study, it is not clear whether the mild bipolarity of the subjects was treated or their borderline lability or a combination of the two.

More recently, Simeon et al. (18), in conjunction with Hollander, conducted an open-label trial of divalproex extended release (ER). This 12-week trial assessed the efficacy of this compound in 20 adults meeting DSM-IV criteria for BPD. None were in any kind of psychiatric treatment. The mean end dose of divalproex was 1350 mg/day. The attrition rate was high (50%). However, the following areas of borderline psychopathology saw significant improvement: overall symptoms, overall functioning, irritability, and aggression.

Lamotrigine

Pinto and Akiskal (19) studied eight DSM-IV borderline outpatients under their clinical care in an open-label trial of lamotrigine. None of the patients had a history of a major mood disorder of a unipolar or bipolar nature. Three of these severely ill patients were judged to be responders. The investigators reported in a series of case reports that the impulsive behaviors of these patients were completely eradicated and that they no longer met criteria for BPD.

Tritt et al. (20) have conducted the only double-blind, placebo-controlled trial of lamotrigine. They assessed 27 female outpatients meeting DSM-IV criteria for BPD, 18 women taking lamotrigine and 9 taking placebo. Over the course of this eight-week trial, the dose of lamotigine was titrated from 50 mg/day during the first two weeks of the trial to 200 mg/day during the final three weeks of the trial. In terms of dropouts, only 6% of those being treated with lamotrigine failed to complete the trial, while 22% of those in the placebo group dropped out prior to trial completion. Tritt et al. found that the active compound was superior to placebo on all five aspects of anger studied: state, trait, inward, outward, and control of anger.

TOPIRAMATE

Nickel et al. (21,22), who are part of the same research team as Tritt et al., conducted two placebo-controlled trials of topiramate. They studied the effects of topiramate versus placebo on the anger of female ($N = 21$ vs. 10) and male ($N = 22$ vs. 22) samples of patients meeting DSM-IV criteria for BPD. The female sample, who participated in an eight-week trial, consisted primarily of outpatients and the male sample, who participated in a 10-week trial, was a combination of outpatients and symptomatic volunteers. The titrated dose for those in both groups was 250 mg/day in the sixth week. Over 90% of those in both groups in both studies completed the trial. They found in both studies that treatment with top-iramate was superior to treatment with placebo on four of the five anger scales studied (i.e., all but anger directed inward). They also found that topiramate-treated subjects lost significantly more weight over the course of the trial than subjects treated with placebo (males = 5 kg and females = 2.3 kg).

The same group conducted a second study of topiramate treatment of females with BPD (23). A somewhat larger sample (28 vs. 28) was studied for 10 weeks with a dose of topiramate that was titrated to 200 mg/day in week 6. Attrition was low for both study groups (4% for active compound and 11% for placebo). It was found that topiramate was superior to placebo on six scales of the SCL-90: somatization, interpersonal sensitivity, anxiety, hostility, phobic anxiety, and global severity. Significant differences were also found on all eight scales of the SF-36 Health Survey (24). In addition, significant differences were found on four of the eight scales of the Inventory of Interpersonal Problems (25): overly autocratic, overly competi-tive, overly introverted, and overly expressive. They also found that topiramate-treated subjects lost significantly more weight over the course of the trial than subjects treated with placebo (4.3 kg).

Other AEDs
Bellino et al. (26) conducted an open-label trial of oxcarbazepine, a medication related to carbamazepine. They studied the effectiveness of this medication in treating 17 outpatients meeting DSM-IV criteria for BPD. None of these subjects had ever met criteria for bipolar I disorder or bipolar II disorder. They found that this medication was broadly effective, with the severity of anxiety symptoms, borderline (including affective instability and general impulsivity) symptoms, and overall symptoms declining significantly over the course of this 12-week trial. The retention rate in this trial was high (76%) and no serious adverse events were reported. The mean daily dose of oxcarbazepine, which was administered twice per day, was 1315 mg.

Limitations of Existing Studies and Directions for Future Research
In general, the methodology of the papers reviewed above is quite good. Firstly, it is particularly important for interpretability that studies either exclude borderline patients with histories of bipolarity or limit themselves to such patients. Secondly, studies involving larger samples would lessen the chances of type II errors. Thirdly, studies may often have included subjects who were not particularly symptomatic in the areas studied and, thus, substantial improvement in these symptoms would be unlikely. In fact, controlled studies of carbamazepine (7) and divalproex sodium (15) were only found to be effective in samples comprising subjects with serious emotional dysregulation and/or impulsive aggression.

CONCLUSIONS

Taken together, the results of these studies suggest several important findings. The first is that most of the AEDs studied in controlled trials were found to be effica-cious. The second finding is that most of these medications were useful in treating symptoms of affective dysregulation and impulsive aggression, which have been suggested as the core dimensions of psychopathology underlying BPD (27). The third finding is that although each of these medications took the edge off of BPD symptomatology, none were curative for BPD. In fact, second-generation antidepressant and antipsychotic agents have also been found to be efficacious but not definitive in the treatment of BPD (28). However, helping borderline patients attain a moment to reflect without swinging into action is no small accomplishment and may set the stage for more adaptive behaviors. It may also allow borderline patients to better engage in psychotherapy. This is particularly important as there are now four forms of therapy that have been found to be efficacious in the treatment of BPD—dialectical behavior therapy (DBT) (29), mentalization-based treatment (MBT) (30), schema-focused therapy (SFT) (31), and transference-focused psychotherapy (TFP) (32).

REFERENCES

1. Bender DS, Dolan RT, Skodol AE, et al. Treatment utilization by patients with personality disorders. Am J Psychiatry 2001; 158(2):295–302.
2. Zanarini MC, Frankenburg FR, Khera GS, et al. Treatment histories of borderline inpatients. Compr Psychiatry 2001; 42(2):144–150.
3. Zanarini MC, Frankenburg FR, Hennen J, et al. Mental health service utilization of borderline patients and axis II comparison subjects followed prospectively for six years. J Clin Psychiatry 2004; 65(1):28–36.
4. Akiskal HS, Chen SE, Davis GC, et al. Borderline: an adjective in search of a noun. J Clin Psychiatry 1985; 46(2):41–48.
5. Gunderson JG, Weinberg I, Daversa MT, et al. Descriptive and longitudinal observations on the relationship of borderline personality disorder and bipolar disorder. Am J Psychiatry 2006; 163(7):1173–1178.
6. Zanarini MC, Frankenburg FR, Hennen J, et al. Axis I comorbidity in patients with borderline personality disorder: 6-year follow-up and prediction of time to remission. Am J Psychiatry 2004; 161(11):2108–2114.
7. Gardner DL, Cowdry RW. Positive effects of carbamazepine on behavioral dyscontrol in borderline personality disorder. Am J Psychiatry 1986; 143(4):519–522.
8. De la Fuente JM, Lotstra F. A trial of carbamazepine in borderline personality disorder. Eur Neuropsychopharmacol 1994; 4(4):479–486.
9. Stein DJ, Simeon D, Frenkel M, et al. An open trial of valproate in borderline personality disorder. J Clin Psychiatry 1995; 56(11):506–510.
10. Coccaro EF, Harvey PH, Kupshaw-Lawrence E, et al. Development of neuropharmacologically based assessments of impulsive aggressive behavior. J Neuropsychiatry 1991; 3(suppl):44–51.
11. Derogatis LR, Lipman RS, Covi L. SCL-90: an outpatient psychiatric rating scale–preliminary report. Psychopharmacol Bull 1973; 9(1):13–28.
12. Wilcox JA. Divalproex sodium as a treatment for borderline personality disorder. Ann Clin Psychiatry 1995; 7(1):33–37.
13. Overall JE, Gorham DR. The brief psychiatric rating scale. Psychol Rep 1962; 10:799–812.
14. Hollander E, Allen A, Lopez RP, et al. A preliminary double-blind, placebo-controlled trial of divalproex sodium in borderline personality disorder. J Clin Psychiatry 2001; 62(3): 199–203.
15. Hollander E, Swann AC, Coccaro EF, et al. Impact of trait impulsivity and state aggression on divalproex versus placebo response in borderline personality disorder. Am J Psychiatry 2005; 162(3):621–624.
16. Frankenburg FR, Zanarini MC. Divalproex sodium treatment of women with borderline personality disorder and bipolar II disorder: a double-blind placebo-controlled pilot study. J Clin Psychiatry 2002; 63(5):442–446.
17. Zanarini MC, Gunderson JG, Frankenburg FR, et al. The revised diagnostic interview for borderlines: discriminating BPD from other axis II disorders. J Personal Disord 1989; 3(1): 10–18.

18. Simeon D, Baker B, Chaplin W, et al. An open-label trial of divalproex extended-release in the treatment of borderline personality disorder. CNS Spectr 2007; 12(6):439–443.
19. Pinto OC, Akiskal HS. Lamotrigine as a promising approach to borderline personality: an open case series without concurrent DSM-IV major mood disorder. J Affect Disord 1998; 51(3): 333–343.
20. Tritt K, Nickel C, Lahmann C, et al. Lamotrigine treatment of aggression in female borderline-patients: a randomized, double-blind, placebo-controlled study. J Psychopharmacol 2005; 19(3):287–291.
21. Nickel MK, Nickel C, Mitterlehner FO, et al. Topiramate treatment of aggression in female borderline personality disorder patients: a double-blind, placebo-controlled study. J Clin Psychiatry 2004; 65(11):1515–1519.
22. Nickel MK, Nickel C, Kaplan P, et al. Treatment of aggression with topiramate in male borderline patients: a double-blind, placebo-controlled study. Biol Psychiatry 2005; 57(5): 495–499.
23. Loew TH, Nickel MK, Muehlbacher M, et al. Topiramate treatment for women with borderline personality disorder: a double-blind, placebo-controlled study. J Clin Psychopharmacol 2006; 26(1):61–66.
24. Bullinger M, Kirchberger I. SF-36 Health Survey. Goettingen, Germany: Hogrefe, 1998.
25. Horowitz LM, Rosenberg SE, Baer BA, et al. Inventory of interpersonal problems: psychometric properties and clinical applications. J Consult Clin Psychol 1988; 56(6):885–892.
26. Bellino S, Paradiso E, Bogetto F. Oxcarbazepine in the treatment of borderline personality disorder: a pilot study. J Clin Psychiatry 2005; 66(9):1111–1115.
27. Siever LJ, Davis KL. A psychobiological perspective on the personality disorders. Am J Psychiatry 1991; 148(12):1647–1658.
28. Zanarini MC. Update on pharmacotherapy of borderline personality disorder. Curr Psychiatry Rep 2004; 6(1):55–70.
29. Linehan MM, Armstrong HE, Suarez A, et al. Cognitive-behavioral treatment of chronically parasuicidal borderline patients. Arch Gen Psychiatry 1991; 48(12):1060–1064.
30. Bateman A, Fonagy P. Effectiveness of partial hospitalization in the treatment of borderline personality disorder: a randomized controlled trial. Am J Psychiatry 1999; 156(10): 1563–1569.
31. Giesen-Bloo J, van Dyck R, Spinhoven P, et al. Outpatient psychotherapy for borderline personality disorder. Arch Gen Psychiatry 2006; 63(6):649–658.
32. Clarkin JF, Levy KN, Lenzenweger MF, et al. Evaluating three treatments for borderline personality: a multiwave study. Am J Psychiatry 2007; 164(6):922–928.

Psychotrophic Mechanisms of Action of Antiepileptic Drugs in Mood Disorder

Robert M. Post
Head, Bipolar Collaborative Network, Bethesda, Maryland, U.S.A.

INTRODUCTION

A number of conundrums complicate the interpretation of which biochemical effects of the antiepileptic drugs (AEDs) may be related to their mood-stabilizing and other psychotropic properties. We outline several of these issues prior to consideration of actions of specific drugs because these are crucial to the interpretation of the data. The first issue to consider is whether the mechanism of action of these agents in the seizure disorders mirrors those in the psychiatric illnesses. There are diverse mechanisms of the AEDs and these may be pertinent to efficacy in different epilepsy syndromes. Some of the AEDs are thought to act by enhancing gamma-aminobutyric acid (GABA)-benzodiazepine receptor inhibition, while others are thought to decrease overexcitation, inhibiting glutamate release, or its postsynaptic receptor effects (Fig. 1).

In either instance, these drugs tend to act against seizures either immediately or as quickly as therapeutic blood levels can be achieved (Fig. 2). In contrast, full antimanic and antidepressant effects are slower to achieve, often requiring days to weeks for mania and two to four weeks for depression, even in those who are eventually highly responsive to carbamazepine, for example (Fig. 3). Thus, the time course of onset of either initial or maximum degree of therapeutic efficacy appears to dissociate the psychotropic from anticonvulsant effects of these agents. Therefore, it would appear that actions of AEDs that require longer time periods or chronic administration in order to be achieved will likely be related to the psychotropic effects, while acute effects are more likely relevant to efficacy in seizure disorders and pain syndromes. However, exceptions are beginning to emerge with very rapid onset of antidepressant effects seen with thyrotropin-releasing hormone (TRH) (1,2), the N-methyl-D-aspartate (NMDA) receptor antagonist ketamine (3), and a specific NR2B subunit antagonist (4).

Another important and perhaps clarifying factor is that all of the AEDs do not appear to possess a similar range of psychotropic effects. Specifically, a number of AEDs do not have acute antimanic efficacy (Table 1). In particular, many of those that increase brain GABA levels (topiramate, gabapentin, tiagabine) are not effective in mania, further dissociating these anticonvulsant and psychotropic effects (Table 2).

There are also a variety of psychiatric illness–related variables that are pertinent to the interpretation of which drug actions are important to their psychotropic profile. That is, a general strategy has been to search for common mechanisms among the mood-stabilizing drugs that appear to exert both antimanic and antidepressant properties and assume that these should be in common with lithium carbonate (5,6). However, while this proposition has some theoretical merit, the issue of subtypes of responsive patients makes it suspect.

Lithium, carbamazepine, and valproate do share the very general psychotropic profile of better antimanic than antidepressant effects, both acutely and, perhaps to a lesser extent, in prophylaxis (7–9). However, considerable evidence suggests that individual patients are differentially responsive to one but not to

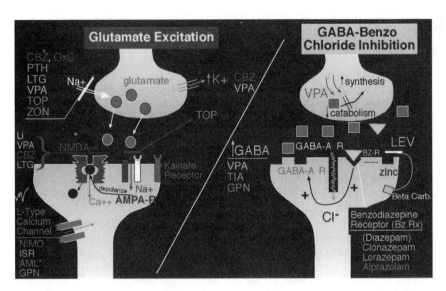

FIGURE 1 Mechanisms of anticonvulsant action. *Abbreviations*: CBZ, carbamazepine; OXC, oxcarbazepine; LTG, lamotrigine; VPA, valproic acid; NMDA, N-methyl-D-aspartate; AMPA, α-amino-3-hydroxy-5-methyl-4-isoxazole proprionic acid; GABA, gamma-aminobutyric acid; PTH, phenytoin; TOP, topiramate; ZON, zonisamide; GPN, gabapentin; TIA, tiagabine; LEV, levetiracetam; NIMO, nimodipine; ISR, isradipine; AML, amlodipine.

another of these drugs (10). For example, lithium-responsive patients are more likely to have classic euphoric manic episodes with discrete well intervals and a lack of anxiety and substance abuse comorbidity, as well as a positive family history for bipolar illness in first-degree relatives (11–13). In contrast, carbamazepine responders appear more likely to be bipolar II, atypical patients with substance abuse comorbidity, schizoaffective presentations, and rapid cycling patterns in the context of a negative family history of bipolar illness in first-degree relatives (13). Valproate responders are characterized by either euphoric or dysphoric mania in contrast to lithium's much greater degree of effectiveness in those with the euphoric compared with dysphoric subtype (14). These differential patient response characteristics suggest that in spite of some common mechanisms, each of these drugs may have biophysical effects that are sufficiently different (Table 2) to account for the differences in profiles of the subtypes of responsive patients.

This caveat is all the more important with respect to lamotrigine, which appears to have effects in the prevention of depressive episodes, and to a lesser extent, manic or mixed episodes. In addition, while several studies have suggested acute antidepressant efficacy (9,15–18), lamotrigine does not possess acute antimanic efficacy. Together, this differential profile of lamotrigine compared with that of lithium, carbamazepine, and valproate further implicates differential mechanisms of action. This conclusion is further supported by the preliminary clinical profiles of patients likely to respond to lamotrigine monotherapy (19–21). Lamotrigine-responsive patients appear more likely to have a positive family history of anxiety disorders in first-degree relatives as well as a personal history of anxiety comorbidity. They are also more likely to have more continuous cyclic courses of illness, as opposed to discrete episodes for lithium.

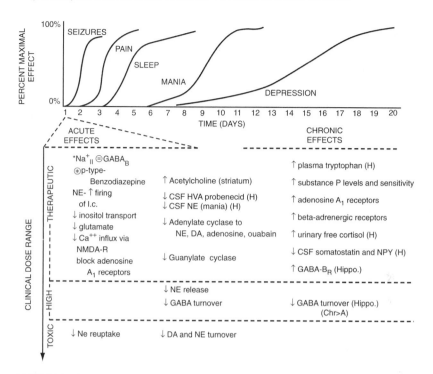

FIGURE 2 Schematic of comparative time course of clinical and biochemical effects of carbamazepine. *Abbreviations*: GABA, gamma-aminobutyric acid; NMDA, *N*-methyl-D-aspartate; HVA, homovanillic acid; NE, norepinephrine (noradrenaline); DA, dopamine; NPY, neuropeptide Y.

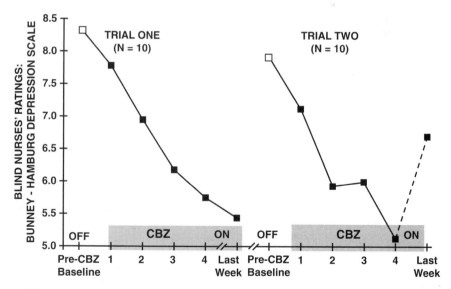

FIGURE 3 Confirmation of antidepressant response to CBZ in off-on-off-on design. *Abbreviation*: CBZ, carbamazepine.

TABLE 1 Spectrum of Psychotropic Action of Anticonvulsants

	Acute Efficacy			Prophylaxis		
	Mania	Depression	Anxiety	Mania	Depression	Other Effects
VPA	+++	++	+++	+++	+++	Migraine, panic, alcohol abstinence (PTSD)
CBZ	+++	++	++	++	+++	Paroxysmal pain syndrome, alcohol withdrawal, (PTSD)
OXC	(+++)	?	?	(++)	(++)	
LTG	0	+++	++	+	+++	(PTSD)
ZNS	(++)	(++)	?	?	?	Bulimia, overweight
PHT	(+++)	(++)	?	?	?	(Pain)
TPM	0	(+)	(+)	?	?	PTSD, bulimia, alcohol and cocaine abstinence, overweight, migraine
GPN	0,−	(+)	+++	(+)	(+)	Panic, social phobia, pain syndromes, alcohol withdrawal
PGN	(0)	(+)	+++	?	?	Panic, social phobia, pain syndromes
TIA	0	(±)	(+)	?	?	[a]May cause new onset seizures
LEV	(+)	(±)	(+)	?	?	
PB	(±)	(±)	+	0	0	(I.V.) anticatatonic effects
BZ	+	+	+	+	+	
FBM	?	?	?	?	?	Refractory seizures, overweight

[a]Adverse effect caution.
Abbreviations: PTSD, posttraumatic stress disorder; VPA, valproic acid; CBZ, carbamazepine; LTG, lamotrigine; OXC, oxcarbazepine; ZNS, zonisamide; PHT, phenytoin; TPM, topiramate; GPN, gabapentin; PGN, pregabalin; TIA, tiagabine; LEV, levetiracetam; PB, phenobarbital; BZ, benzodiazepine; FBM, felbamate.
+++, highly effective, placebo controlled data; ++, effective, substantial literature; +, likely effective; ±, possibly effective; (), ambiguous result; 0, no effect; −, worse.

Such distinctions are likely to be mechanistically relevant. For example, Du et al. (22) found that lamotrigine and riluzole, which are predominately antidepressant, enhanced surface expression of α-amino-3-hydroxy-5-methylisoxazole-4-propionic acid (AMPA) GluR1 and GluR2 receptors in cultured hippocampal neurons. Conversely, the predominately antimanic drug, valproate, significantly reduced expression of GluR1 and GluR2 subunits. Such divergent actions may ultimately be useful in the targeting and development of novel drugs with phase-selective effects.

Perhaps the most serious complicating factor is the lack of suitable animal models of manic-depressive illness in particular and only very cumbersome models for examining antidepressant actions. This contrasts with the situation in the epilepsies where a wide range of readily available animal models have been delineated for different seizure subtypes, further implying differences in mechanisms of action. Until this deficiency is ameliorated, it is highly likely that we will have to remain satisfied with only rough inferences about potential mechanisms of action related to psychotropic effects.

Lastly, a caveat about lithium's potential mechanisms of action would appear appropriate in this regard. It had been widely assumed that understanding lithium's mechanisms of action in manic-depressive illness would rapidly be converted to a better understanding of the pathophysiology of the disorder. This has not happened and, instead, lithium has been found to have a panoply of biochemical effects, none of which has been definitely linked to its psychotropic properties. It is of historical interest that lithium's actions in manic-depressive illness were first assumed to reside at the level of ion channels; then on neurotransmitter release and reuptake mechanisms presynaptically; later at postsynaptic

TABLE 2 Mechanism of Action of Anticonvulsants

	GABA levels	GABA$_A$R (indirect)	↓Na$^+$	Voltage-gated Ca^{2+} T	N	P	L	NMDA Ca^{2+}	Other mechanisms
VPA	↑		+	T			✓	→	↑ Inositol monophosphase; ↑ GABA synthesis and ↓ catabolism; ↑ K efflux; ↓ folate; ↑GABA$_B$R$_{(hippo)}$; ↑Bcl-2; ↓ histone deacetylase; ↓ aspartate; ↑ Homocysteine
CBZ			++				✓?	(↓)	↑ Striatal choline; ↑5HT$_{hippo}$; ↓NE release; ↑ AVP; ↑Sub P; ↓ SRIF; ↓ DA T.O.; ↓ α4 subunit muscarinic Ach-R; ↑ K efflux; ↑ GABA$_B$ R $_{(hippo)}$, ↓ Adenosine A$_1$R; GABA$_A$Rα_1 ↓ Histone deacetylase; ↑ BDNF; ↓AA T.O.
OXC		++	++		N,	P			↑ K efflux
LTG	(↑)26%	(↓)	++		N,	P			Amygdala slice,↓ glutamate and ↓ GABA; ↑ K efflux (weak ↓ folate)
ZNS	↑	↑	++	T		(P/Q)	L	(↓)	↓↓ CA (carbonic anhydrase inhibition), ↑,↓ DA and 5HT T.O., free radical scavenger; ↑glutamate, and ↓ GABA transporters
PHT	↑	↑	++	(T)			✓		↓ SRIF
TPM	↑	↑	++				↓R		↓↓ CA; ↓ AMPA/Kainate R; binds GluR$_5$ subunit K$_R$
GPN^a	↑	↑	+				(L)		↓ Strychnine insensitive glycine receptors; ↓ glutamate; ↓L-amino acid transporter; α$_2$ δ subunit of L-type Ca^{2+} channel
PGN^b	↑	↑					(L)		↓α$_2$ δ subunit of L-type Ca^{2+} calcium channel
TIA	↑	↑							GABA reuptake inhibitor
LEV		↑			N,	(P/Q)	✓		↓ Zn^{2+} and βcarboline negative modulation of GABA$_A$R; own CNS binding site (SV2-A); ↓ Delayed K$^+$ rectifier
PB		↑ duration open time		+					
BZ		↑ frequency open time		+					
FBM	↑	↑		++			✓	↓↓	Glycine; ↓ NR-1A and ↓ NR-2B subunits of NMDAR

Note: ✓ indicates VACC high voltage activated calcium channel.
a and b Act at α2 δ subunit of L-type calcium channel.

Abbreviations: GABA, gamma-aminobutyric acid; AMPA, α-amino-3-hydroxy-5-methylisoxazole-4-propionic acid; BDNF, brain-derived neurotrophic factor; T.O., turnover; VPA, valproic acid; CBZ, carbamazepine; LTG, lamotrigine; OXC, oxcarbazepine; ZNS, zonisamide; PHT, phenytoin; TPM, topiramate; GPN, gabapentin; TIA, tiagabine; LEV, levetiracetam; PB, phenobarbital; BZ, benzodiazepine; FBM, felbamate; DA, dopamine; AA, arachidonic acid; NR, NMDA receptor. [Types of calcium channels: T, transient; N, neither nor; P, purkinje cell; L, long lasting] receptors, second messengers, protein kinases, transcription factors; and ultimately at a variety of effects on gene expression, with most recent interest in its potential neurotrophic and neuroprotective effects.

Thus, candidate mechanisms for lithium's psychotropic actions have generally followed our increasingly detailed understanding of synaptic and intracellular transduction mechanisms and those of gene expression, but even this sequence has not necessarily propelled us to a more definitive relationship of a specific mechanism to a specific psychotropic effect. It therefore would appear prudent to be similarly cautious in our assumptions about what precise mechanisms underlie the psychotropic actions of the AEDs. We should continue to examine potential candidate mechanisms as important for clinical hypothesis testing (5), but should remain skeptical that we have as yet definitely identified the critical actions of any single drug.

PRESUMPTIVE ANTICONVULSANT MECHANISMS

As outlined in Table 2, among the AEDs there are a series of actions that appear to be pertinent for many members of a given subclass. Thus, many AEDs are blockers of type II bratrachotoxin-sensitive sodium channels. This property is thought to be related to their effects on complex partial and major motor seizures. Mishory and colleagues (23) have postulated that it is this set of actions of the AEDs that most likely underlies their antimanic efficacy. However, weighing against this proposition are the findings that lamotrigine and topiramate are sodium channel blockers but have no efficacy in mania.

A series of AEDs enhance chloride influx directly or indirectly via their effects on GABA$_A$ or benzodiazepine receptors. The high potency benzodiazepines such as clonazepam, lorazepam, and alprazolam are clearly anticonvulsant moieties, but the antimanic effects of the first two compounds remain somewhat ambiguous, and alprazolam can induce mania in isolated cases as opposed to treating or preventing it (24).

Drugs that exert major actions on GABA metabolism, brain GABA levels, or GABA$_A$ receptors directly are not necessarily antimanic. It had been hoped that since valproate increases brain GABA levels in animals and humans, enhances GABA synthesis, and decreases GABA breakdown, other GABA-active drugs might share its excellent profile in acute mania. This has not proven to be the case. Gabapentin does not have acute antimanic efficacy over placebo when used as an adjunct to lithium and/or valproate (25) or when used in high-dose monotherapy in treatment-refractory (predominantly bipolar) affectively ill patients (16,17).

Tiagabine is a relatively selective reuptake inhibitor of GABA that enhances intrasynaptic levels of GABA, and also increases brain GABA levels in animals and humans. Not only does it not appear to have acute antimanic efficacy, but, paradoxically, several psychiatric patients without a history of seizure disorders experienced seizures on this drug (26,27).

Convergent with this theme are the ambiguous antimanic effects of levetiracetam, which is thought to enhance the GABA/benzodiazepine receptor chloride ionophore indirectly (28). At this site, it blocks the actions of zinc and β carboline, which are endogenous negative modulators, thus indirectly potentiating actions at this ionophore. However, levetiracetam also has its own binding site in brain, which has recently been identified as the synaptic vesicle protein 2A component of the calcium-sensitive release mechanisms closely linked to synaptophysin or synaptotagmin. This mechanism could account for the drug's somewhat mysterious anticonvulsant properties where it fails to exert efficacy in standard models for grand mal and petit mal seizures, such as maximal electroshock and pentylentetrazol seizures, respectively (29–31).

Interestingly, levetiracetam, in concert with valproate and the high potency benzodiazepines, blocks both the development and fully expressed phases of amygdala-kindled seizures (Fig. 4). In contrast, carbamazepine, lamotrigine, and

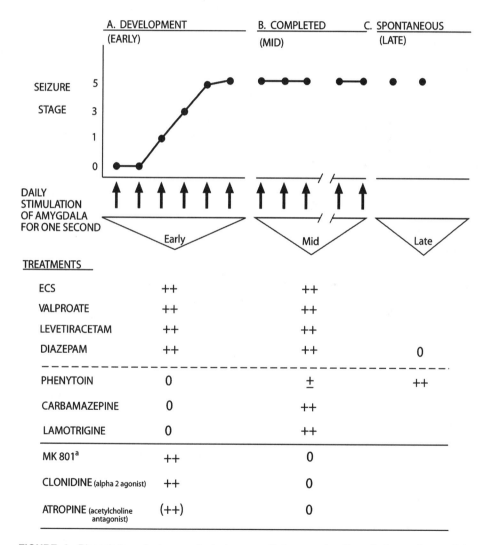

FIGURE 4 Dissociation of pharmacological responsivity as a function of phase of amygdala kindling evolution. [a]indicates glutamate NMDA R antagonist. *Abbreviations*: NMDA, *N*-methyl-D-aspartate; ++, highly effective, ±, ambiguous; 0, not effective; (), inconsistent data.

phenytoin do not block the early development phase and are only effective on completed or full-blown kindled seizures (32). Given its so far ambiguous psychotropic profile and the indirect enhancement of benzodiazepine GABA receptors, it would appear that further exploration of levetiracetam's potential antianxiety effects would be warranted even in the absence of a clear-cut demonstration of its antimanic efficacy.

Zonisamide has not been adequately tested for its acute antimanic efficacy in controlled clinical trials, but open studies suggest its promising effects in acute mania and a potentially useful side-effect profile regarding weight loss (33,34). Not only does it share this latter property with topiramate, but both drugs are also carbonic anhydrase inhibitors, which is thought to relate to their approximately 1% incidence of renal calculi, and dysaesthesias in a larger percentage of patients.

CONVERGENT MECHANISMS OF LITHIUM AND THE ANTICONVULSANT MOOD STABILIZERS, CARBAMAZEPINE AND VALPROATE

If one examines common mechanisms attributable to all three drugs (lithium, carbamazepine, and valproate) that are more effective in acute mania than in depression, one recognizes a series of potential candidates for their psychotropic effects (Table 3). These include: the ability to reduce dopamine turnover (35); to increase GABA$_B$ receptors in the hippocampus upon chronic, but not acute, administration (36); to acutely block the inositol transporter (37); and to moderately inhibit calcium influx through the NMDA receptor (38). It is of interest that this last mechanism is also shared by lamotrigine.

TABLE 3A Common Actions of Mood Stabilizers

	Li	VPA	CBZ	LTG
Common to Li and ACs				
↓ Inositol transport	+	+	+	?
↑ GABA$_B$R$_{hippo}$	+	+	+	?
↓ DA turnover	+	+	+	?
↓ Phospholipase A$_2$ and AA cascade	+	+	+	?
↓ Ca^{2+} influx via NMDA R	+	+	+	?
↑ BDNF	+	+	+	?
stroke neuroprotection	+	+	+	+
↓ GSK-3β	+	+	+	?
Common to two				
↓ PKC	+	+		
↑Bcl-2	+	+		
↓ β catenin	+	+		
↓ ras-erk-pathway	+	+		
↑ Akt	+	+		
↑ AP-1	+	+		
Block C-Amp	+		+	
↑ Substance P (striatum)	+		+	

Abbreviations: NMDA, *N*-methyl-D-aspartate, BDNF, brain-derived neurotrophic factor; GABA, gamma-aminobutyric acid; AMPA; VPA, valproic acid; CBZ, carbamazepine; LTG, lamotrigine; DA dopamine; AA, arachidonic acid; PKC, protein kinase C; +, positive effect; −, no effect; ↑, increase; ↓, decrease; ( ), ambiguous data.

TABLE 3B Common Actions of Anticonvulsant Mood Stabilizers

	Li	VPA	CBZ	LTG
Block Na⁺ influx		(+)	+	+
↑ K⁺ efflux		+	+	+
↓ Histone deacetylase		+	+	

Abbreviations: Li, lithium, VPA, valproic acid; CBZ, carbamazepine; LTG, lamotrigine.

TABLE 3C Divergent Actions of Mood Stabilizers

	Li	VPA	CBZ	LTG
Inositol monophosphotase	↓	↑	–	?
Absence seizures	–	↓	↑	↓
GABA levels	( )	↑	–	(↑)₂₆%
AMPA receptor subunits Glu R1 and R2[a]		↓		↑

[a]From Ref. 22
Abbreviations: GABA, gamma-aminobutyric acid; Li, lithium, VPA, valproic acid; CBZ, carbamazepine; LTG, lamotrigine.

TABLE 3D Unique Effects of Mood Stabilizers

Lithium	CBZ	VPA	LTG
↑ NAA[a]	↓ SRIF[a]	↑ ER stress protein	↓ GABA release
↑ Grey Matter[a]	↓ choline (striatum)	GRP 78 & 94	
↓ BAX, P53	↓ Adenosine		
pilocarpine	A₁ receptors		
seizures and	↓ p-type Bz R		
↓sprouting	↓ Ne β R		
↓ CAMK-IV	↑ 5HT_hippo.		
↓ CAMK-II	α4subunit Ach R		
	(↑ GRP78) ±		

[a] in patients.
Abbreviations: NAA, *N*-acetylaspartate; GABA, gamma-aminobutyric acid; VPA, valproic acid; CBZ, carbamazepine; LTG, lamotrigine; ER, estrogen receptor.

The examination of the comparative effects of lithium and valproate are particularly intriguing from the perspective of potential neurotrophic and neuroprotective effects (Table 4, Fig. 5). Both of these agents increase brain-derived neurotrophic factor (BDNF) and Bcl-2 (39); lithium also decreases cell death factors Bax and p53 (40). Both seem to activate many elements of the mitogen-activated protein (MAP) kinase pathway (41), but valproate has the additional effects of being a histone deacetylase inhibitor (42). It is of interest that recently carbamazepine has been shown to exert this same activity (43), and this action could account for more readily available changes in gene expression based on altered DNA conformation.

Lithium and carbamazepine also have interesting shared mechanisms, including the ability to inhibit noradrenergic-stimulated adenylate cyclase and to increase substance P levels and substance P receptor sensitivity in the striatum and nucleus accumbens (NAcc).

Carbamazepine has unique effects in decreasing somatostatin levels in cerebrospinal fluid (CSF) and in acting as an indirect potentiator of vasopressin receptors. Additionally, it inhibits the release of corticotropin-releasing hormone (CRH)

TABLE 4 Neurotropic and Protective Effects of Psychotropic Drugs

	Lithium	Valproate	Antidepressants	Electro convulsive therapy	Atypical antipsychotic
In vitro					
Sprouting	↑	↑		↑	
Neurogenesis	↑		↑	↑	
BDNF	↑	↑	↑	↑	
Prevention of ↓ BDNF with stress			+a	+	+
↑ Bcl-2	↑	↑		↑	
Gliogenesis	↑	↑		↑	↓
In vivo NAA (neuronal integrity)					
Pfc (H)	↑	–			
Temporal lobe (H)	↑	↑			
Gray matter (MRI) Pfc and B25 (H)	↑				
Stroke neuroprotection	↑b/a	↑b/a		(↑)	
Hippocampal volume protection (in depressed patients) (H)			↑		

[a]Pramipexole.
Abbreviations: H, humans; b/a, before and after insult; BDNF, brain-derived neurotrophic factor; NAA, N-acetylaspartate.

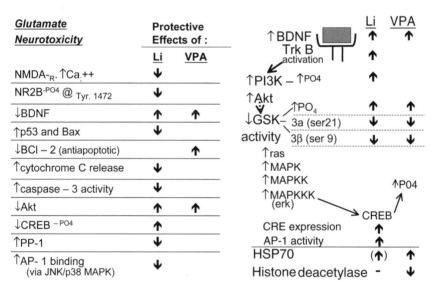

FIGURE 5 Lithium and valproate block glutamate toxicity and enhance growth factors. *Abbreviations*: VPA, valproic acid; NMDA, N-methyl-D-aspartate; BDNF, brain-derived neurotrophic factor. *Source*: From refs. 39–41.

from the hypothalamus and is uniquely able to increase 24-hour urinary free cortisol levels and produce false-positive escape from dexamethasone suppression.

Carbamazepine and valproate share the ability to enhance potassium channel–mediated efflux, and as noted previously, block batrachotoxin type II sodium channels.

Lithium is an inositol 1-monophosphate inhibitor and is capable of decreasing membrane inositol and inhibiting phosphoinositol turnover. Valproate is without effect on this system, and carbamazepine may have opposing effects (44,45), again highlighting potentially very different mechanisms of these drugs which could, in part, account for their differential profiles of clinical efficacy within individual patients.

Clinical Implications of the Mechanistic Differences Among the Antiepileptics

Since lamotrigine and carbamazepine share the ability to potently inhibit sodium influx through the type II channel, it is apparent that some other mechanism of action of lamotrigine must underlie its profile of being a better antidepressant than antimanic agent. In addition to blocking glutamate release (via the sodium channel blockade similar to that of carbamazepine), lamotrigine has the ability to inhibit GABA release. It also has effects on N- and P-type calcium channels that do not appear to be shared by carbamazepine.

However, if one is considering augmenting lamotrigine with another mood stabilizer, using lithium or valproate with their very different mechanistic profiles would be more worthy of consideration than adding carbamazepine, given the considerable mechanistic overlap between lamotrigine and carbamazepine. If valproate is used with lamotrigine, however, lamotrigine doses should be reduced by one half because valproate can double lamotrigine levels and increase the risk of rash. Nonetheless, when the two are used in combination in refractory seizure disorders, they appear to be particularly well tolerated.

Lithium and valproate are widely used together, but this combination poses increased risk from potentially additive side effects such as gastrointestinal distress, tremor, and weight gain. These are not particularly prominent side effects of carbamazepine or lamotrigine, and avoidance of side effects may provide an alternate rationale to therapeutic mechanistic considerations in the choice of agents.

Since the U.S. Food and Drug Administration (FDA) approval of new drugs is almost exclusively based on placebo-controlled, parallel group study designs which cannot distinguish individually responsive patients from nonresponders (46), there is great underappreciation in the literature that patients respond differentially to the mood stabilizers in general and the AEDs in particular. Each of the AEDs carries an approximately 50% response rate in uncomplicated patients, but unless one examines individual patients on a series of drugs or in an on-off-on fashion, one is not able to ascertain individual patient responsiveness or unique responsiveness to one compound and not another. Using more clinician-friendly longitudinal clinical designs, we have consistently seen that some patients respond to valproate and not to carbamazepine, while others showed good responses to carbamazepine but not to valproate (10).

In the past decade, valproate has surpassed lithium for a larger market share for first treatment of manic patients, but with the recent approval of a long-acting carbamazepine preparation, the clinician may also want to consider carbamazepine as a reasonable option for the patient inadequately responsive or intolerant to other agents. The extended-release capsule is suitable for single h.s. dosing, at least in bipolar illness, although not in those with epilepsy. There are only a few preliminary clinical hints of which patient may respond to which agent, as noted above, so one looks forward to the use of currently available single nucleotide polymorphism (SNP) profiling techniques to more formally and quantitatively help predict individual patient's likelihood of clinical response or severe side effects.

Oxcarbazepine is structurally similar to carbamazepine, differing only by a keto oxygen molecule in the middle ring instead of a double bond between carbon atoms in carbamazepine. It is thought to have a generally similar clinical profile and mechanism of action to carbamazepine, but has been much less well studied. Ambiguities about its range of efficacy are further supported by the negative study of Wagner et al. (47) in child and adolescent mania. The ability of oxcarbazepine to substitute for carbamazepine in psychiatric illness therefore requires further evaluation. It is a less potent inducer of hepatic enzymes, but more likely to cause hyponatremia. It does not have a black box warning for hematological side effects and may be an appropriate drug to explore clinically in those who do not wish to risk these very rare, but serious side effects.

POTENTIAL NEUROTROPHIC AND NEUROPROTECTIVE EFFECTS OF LITHIUM, VALPROATE, AND THE UNIMODAL ANTIDEPRESSANTS

Recent data indicate that all of the antidepressant modalities, as well as the mood stabilizers lithium, carbamazepine, and valproate, are capable of increasing both BDNF and neurogenesis (48,49) (Table 4). For example, Sheline and colleagues (50) found that depressed patients treated with antidepressants more of the time had no evidence of hippocampal atrophy compared with those with less antidepressant treatment. Taken together with preclinical data, these findings suggest that antidepressants may be pertinent to sustaining hippocampal volume in unipolar depressed humans, possibly by enhancing neural production and survival via increasing BDNF (49).

Preliminary evidence also suggests that lithium not only increases N-acetyl aspartate (NAA), a marker of neuronal integrity, but also increases gray matter volume in patients with bipolar disorder (but not in normal controls) (51,52). These findings raise the possibility that enhancing neurogenesis and gliogenesis and changing the ratio of cell survival factors (BDNF and Bcl-2) to cell death factors (Bax and p53) in favor of survival factors could be important to the therapeutic action of these drugs (40).

There is considerable evidence, as summarized in Figure 6, for deficits in prefrontal cortical neuronal and glial elements, biochemistry, and physiology in recurrent mood disorder. The extent to which some of our therapeutic agents could either help reverse these deficits or prevent their progression raises an entirely new perspective about long-term prophylaxis of bipolar illness. It is not only possible that these treatments could help decrease recurrence of both manic and depressive episodes, but they might also reverse or prevent progression of some of the biochemical and physiological alterations associated with the recurrent mood episodes as well as the underlying affective illness.

A number of the pathological findings in both unipolar and bipolar mood disorders have been shown to vary either as a function of illness duration or prior number of episodes (53,54). While it is unclear as to whether greater degrees of abnormalities are causally linked to a more adverse course of illness or whether a more adverse course of illness is etiologically involved in more severe biochemical abnormalities, the findings at least raise the question of whether episode

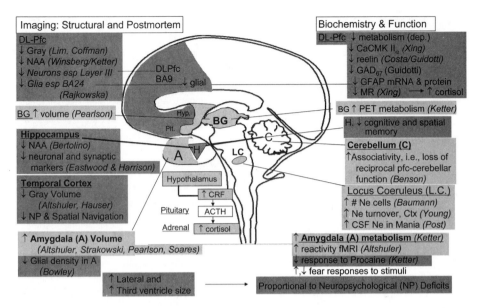

FIGURE 6 Convergence of structural, biochemical, and functional abnormalities in bipolar illness. *Source*: From Ref. 84.

prophylaxis with these agents may also alter the underlying neurobiology of the illness.

The bulk of the literature supports the clinical validity of the sensitization and kindling hypothesis which postulates that having recurrent mood episodes increases the vulnerability to subsequent episodes and to their occurring more autonomously from psychosocial stressors (54–56). This evidence, along with findings that patients with greater numbers of prior episodes and more rapid-cycling forms of the illness are, in general, more refractory to most treatments for bipolar disorder, further raises the urgency of attempting to initiate effective prophylaxis earlier in the course of illness.

At the least, the benefit of acting on this proposition would be a reduction in number of episodes. On the basis of the sensitization and kindling hypothesis and the data alluded to here, the maximal benefit would be to also alter some of the biochemical consequences of illness recurrence, decrease sensitization phenomenon, reduce vulnerability to recurrences, and potentially change the course of illness. This might be associated with not only fewer neurobiological alterations but a less treatment-refractory type of illness. Even if the sensitization and kindling notions of progressive changes associated with recurrent episodes are not entirely validated, the patient and clinician have little to lose and much to gain from earlier and concerted attempts at episode prophylaxis (Table 5).

However, early and sustained prophylactic intervention in bipolar illness is neither readily achieved nor high in the public health consciousness of many physicians and patients in the United States. The lag from illness onset to first treatment averaged 10 years in our large outpatient series (57,58) and was inversely associated with age of onset (59). Moreover, those with the earliest ages of onset

TABLE 5 Testable Clinical Predictions About Therapeutic Approaches to Tolerance Development to be Explored Based on the Preclinical Model

Preclinical study findings in amygdala-kindled seizures	Future studies: Are there parallel findings for clinical tolerance in affective illness?
A. Tolerance to anticonvulsant effects slowed by: higher doses (except with LTG)	A. Would tolerance be slowed by: maximum tolerated doses rather than minimally effective doses
not escalating doses	stable dosing
more efficacious drugs (VPA > CBZ)	valproate compared with carbamazepine
treatments initiated early in course of kindled seizures	early treatment more effective (as observed with lithium)[a]
combination treatment (CBZ + VPA)	combination treatment rather than monotherapy
reducing illness drive (stimulation intensity)	treatment or prevention of comorbidities and concomitant stressors
B. Treatment response in tolerant animals restored by: period of drug discontinuation, then re-exposure	B. Would treatment response be restored by: period of time off-CBZ in tolerant patients (randomized study of discontinuation and re-treatment needed)
agents with different mechanisms of action, i.e., no cross tolerance	anticonvulsant cross tolerances (as summarized in Table 6A) may or may not be predictive of cross tolerances in affective illness

[a]Supported by clinical studies.
Abbreviations: VPA, valproic acid; CBZ, carbamazepine; LTG, lamotrigine.

were at highest risk for an adverse course of bipolar illness, as assessed both retrospectively in the Systematic Treatment Enhancement Program for Bipolar Disorder (STEP-BD) network (60) and prospectively in our collaborative network (53,54). These are the very patients who have the longest time between first symptoms with dysfunction and first treatment for manic or depressive illness.

Indeed, in our subgroup of patients with illness onset prior to age 13 years, the lag to first treatment averaged about 15 years (59). This inverse relationship between age of onset and lag time to first treatment was also found in the epidemiological studies of Kessler and colleagues (61). Together, these data speak to the importance of earlier recognition of the illness and institution of more effective treatment in the hope of altering what can otherwise be a very difficult illness course, including one associated with a relatively high rate of lethality. These data and implications contrast somewhat with those of Baldessarini et al. (62) who found that delay to initiating prophylaxis (with lithium) was not associated with differential outcome. However, their sample was from Italy and Germany where universal health care is available, prophylaxis (rather than acute treatment) was examined, lithium was used in more than 90% of patients, and shorter time to institute prophylaxis was confounded by increased severity of baseline psychopathology. Thus, their (62) findings may not generalize to other populations.

Fortunately, there appears to be increased recognition of early-onset bipolar illness in children and adolescents. Lange and McInnis (63) analyzed the literature on this issue and concluded that there is substantial evidence for both cohort (year of birth) and anticipation (generational) effects. Together, the cohort and anticipation effects convey a greater incidence and earlier age of onset of both unipolar and bipolar illness in each generation since World War I. Given this increasing recognition of childhood-onset bipolar illness, one needs to raise a further caveat about the mechanism of action of AEDs. It is not at all clear whether the same degree of clinical responsivity occurs in children as it does in adults. This could be partially attributable to differences in maturity of various aspects of the developing central nervous system (CNS). Pertinent to this point are the observations that the GABA$_B$ antagonist baclofen is effective as an anticonvulsant in very young animals, but not in older animals, and the considerable evidence for altered GABAergic function across different stages of development (64). In the youngest animals, for example, GABA receptor activity is paradoxically associated with excitation, and only later in development do alterations in GABAergic tone convey their inhibitory properties.

Thus, how the mechanisms of action of GABAergic and other mechanistically acting drugs play out in relationship to efficacy in children remains a further conundrum, and one that requires new reassessment of the efficacy of each drug in children and adolescents to see whether or not it parallels that observed in adults.

Finally, as one moves toward notions of identifying those at highest risk and beginning to intervene very early in the course of illness (secondary prevention), and even prior to illness onset (i.e., primary prevention), one also needs to consider the possibility, on the basis of the striking data evident in the kindling model, that different agents may be effective in different phases of illness evolution and that what works against fully developed episodes may not prevent their initial developmental stages. Carbamazepine, lamotrigine, and phenytoin are potent against fully developed seizures, but ineffective against their development (Fig. 4). By contrast, valproate, diazepam, and levetiracetam are effective in the developmental stage of kindling. Perhaps in the most remarkable dissociation, the high potency benzodiazepines are effective in the early (or developmental) and mid (or completed) stages of kindling, but are not effective in the late, spontaneous seizures associated with kindling (65). Conversely, phenytoin is ineffective in preventing the development of kindling, has mixed effects on fully kindled seizures, but is highly effective in preventing the spontaneous variety. Thus, the psychotropic drugs and their associated mechanistic properties that are associated with prevention of the development of syndromal unipolar and bipolar illness may be different from those that are effective in the mid phases of the illnesses or even, again, in the very latest (or spontaneous) phases, where there appears to be the greatest amount of automaticity and rapid cycling independent of specific psychosocial stressors.

Lastly, one must caution patients and family members that effectiveness of a treatment regimen in the short or intermediate term (e.g., two years) may not guarantee long-term freedom from illness burden, even with excellent compliance. A subset of patients (perhaps from 25% to 35% of those with initially highly treatment-responsive presentations) may begin to show a progression of minor intermittent to more frequent and major breakthrough episodes in a fashion that suggests the development of pharmacodynamic tolerance. This should not be used as a "negative" with patients, but as a "positive" in helping them maintain long-term full or steady-dose prophylaxis, since lowering doses appears to enhance the onset and likelihood of tolerance development (Table 5).

In addition, from a mechanistic perspective, the development of inefficacy through drug tolerance may show cross tolerance to some, but not to other AEDs (32,66) (Table 6). Moreover, it is unknown whether one can directly extrapolate via drug classes and/or mechanisms from AED tolerance to psychotropic tolerance (Table 5,6), but using drugs clinically which do not show cross tolerance in the

TABLE 6A   Cross-Tolerance Patterns in Contingent Anticonvulsant Effects on Amygdala-Kindled Seizures

Drug; tolerance from	Cross tolerance to	No cross tolerance to
CBZ	PK11195 CBZ-10,11-epoxide Valproate[a]	Clonazepam Diazepam Phenytoin LEV[b]
LTG	CBZ	Valproate MK801a Gabapentin[c]
LEV	CBZ[a]	

[a]Cross tolerance from CBZ to valproate may occur because of the observed failure to upregulate the $\alpha 4$ subunit of the $GABA_A$ receptor during CBZ tolerance.
[b]Unidirection cross tolerance from LEV to CBZ, not CBZ to LEV.
[c]These drugs slow the development of tolerance to LTG.
Abbreviations: GABA, gamma-aminobutyric acid; CBZ, carbamazepine; LTG, lamotrigine; LEV, levetiracetam.

TABLE 6B   Differential Effects of CBZ and LTG on Anticonvulsant Tolerance Development

	CBZ (15 mg/kg)	LTG (15 mg/kg)
Rapid tolerance to anticonvulsant effects (amygdala kindling)	+++	+++
Cross tolerance	+++	+++
Duration of "time-off" effect (seizures enhance efficacy)	4–5 days	4–5 days
Seizure threshold change with tolerance	Decrease	Increase (possible residual drug effect)
Using high doses	Slows tolerance	Speeds tolerance and are proconvulsant
Alternating high and low doses	?	Slows tolerance
Chronic noncontingent drug dosing	Slows tolerance	?
MK801 on tolerance development	No effect	Slows (NMDA implicated)
Cross tolerance to valproate	Yes	No
Valproate combination	Slows tolerance	?
Gabapentin augmentation (2 hr pretreatment)	?	Slows tolerance
(½ hr pretreatment)	No effect	↓ Stage VI seizures
(Tolerance reversal)	?	+++

Abbreviations: LTG, lamotrigine; CBZ, carbamazepine; NMDA, *N*-methyl-D-aspartate.

kindled seizure model may be a more appropriate first approximation for a given individual than crossing over to a drug with known AED cross tolerance. If this proposition is proven empirically in the clinic, it may be one other reason to consider presumptive mechanisms of action in choice of a therapeutic agent.

Electroconvulsive therapy (ECT) is not only acutely effective in depression and mania, it is also a potent anticonvulsant (67). Recent data, however, indicate that depressive relapses/remissions occur rapidly after the last ECT treatment, at a rate of 4% per day over the first 10 days (68,69). These data suggest that mechanisms induced even by ECT only convey therapeutic effects in the short-term.

TABLE 7 Topiramate: Not Antimanic but Potentially Useful in Comorbidities

Comorbidities	Study (Refs.)
Alcohol use	Johnson et al., 2007; Johnson 2004 (78,79)
Cocaine use	Johnson, 2005 (80)
PTSD	Berlant, 2002; Berlant, 2001; (74,75) Tucker et al., 2007 (85)
Bulimia	McElroy et al., 2007; McElroy et al., 2004 (73,81)
Weight Loss	McElroy et al., 2007 (73)
Depression	McIntyre et al., 2002 (82)
Migraine	Dahlof et al., 2007 (83)
Side effects	
Renal calculi and parasthesia related to carbonic anhydrase inhibition	
Decreased word retrieval/memory probably related to blockage of AMPA receptors	

By contrast, vagal nerve stimulation (VNS) is an adjunctive anticonvulsant modality for refractory epilepsy and appears unique in both seizure disorders and affective illness in that effectiveness increases progressively over the first year of treatment (70,71). Thus, changes occurring over the long-term may be most pertinent to its therapeutic effectiveness. How these (72) interact with the diverse pharmacotherapies with which it is typically administered require further study. While there are ambiguities about the magnitude of VNS effects in both seizure disorders and affective illness, the trend for increasing effectiveness over time, in contrast to ECT and most other long-term treatments in bipolar illness, suggest active effects that are likely not placebo effects.

Bipolar illness is also associated with a multiplicity of comorbid conditions, and some AEDs that lack antimanic or mood-stabilizing effects may nonetheless be helpful in treating a co-occurring syndrome. In this fashion, topiramate shows substantial evidence for decreasing alcohol and cocaine use in those with these primary substance use disorders (Table 7). It is also effective in binge eating disorder and bulimia nervosa (73) and may be helpful in posttraumatic stress disorder (PTSD) (74,75). These actions of the drug may thus be dissociated from those that are required for effective mood stabilization.

Similarly, gabapentin and pregabalin have a range of effects in anxiety syndromes, such as panic disorder and social phobia and are particularly effective in pain syndromes (76,77). Whether these effects are based on their ability to increase brain GABA levels or to inhibit the α_2-δ subunit of the L-type calcium channel requires further investigation.

The therapeutics of bipolar illness have progressed over the past 50 years from just one or two effective agents to an entire range of agents from multiple classes with multiple drugs within each class. We have some preliminary understanding of the mechanisms of action of the AEDs, but much work remains in identifying those crucially related to a given syndrome and to individual clinical responsivity. We look forward to this phase of individualized medicine rapidly becoming realized so that bipolar patients can be more readily treated with the most appropriate therapeutic regimens right from the outset, thus sparing many individuals from the very considerable morbidity and dysfunction associated with the recurrent affective disorders in general, and bipolar illness in particular.

REFERENCES

1. Marangell LB, George MS, Callahan AM, et al. Effects of intrathecal thyrotropin-releasing hormone (protirelin) in refractory depressed patients. Arch Gen Psychiatry 1997; 54:214–222.
2. Szuba MP, Amsterdam JD, Fernando AT III, et al. Rapid antidepressant response after nocturnal TRH administration in patients with bipolar type I and bipolar type II major depression. J Clin Psychopharmacol 2005; 25:325–330.
3. Maeng S, Zarate CA Jr., Du J, et al. Cellular mechanisms underlying the antidepressant effects of ketamine: role of alpha-amino-3-hydroxy-5-methylsoxazole-4-propionic acid receptors. Biol Psychiatry 2008; 63(4):349–352.
4. Preskorn SD, Baker B, Omo K, et al. A placebo- controlled trial of the NR2B specific NMDA antagonist CP-101, 606 plus paroxetine for treatment resistant depression. 160th Annual Meeting of the American Psychiatric Association, San Diego, CA, 2007 (New Research Abstracts No.362).
5. Manji HK, Duman RS. Impairments of neuroplasticity and cellular resilience in severe mood disorders: implications for the development of novel therapeutics. Psychopharmacol Bull 2001; 35:5–49.
6. Zarate CA Jr., Singh JB, Carlson PJ, et al Efficacy of a protein kinase C inhibitor (tamoxifen) in the treatment of acute mania: a pilot study. Bipolar Disord 2007; 9:561–570.
7. Post RM, Speer AM, Obrocea, GV, et al Acute and prophylactic effects of anti-convulsants in bipolar depression. Clin Neurosci Res 2002; 2:228–251.
8. Geddes JR, Burgess H, Hawton K, et al. Long-term lithium treatment therapy for bipolar disorder: systemic review and meta-analysis of randomized controlled trials. Am J Psychiatry 2004; 161(2): 217–22.
9. Cipriani A, Smith K, Burgess S, et al. Lithium versus antidepressants in the long-term treatment of unipolar affective disorder. Cochrane Database Syst Rev 2006; 168(4):CD003492.
10. Post RM, Berrettini W, Uhde TW, et al. Selective response to the anticonvulsant carbamazepine in manic–depressive illness: a case study. J Clin Psychopharmacol 1984; 4: 178–185.
11. Greil W, Kleindienst N. Lithium versus carbamazepine in the maintenance treatment of bipolar II disorder and bipolar disorder not otherwise specified. Int Clin Psychopharmacol 1999; 14(5):283–285.
12. Greil W, Kleindienst N. The comparative prophylactic efficacy of lithium and carbamazepine in patients with bipolar I disorder. Int Clin Psychopharmacol 1999; 14(5):277–281.
13. Greil W, Kleindienst N, Erazo N, et al. Differential response to lithium and carbamazepine in the prophylaxis of bipolar disorder. J Clin Psychopharmacol 1998; 18:455–460.
14. Bowden CL. Predictors of response to divalproex and lithium. J Clin Psychiatry 1995; 56(suppl 3):25–30.
15. Calabrese JR, Fatemi SH, Woyshville MJ. Antidepressant effects of lamotrigine in rapid cycling bipolar disorder. Am J Psychiatry 1996; 153:236.
16. Frye MA, Ketter TA, Kimbrell TA, et al. A placebo-controlled study of lamotrigine and gabapentin monotherapy in refractory mood disorders. J Clin Psychopharmacol 2000; 20:607–614.
17. Obrocea GV, Dunn RM, Frye MA, et al. Clinical predictors of response to lamotrigine and gabapentin monotherapy in refractory affective disorders. Biol Psychiatry 2002; 51: 253–260.
18. van der Loos ML, Kolling P, Knoppert-van der Klein EA et al. Lamotrigine as add-on to lithium in bipolar depression, 160th Annual Meeting American Psychiatric Association, San Diego, CA, New Research Abstract No.286, p.20.
19. Passmore MJ, Garnham J, Duffy A, et al. Phenotypic spectra of bipolar disorder in responders to lithium versus lamotrigine. Bipolar Disord 2003; 5:110–114.
20. Alda M. The phenotypic spectra of bipolar disorder. Eur Neuropsychopharmacol 2004; 14(suppl 2): S94–S99.
21. Grof P. Selecting effective long-term treatment for bipolar patients: monotherapy and combinations. J Clin Psychiatry 2003; 64(suppl 5):53–61.
22. Du J, Suzuki K, Wei Y, et al. The anticonvulsants lamotrigine, riluzole, and valproate differentially regulate AMPA receptor membrane localization: relationship to clinical effects in mood disorders. Neuropsychopharmacology 2007; 32:793–802.

23. Mishory A, Yaroslavsky Y, Bersudsky Y, et al. Phenytoin as an antimanic anticonvulsant: a controlled study. Am J Psychiatry 2000; 157:463–465.
24. Post RM, Speer AM. A brief history of anticonvulsant use in affective disorders. In: Trimble MR, Schmitz B, eds. Seizures, Affective Disorders and Anticonvulsant Drugs. Surrey, UK: Clarius Press, 2002:53–81.
25. Pande AC, Crockatt JG, Janney CA, et al. Gabapentin in bipolar disorder: a placebo-controlled trial of adjunctive therapy. Gabapentin Bipolar Disorder Study Group. Bipolar Disord 2000; 2(3 pt 2):249–255.
26. Grunze H, Erfurth A, Marcuse A, et al. Tiagabine appears not to be efficacious in the treatment of acute mania. J Clin Psychiatry 1999; 60:759–762.
27. Suppes T, Chisholm KA, Dhavale D, et al. Tiagabine in treatment-refractory bipolar disorder: a clinical case series. Bipolar Disord 2002; 4:283–289.
28. Post RM, Altshuler LL, Frye MA, et al. Preliminary observations on the effectiveness of levetiracetam in the open adjunctive treatment of refractory bipolar disorder. J Clin Psychiatry 2005; 66:370–374.
29. Rigo JM, Hans G, Nguyen L, et al. The anti-epileptic drug levetiracetam reverses the inhibition by negative allosteric modulators of neuronal GABA- and glycine-gated currents. Br J Pharmacol 2002; 136:659–672.
30. Klitgaard H. Levetiracetam: the preclinical profile of a new class of antiepileptic drugs? Epilepsia 2001; 4:13–18.
31. Klitgaard H, Matagne A, Gobert J, et al. Evidence for a unique profile of levetiracetam in rodent models of seizures and epilepsy. Eur J Pharmacol 1998; 353(2–3):191–206.
32. Post RM. Animal models of mood disorders: kindling as a model of affective illness progression. In: Schachter S, Holmes G, Kasteleijn-Nolst Trenité D, eds. Behavioral Aspects of Epilepsy: Principles and Practice. New York, NY: Demos Medical Publishing, 2008.
33. McElroy SL, Suppes T, Keck PE Jr., et al. Open-label adjunctive zonisamide in the treatment of bipolar disorders: a prospective trial. J Clin Psychiatry 2005; 66(5):617–624.
34. McElroy SL, Kotwal R, Guerdjikova AI, et al. Zonisamide in the treatment of binge eating disorder with obesity: a randomized controlled trial. J Clin Psychiatry 2006; 67(12):1897–1906.
35. Maitre M, Mandel P. [Properties allowing the attribution to gamma-hydroxybutyrate the quality of neurotransmitter in the central nervous system] C R Acad Sci III 1984; 298(12):341–345.
36. Motohashi N, Ikawa K, Kariya T. GABA_B receptors are up-regulated by chronic treatment with lithium or carbamazepine: GABA hypothesis of affective disorders. Eur J Pharmacol 1989; 166:95–99.
37. van Calker D, Belmaker RH. The high affinity inositol transport system–implications for the pathophysiology and treatment of bipolar disorder. Bipolar Disord 2000; 2(2):102–107.
38. Hough CJ, Irwin RP, Gao XM, et al. Carbamazepine inhibition of N-methyl-D-aspartate-evoked calcium influx in rat cerebellar granule cells. J Pharmacol Exp Ther 1996; 276(1):143–149.
39. Manji HK, Moore GJ, Rajkowska G, et al. Neuroplasticity and cellular resilience in mood disorders. Mol Psychiatry 2000; 5(6):578–593.
40. Chuang DM, Chen RW, Chalecka-Franaszek E, et al. Neuroprotective effects of lithium in cultured cells and animal models of diseases. Bipolar Disord 2007; 4(2):129–136.
41. Einat H, Yuan P, Gould TD, et al. The role of the extracellular signal-regulated kinase signaling pathway in mood modulation. J Neurosci 2003; 13; 23(19):7311–7316.
42. Chen PS, Wang CC, Bortner CD, et al. Valproic acid and other histone deacetylase inhibitors induce microglial apoptosis and attenuate lipopolysaccharide-induced dopaminergic neurotoxicity. Neuroscience 2007; 149(1):203–212.
43. Beutler AS, Li S, Nicol R, et al. Carbamazepine is an inhibitor of histone deacetylases. Life Sci 2005; 76(26):3107–3115.
44. Sherman WR, Leavitt AL, Honchar MP, et al. Evidence that lithium alters phosphoinositide metabolism: chronic administration elevates primarily D-myo-inositol-1-phosphate in cerebral cortex of the rat. J Neurochem 1981; 36:1947–1951.

45. Post RM, Weiss SRB, Clark M, et al. Lithium, carbamazepine and valproate in affective illness. In Manji HK, Bowden CL, Belmaker RH, eds. Bipolar Medications: Mechanisms of Action. Washington, DC: Am Psychiatric Press, Inc., 2000:219–248.
46. Post RM, Luckenbaugh DA. Unique design issues in clinical trials of patients with bipolar affective disorder. J Psychiatr Res 2003; 37(1):61–73 (review).
47. Wagner KD, Kowatch RA, Emslie GJ, et al. A double-blind, randomized, placebo-controlled trial of oxcarbazepine in the treatment of bipolar disorder in children and adolescents. Am J Psychiatry 2006; 163(7):1179–1186.
48. Duman RS, Monteggia LM. A neurotrophic model for stress-related mood disorders. Biol Psychiatry 2006; 59(12):1116–1127.
49. Post RM. Role of BDNF in bipolar and unipolar disorder: clinical and theoretical implications. J Psychiatr Res 2007; 41(12):979–990.
50. Sheline YI, Wang PW, Gado MH, et al. Hippocampal atrophy in recurrent major depression. Proc Natl Acad Sci U S A 1996; 93(9):3908–3913.
51. Moore GJ, Bebchuk JM, Wilds IB, et al. Lithium-induced increase in human brain grey matter. Lancet 2000; 356:1241–1242.
52. Bearden CE, Thompson PM, Dalwani M, et al. Reply: lithium and Increased Cortical Gray Matter-More Tissue or More Water? Biol Psychiatry 2008; 63(3):E19.
53. Post RM, Denicoff KD, Leverich GS, et al. Morbidity in 258 bipolar outpatients followed for one year with daily prospective ratings on the NIMH-Life Chart Method. J Clin Psychiatry 2003; 64:680–690.
54. Post RM. Kindling and sensitization as models for affective episode recurrence, cyclicity, and tolerance phenomena. Neurosci Biobehav Rev 2007; 31(6):858–873.
55. Post RM. Transduction of psychosocial stress into the neurobiology of recurrent affective disorder. Am J Psychiatry 1992; 149: 999–1010.
56. Post RM, Leverich GS. The role of psychosocial stress in the onset and progression of bipolar disorder and its comorbidities: the need for earlier and alternative modes of therapeutic intervention. Dev Psychopathol 2006; 18:1181–1211.
57. Leverich GS, McElroy SL, Suppes T, et al. Early physical and sexual abuse associated with an adverse course of bipolar illness. Biol Psychiatry 2002; 51(4):288–297.
58. Leverich GS, Altshuler LL, Frye MA, et al. Factors associated with suicide attempts in 648 patients with bipolar disorder in the Stanley Foundation Bipolar Network. J Clin Psychiatry 2003; 64(5):506–515.
59. Leverich GS, Post RM, Keck PE Jr., et al. The poor prognosis of childhood-onset bipolar disorder. J Pediatr 2007; 150: 485–490.
60. Perlis RH, Miyahara S, Marangell LB, et al. Long-Term implications of early onset in bipolar disorder: data from the first 1000 participants in the systematic treatment enhancement program for bipolar disorder (STEP-BD). Biol Psychiatry 2004; 55(9):875–881.
61. Kessler RC, Berglund P, Demler O, et al. Lifetime prevalence and age-of-onset distributions of DSM-IV disorders in the National Comorbidity Survey Replication. Arch Gen Psychiatry 2005; 62(6):593–602.
62. Baldessarini RJ, Tondo L, Baethge CJ, et al. Effects of treatment latency on response to maintenance treatment in manic-depressive disorders. Bipolar Disord 2007; 9(4): 386–393.
63. Lange KJ, McInnis MG. Studies of anticipation in bipolar affective disorder. CNS Spectr 2002; 7(3):196–202.
64. Velísek L, Velíshková J, Ptachewich Y, et al. Age-dependent effects of gamma-aminobutyric acid agents on flurothyl seizures. Epilepsia 1995; 36(7): 636–643.
65. Pinel JP. Kindling-induced experimental epilepsy in rats: cortical stimulation. Exp Neurol 1981; 72(3):559–569.
66. Weiss SR, Clark M, Rosen JB, et al. Contingent tolerance to the anticonvulsant effects of carbamazepine: relationship to loss of endogenous adaptive mechanisms. Brain Res Rev 1995; 20:305–325.
67. Post R, Uhde T, Kramlinger K, et al. Carbamazepine treatment of mania: clinical and biochemical aspects. Clin Neuropharmacol 1986; 4:547–549.
68. Prudic J, Olfson M, Marcus SC, et al. Effectiveness of electroconvulsive therapy in community settings. Biol Psychiatry 2004; 55(3):301–312.

69. Sackeim HA, Prudic J, Olfson M. Response to Drs Abrams and Kellner: the cognitive effects of ECT in community settings. J ECT 2007; 23(2):65–67.
70. Rush AJ, Sackeim HA, Marangell LB, et al. Effects of 12 months of vagus nerve stimulation in treatment-resistant depression: a naturalistic study. Biol Psychiatry 2005; 58(5): 355–363.
71. Rush AJ, Marangell LB, Sackeim HA, et al. Vagus nerve stimulation for treatment-resistant depression: a randomized, controlled acute phase trial. Biol Psychiatry 2005; 58(5):347–354.
72. Nemeroff CB, Mayberg HS, Krahl SE, et al. VNS therapy in treatment-resistant depression: clinical evidence and putative neurobiological mechanisms. Neuropsychopharmacology 2006; 31(7):1345–1355.
73. McElroy SL, Hudson JI, Capece JA, et al. Topiramate for the treatment of binge eating disorder associated with obesity: a placebo-controlled study. Biol Psychiatry 2007; 61(9): 1039–1048.
74. Berlant JL. Topiramate in posttraumatic stress disorder: preliminary clinical observations. J Clin Psychiatry 2001; 62(suppl 17):60–63.
75. Berlant J, van Kammen DP. Open-label topiramate as primary or adjunctive therapy in chronic civilian posttraumatic stress disorder: a preliminary report. J Clin Psychiatry 2002; 63(1):15–20.
76. Pande AC, Davidson JR, Jefferson JW, et al. Treatment of social phobia with gabapentin: a placebo-controlled study. J Clin Psychopharmacol 1999; 19(4):341–348.
77. Pande AC, Pollack MH, Crockatt J, et al. Placebo-controlled study of gabapentin treatment of panic disorder. J Clin Psychopharmacol 2000; 20:467–471.
78. Johnson BA. Uses of topiramate in the treatment of alcohol dependence. Expert Rev Neurother 2004; 4(5):751–758.
79. Johnson BA, Rosenthal N, Capece JA, et al. Topiramate for treating alcohol dependence: a randomized controlled trial. JAMA 2007; 298(14):1641–1651.
80. Johnson BA. Recent advances in the development of treatments for alcohol and cocaine dependence: focus on topiramate and other modulators of GABA or glutamate function. CNS Drugs 2005; 19(10):873–896.
81. McElroy SL, Shapira NA, Arnold LM, et al. Topiramate in the long-term treatment of binge-eating disorder associated with obesity. J Clin Psychiatry 2004; 65(11):1463–1469.
82. McIntyre RS, Mancini DA, McCann S, et al. Topiramate versus bupropion SR when added to mood stabilizer therapy for the depressive phase of bipolar disorder: a preliminary single-blind study. Bipolar Disord 2002; 4(3):207–213.
83. Dahlof C, Loder E, Diamond M, et al. The impact of migraine prevention on daily activities: a longitudinal and responder analysis from three topiramate placebo-controlled clinical trials. Health Qual Life Outcomes 2007; 5(1):56.
84. Post RM, Speer AM, Hough CJ, et al. Neurobiology of bipolar illness: implications for future study and therapeutics. Ann Clin Psychiatry 2003; 15:85–94.
85. Tucker P, Trautman RP, Wyatt DB, et al. Efficacy and safety of topiramate monotherapy in civilian posttraumatic stress disorder: a randomized, double-blind, placebo-controlled study. J Clin Psychiatry 2007; 68(2):201–206.

Abbreviations

ACTH: adrenocorticotropic hormone

ADHD: attention deficit hyperactivity disorder

ADHD: hyperactivity disorder

AEDs: antiepileptic drugs

ALT: alanine aminotransferase

AMPA: α-amino-3 hydroxy-5-methyl-4-isoxazole propionic acid

API: Acute Panic Inventory

ASPD: antisocial personality disorder

AST: aspartate aminotransferase

AZM: Acetazolamide

BA: Brodmann area

BAI: Beck Anxiety Inventory

bcl-2:   B-cell lymphoma/leukemia-2 gene

BDI: Beck Depression Inventory

BDNF: brain-derived neurotrophic factor

BED: binge eating disorder attention deficit

BMI: body mass index

BPD: borderline personality disorder

BPRS: Brief Psychiatric Rating Scale

BSPS: Brief Social Phobia Scale

BZ: benzodiazepine

CAPS: Clinician-Administered PTSD Scale

CBZ: carbamazepine

CCK-4: cholecystokinin-tetrapeptide

CD: conduct disorder

CGI: Clinical Global Impression

CGI-BP: Clinical Global Impressions Scale modified for bipolar disorder

CGI-C: Clinical Global Impression of Change

CGI-I: Clinical Global Impression of Improvement

CGI-S: Clinical Global Impression-Severity

CI: confidence interval

CIWA-Ar: Clinical Institute Withdrawal Assessment for Alcohol-Revised

CNS: central nervous system

CRH: corticotropin-releasing hormone

CSF: cerebrospinal fluid

DA: dopamine

DALYs: disability-adjusted life years

DBT: dialectical behavior therapy

DGRP: Duke Global Rating for PTSD

DIB-R: revised Diagnostic Interview for Borderlines

DSM-III: Diagnostic and Statistical Manual of Mental Disorders III

DSM-III-R: Diagnostic and Statistical Manual of Mental Disorders-Third Edition, Revised

DSM-IV: Diagnostic and Statistical Manual of Mental Disorders IV

DSM-IV-TR: Diagnostic and Statistical Manual of Mental Disorders IV-Text Revision

DTS: Davidson Trauma Scale

ER: extended release

ERK: extracellular signal-regulated kinase

ERP: event-related potential

ESM: ethosuximide

FBM: felbamate

FDA: Food and Drug Administration

FMRI: functional magnetic resonance imaging

GABA: gamma-aminobutyric acid

GABAA: gamma-aminobutyric acid type-A

GABA-T: GABA transaminase

GAD: generalized anxiety disorder

GAD: glutamic acid decarboxylase

GAF: global assessment function

GBP: gabapentin

GSK-3: glycogen synthase kinase 3

GTP: gammaglutamyltranspeptidase

HAM-A: Hamilton Anxiety Scale

HAM-A: Hamilton Rating Scale for Anxiety

HAM-D: Hamilton Depression Rating Scale

HVA: homovanillic acid

ICDs: impulse control disorders

IED: explosive disorder

IES-R: Impact of Event Scale-Revised

ITT: intent-to-treat

LEV: levetiracetam

LOCF: last observation carried forward

LSAS: Liebowitz Social Anxiety Scale

LTG: lamotrigine

MADRS: Montgomery-Asberg Depression Rating Scale

MAOIs: monoamine oxidase inhibitors

MAP: mitogen-activated protein

MBT: mentalization-based treatment

MGlu: metabotropic glutamate

MMRM: mixed models repeated-measures

MRI: magnetic resonance imaging

MRS: Mania Rating Scale

NAA: *N*-acetylaspartate

Nacc: nucleus accumbens

NE: norepinephrine (noradrenaline)

NMDA: *N*-methyl-D-aspartate

NPO: nothing-by-mouth

NPY: neuropeptide Y

NYSOMH: New York State Office of Mental Health

OAS-M: Overt Aggression Scale-Modified

OCD: obsessive-compulsive disorder

OFC: orbitofrontal cortex

OXC: oxcarbazepine

PANSS: Positive and Negative Syndrome Scale

PAS: Panic and Agoraphobia Scale

PB: phenobarbital

PCL-C: PTSD Checklist-Civilian Version

PDS: Posttraumatic Diagnostic Scale

PFC: prefrontal cortex intermittent

PGL: Pregabalin

PHT: phenytoin

PKC: protein kinase C

POMS: Profile of Mood State

PTSD: posttraumatic stress disorder

PWS: Prader-Willi syndrome

rCBF: regional cerebral blood flow

RIMAs: reversible inhibitors of monoamine oxidase-A

SCID: Structured Clinical Interview for DSM-IV

SCL-90: Symptom Checklist-90

SDS: Sheehan Disability Scale

SEP: somatosensory evoked potentials

SFT: schema-focused therapy

SGRI: selective GABA reuptake inhibitor

SIB: self-injurious behavior

SNP: single nucleotide polymorphism

SNRIs: serotonin-norepinephrine reuptake inhibitors

SPIN: Social Phobia Inventory

SR: slow release

SRI: serotonin reuptake inhibitor

SSRI: selective serotonin reuptake inhibitor

STAXI: State Trait Anger Expression Inventory

STEP-BD: Systematic Treatment Enhancement Program for Bipolar Disorder

TFP: transference-focused psychotherapy

TGB: Tiagabine

TLFB: Timeline Follow Back

TOP: Treatment Outcome PTSD scale

TPM: topiramate

TRH: thyrotropin-releasing hormone

VAMS: Visual Analogue Mood Scale

VAS: Visual Analogue Scale

VGB: vigabatrin

VNS: vagal nerve stimulation

VPA: valproate

YBOCS-PG: Yale-Brown Obsessive-Compulsive Scale Modified for Pathological Gambling

YMRS: Young Mania Rating Scale

ZNS: zonisamide